Imaging for Surgeons

Imaging for Surgeons

A CLINICAL GUIDE

SECOND EDITION

David A. Lisle MBBS, FRACR

Consultant Radiologist with Queensland Diagnostic Imaging, based at the Holy Spirit Hospital, Brisbane. Visiting Radiologist, Royal Children's Hospital, Brisbane. Clinical Lecturer in Radiology, University of Queensland. Lecturer in Medical Imaging, Queensland University of Technology

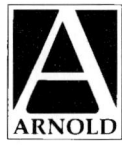

A member of the Hodder Headline Group
LONDON • SYDNEY • AUCKLAND
Co-published in the USA by
Oxford University Press Inc., New York

First published in Great Britain in 1999 by
Arnold, a member of the Hodder Headline Group,
338 Euston Road, London NW1 3BH
http://www.arnoldpublishers.com

Co-published in the United States of America by
Oxford University Press, Inc.,
198 Madison Avenue, New York, NY10016
Oxford is a registered trademark of Oxford University Press

British Library Cataloguing in Publication Data
A catalogue record for this book is available from the British Library

Library of Congress Cataloging-in-Publication Data
A catalog record for this book is available from the Library of Congress

ISBN 0 340 69267 7

1 2 3 4 5 6 7 8 9 10

Publisher: Georgina Bentliff
Production Editor: James Rabson
Production Controller: Sarah Kett
Cover designer: Mouse Mat Design
Composition by Scribe Design, Gillingham, Kent
Printed and bound in Great Britain by The Bath Press, Bath

What do you think about this book? Or any other Arnold title?
Please send your comments to feedback.arnold@hodder.co.uk

Everything should be made as simple as possible, but not simpler.

ALBERT EINSTEIN (1879–1955)

To my wife Lyn and my daughter Victoria

Contents

Preface

Since the publication of *Imaging for Surgeons* in 1993, technological advances in the practice of medicine have continued apace. Several radiological advances have impacted significantly on surgical practice. The most significant of these has been helical CT. Other recent developments have included better quality ultrasound equipment, new pharmaceutical agents for scintigraphy such as sestamibi, and more widespread application of interventional radiology.

At the same time, surgical advances have influenced the practice of radiology. These include laparoscopic surgery, especially laparoscopic cholecystectomy, which has pushed the development of new non-invasive techniques for imaging the biliary tree. Other developments in endocrine and transplantation surgery have presented new sets of challenges to radiologists.

The text for the second edition has been expanded to include the above advances in surgery and radiology. Images and diagrams have been replaced and updated to reflect these changes, and in particular, to highlight the increasing role of CT in general surgical practice.

This book is intended for surgical trainees and junior surgeons. Emergency physicians may also find it useful. As with the first edition, Chapter 1 is a brief introduction to the basic physics of each of the imaging modalities. It is hoped that this will provide a foundation for the understanding of terms used in the remainder of the text and for interpretation of images.

The remaining chapters are set out in what I hope is a reasonably logical sequence with priority given to abdominal topics and trauma. Some of the topics covered may seem a little incongruous to a general surgical readership. However, based on my own experience in British and Australian teaching hospitals, I have included topics such as subarachnoid haemorrhage; the emergency physician is usually the first to see such patients and is often required to organise appropriate investigations prior to specialist consultation.

Let me finish by saying what this book isn't. It is not a clinical textbook. This is an imaging book designed to guide surgeons to the appropriate use of imaging technology in the investigation of common clinical problems. Some variation in the use of imaging techniques will be encountered due to local expertise and availability of equipment.

Acknowledgements

Many people have helped me in the preparation of this book. I would like to thank the following colleagues who donated images:

Dr John Andersen, Princess Alexandra Hospital, Brisbane.

Dr Darryl Burstow, Prince Charles Hospital, Brisbane.

Dr Sutherland MacKechnie, Queensland Diagnostic Imaging.

Dr Ken Mitchell, Queensland Diagnostic Imaging.

Dr John Ratcliffe, Royal Children's Hospital, Brisbane.

Dr Jane Reasbeck, Queensland Diagnostic Imaging.

Dr Frank Smith, Aberdeen Royal Infirmary.

Dr Elizabeth Stockdale, Aberdeen Royal Infirmary.

I would like also to express my appreciation to the following friends and mentors for their continued teaching and inspiration: Dr John Earwaker, Dr Craig Hunter, Dr John Masel and Dr John Ratcliffe.

Finally, my eternal gratitude goes to Miss Esther Dragt for her invaluable and tireless assistance in the typing and setting out of the manuscript.

1   Introduction to medical imaging

Conventional radiography (X-rays; plain films)

X-rays are a form of electromagnetic radiation; their frequency and energy are much greater than visible light. X-rays are produced in an X-ray tube by focusing a beam of high-energy electrons on to a tungsten target. They are able to pass through a patient and on to X-ray film thus producing an image (*Fig. 1.1*).

In passing through a patient the X-ray beam is decreased according to the density and atomic number of the various tissues in a process known as

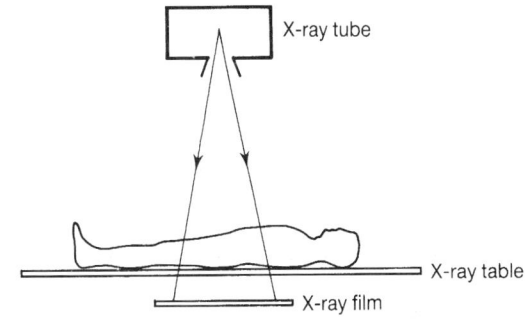

Figure 1.1 *Conventional radiography.*

attenuation. X-rays turn X-ray film black. Therefore the less dense a material, the more X-rays get through and

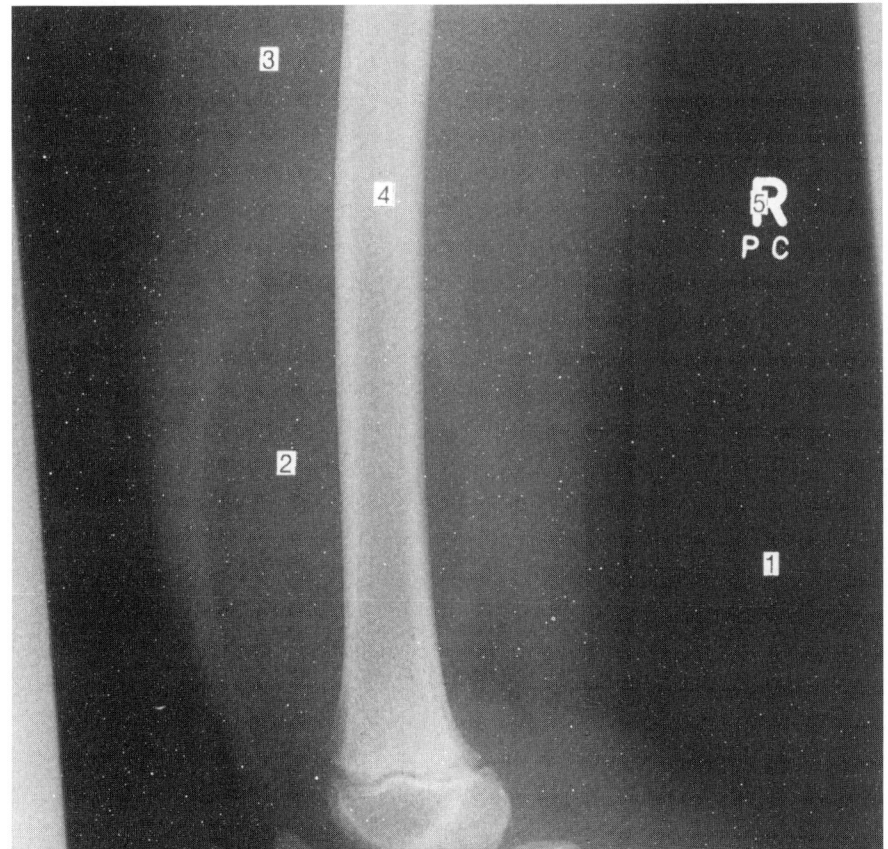

Figure 1.2 *The 5 principal radiographic densities. This plain film of a benign lipoma in a child's thigh demonstrates nicely the 5 basic radiographic densities:*
1. *air*
2. *fat*
3. *soft tissue*
4. *bone*
5. *metal.*

the blacker the film, i.e. materials of low density appear darker than objects of high density.

Five principal densities are recognised on plain X-ray films. They are listed here in order of increasing density:

1. Air/gas: black (e.g. lungs, bowel, stomach).

2. Fat: dark grey (e.g. subcutaneous tissue layer, retroperitoneal fat).

3. Soft tissues/water: light grey (e.g. solid organs, heart, blood vessels, muscle, fluid-filled organs such as bladder).

4. Bone: off-white.

5. Contrast material/metal: bright white (*Fig. 1.2*).

An object will be seen with conventional radiography if its borders lie beside tissue of different density. For example, the right heart border is seen because it lies against aerated lung which is less dense (*Fig. 1.3*); should that part of the lung (right middle lobe) be collapsed or consolidated, it then has soft tissue density and the right heart border is no longer seen (*Fig. 1.4*). Similarly, the psoas muscle margin is seen on a plain abdominal film owing to the lower density of fat lying against it; retroperitoneal fluid or soft tissue mass lead to loss of visualisation of the psoas margin (*Fig. 1.5*). These comments apply to all radiographically visible anatomical interfaces in the body.

Conventional tomography

Conventional tomography or sectional radiography may be used where an object is obscured by overlying or underlying structures. A good example is during intravenous pyelogram (IVP) where the kidneys may be obscured by overlying bowel loops.

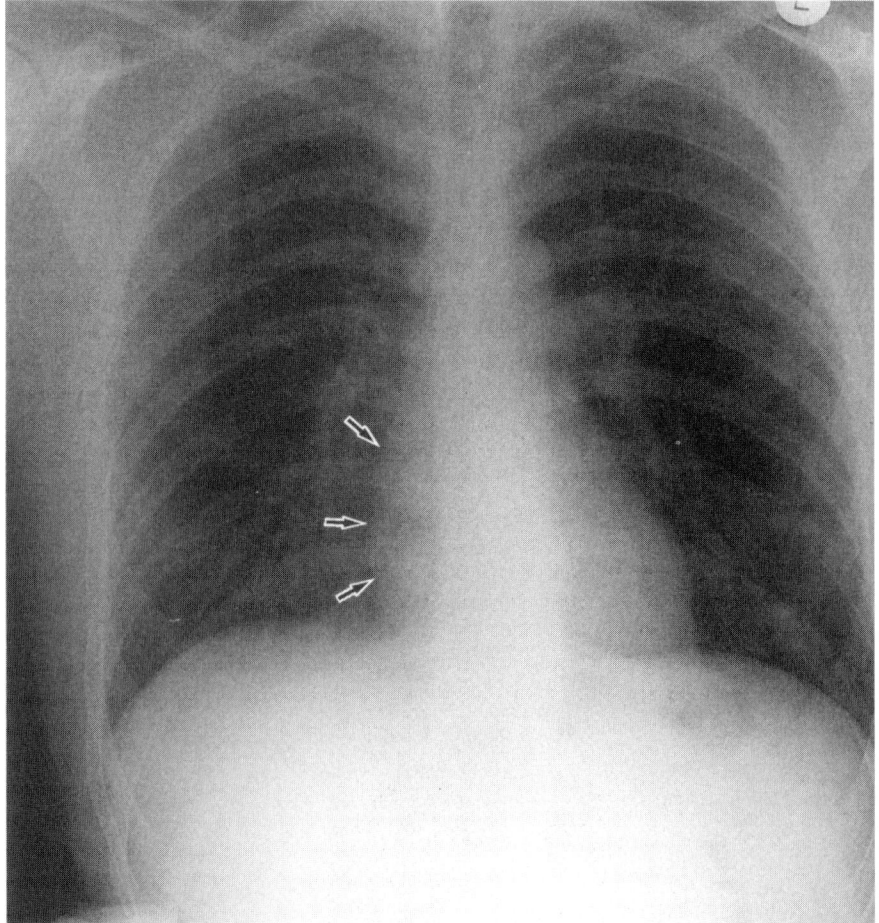

Figure 1.3 *Normal chest X-ray.*
The right heart border (arrows) (and all the other normal interfaces) is clearly seen.

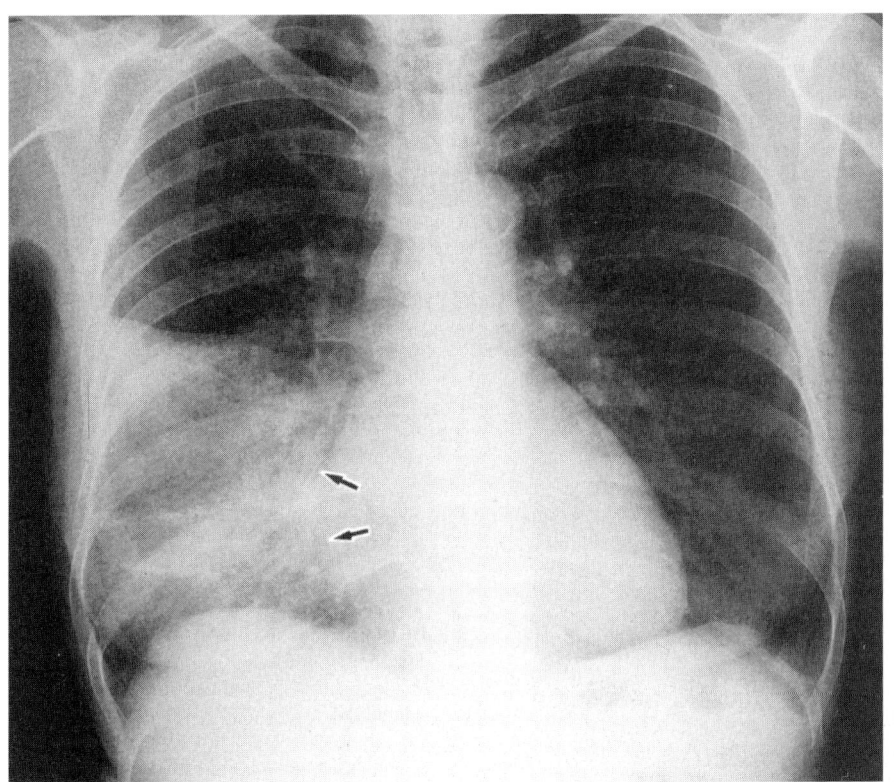

Figure 1.4 *Right middle lobe consolidation. There is non-visualisation of the right heart border (arrows) due to consolidation of the right middle lobe.*

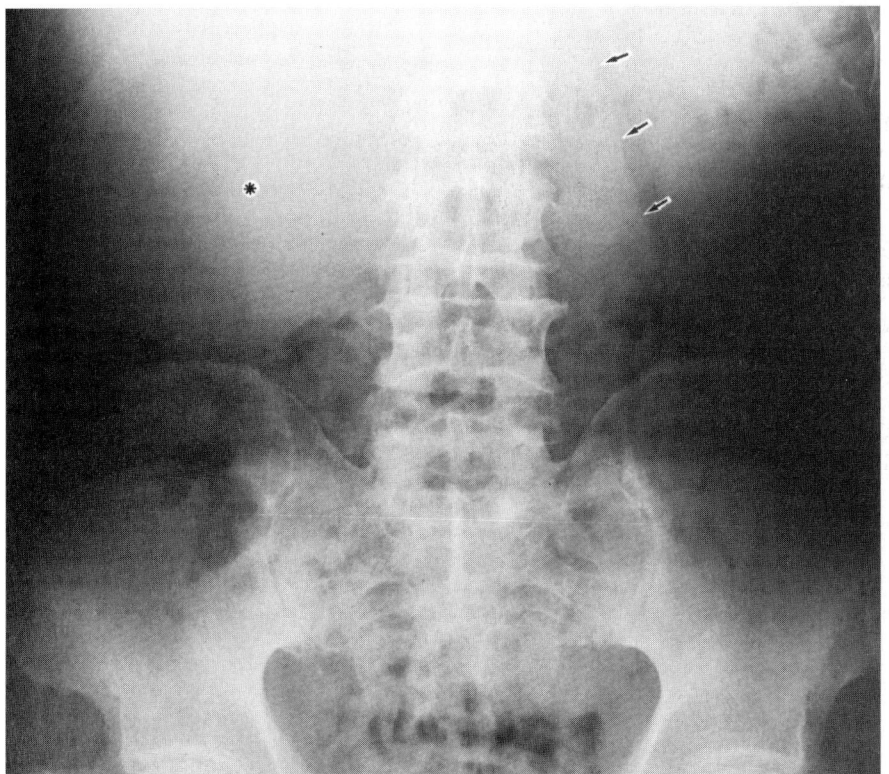

Figure 1.5 *Retroperitoneal mass. The left psoas margin is well defined (arrows). The right psoas margin is lost due to a large renal cell carcinoma (*).*

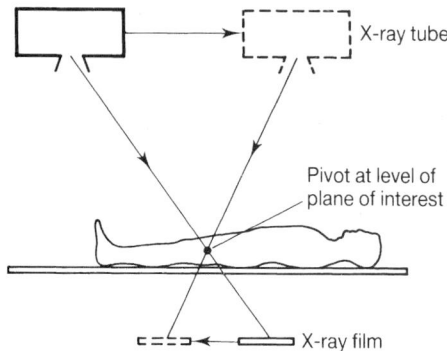

Figure 1.6 *Conventional tomography.*
The X-ray tube and X-ray film move about a pivot, the
level of which is set at the desired plane of interest.

With conventional tomography, the X-ray tube and X-ray film move about a pivot set at a desired level of interest (*Fig. 1.6*). Objects above and below the plane of pivot are blurred by the motion of tube and film, while objects in the plane of interest are seen in sharper relief (*Fig. 1.7*).

Conventional tomography is used less in modern practice since the advent of cross-sectional imaging techniques (ultrasound, CT, MRI), though it still finds application in IVP, as above, and in some complex orthopaedic problems.

Fluoroscopy

Fluoroscopy refers to the technique of examination of the anatomy and motion of internal structures by a constant stream of X-rays. The term 'fluoroscopy' is derived from the ability of X-rays to cause fluorescence. Uses of fluoroscopy include:

1. Barium studies of the gastrointestinal tract.

2. Angiography and interventional radiology.

3. General surgery: operative cholangiography, colonoscopy, etc.

4. Orthopaedic surgery: reduction and fixation of fractures, joint replacement, etc.

5. Airway screening in children for tracheomalacia; diaphragm screening.

The original fluoroscopes were rather primitive and consisted of an X-ray tube, fluorescent screen, and X-

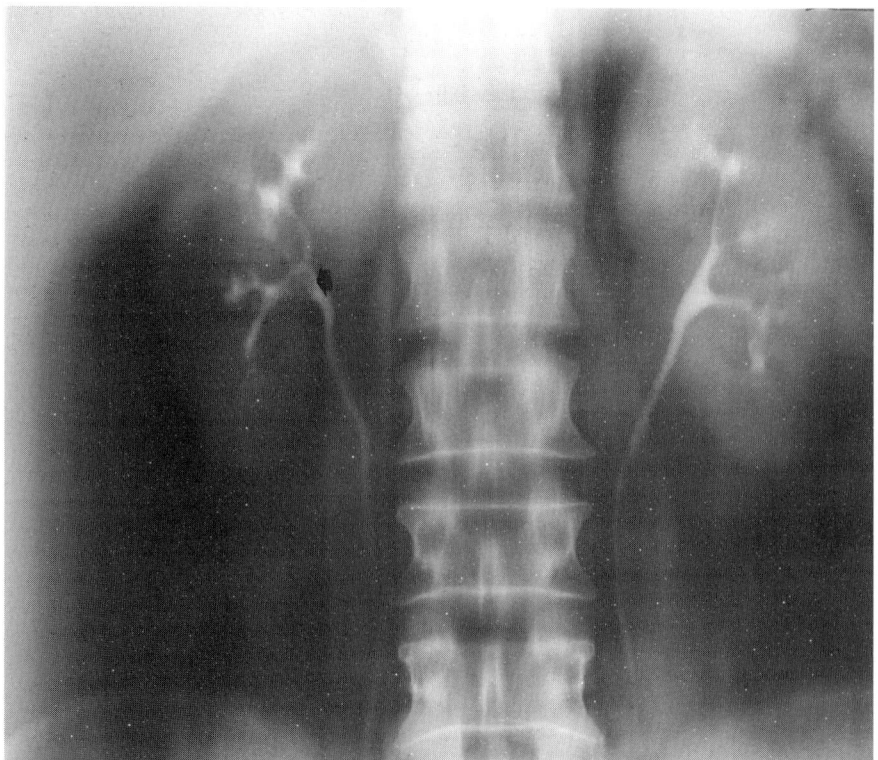

Figure 1.7 *Conventional tomography.*
A tomogram at the level of the kidneys 'removes' overlying bowel loops from view. Note that the spine is also blurred. A calculus is clearly seen in the right renal pelvis (arrow).

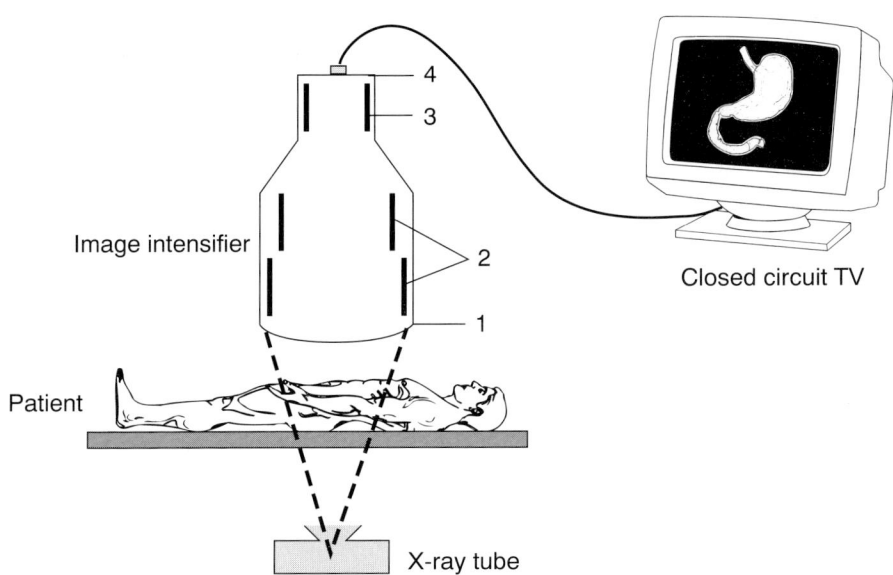

Figure 1.8
Fluoroscopy.
Note the components of
the image intensifier:
1. input fluorescent
    screen and
    photocathode
2. electrostatic lens
3. accelerating anode
4. output fluorescent
    screen.

Image intensifier

Patient

X-ray tube

Closed circuit TV

ray table. The radiologist directly viewed the image on the fluorescent screen. The images were very faint; examinations were performed in a darkened room by a radiologist with dark adapted vision. Dark adaptation was achieved by wearing red goggles for 30 minutes.

Fluoroscopy was revolutionised in the 1950s by the development of the image intensifier. An image intensifier consists of the following:

- Vacuum tube.
- Input fluorescent screen.
- Photocathode.
- Accelerating anode.
- Electrostatic focusing lens.
- Output fluorescent screen.

The fluoroscopic image is produced in the following way:

- X-ray beam passes through the patient and enters the image intensifier vacuum tube.
- X-rays strike the input fluorescent screen and produce light photons.
- Light photons strike the photocathode producing electrons.
- Electrons are drawn away from the photocathode

by the accelerating anode and focused by the electrostatic lens.

- Focused electrons strike the output fluorescent screen producing the fluoroscopic image (*Fig. 1.8*).

The fluoroscopic image is usually viewed via a closed circuit television chain. Images may be recorded in a number of ways:

- X-ray 'spot' films performed during screening.
- Light image from output fluorescent screen recorded by photospot or cine camera.
- Electronic image from television camera recorded in digital format on magnetic tape, magnetic disc, or optical disc.

Ultrasound (US)

Physics and terminology

Ultrasound imaging uses ultra-high frequency sound waves to produce cross-sectional images of the body. The basic component of the ultrasound probe is the *piezoelectric crystal*. Excitation of this crystal by electrical signals causes it to emit ultra-high frequency sound waves: this is the *piezoelectric effect*. Sound waves are reflected back to the crystal by the various

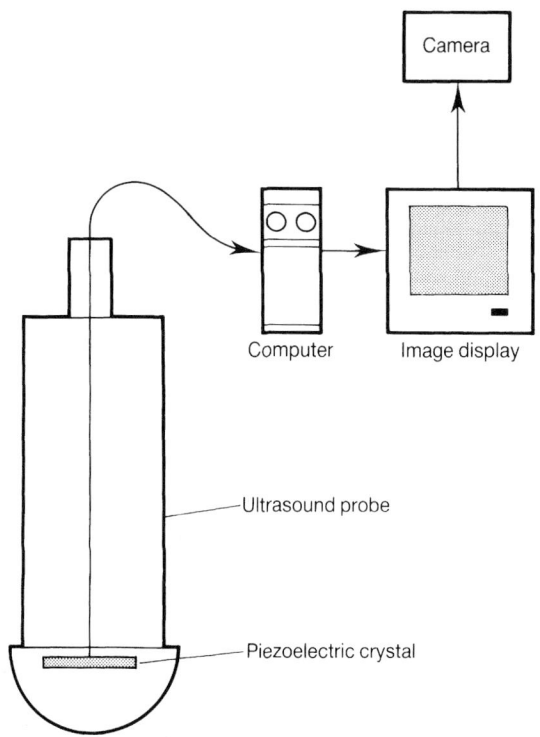

Figure 1.9 *Ultrasound.*
The piezoelectric crystal in the ultrasound probe is used to both transmit and receive the ultrasound waves. The returned signal is analysed by computer and displayed as an image.

tissues of the body. These sound waves act on the piezoelectric crystal in the ultrasound probe to produce an electric signal, again by the piezoelectric effect. Analysis of this electric signal by a computer produces a cross-sectional image (*Fig. 1.9*).

Assorted body tissues produce various degrees of sound wave reflection and are said to be of different echogenicity. A tissue of high echogenicity reflects more sound than a tissue of low echogenicity. The terms *hyperechoic* and *hypoechoic* are used to describe tissues of high and low echogenicity respectively. In producing an image hyperechoic tissues are shown as white or light grey, compared with hypoechoic tissues which are seen as dark grey. Examples of hyperechoic tissues include fat-containing masses and liver haemangiomas; lymphoma and fibroadenoma of the breast are examples of hypoechoic tissues.

Pure fluid reflects virtually no sound and is said to be anechoic. Fluid is seen on ultrasound images as black. Furthermore, because virtually all sound is transmitted through a fluid containing area, tissues distal to such an area receive more sound and hence appear lighter. This effect is known as *acoustic enhancement* and is seen in tissues distal to the gallbladder, the urinary bladder, and simple cysts (*Fig. 1.10*). The reverse effect occurs with areas of sharply increased echogenicity where distal tissues receive little sound and are thus perceived as black. This phenomenon is known as

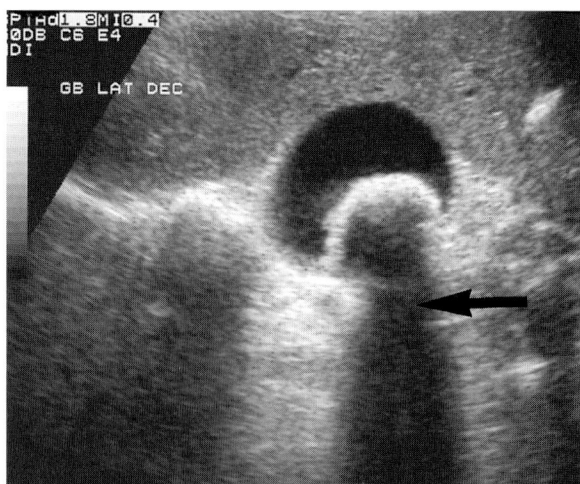

Figure 1.10 *Acoustic enhancement – simple cyst.*
A well defined area of increased echogenicity or brightness is seen deep to a simple cyst of the breast. This is an area of acoustic enhancement (arrows).

Figure 1.11 *Acoustic shadow – gallstone.*
Prominent acoustic shadow (arrow) deep to a large gallstone.

acoustic shadow and is seen distal to gas-containing areas, as well as gallstones, renal stones, and other areas of calcification (*Fig. 1.11*).

Further developments

1. Doppler US

Anyone who has heard a police or ambulance siren speed past will be familiar with the Doppler effect, which describes the influence of a moving object on sound waves. An object travelling towards the listener causes sound waves to be compressed giving a higher frequency; an object travelling away from the listener gives a lower frequency.

The Doppler effect has been applied to ultrasound imaging. Flowing blood causes an alteration to the frequency of sound waves returning to the ultrasound probe. This frequency change or shift is calculated allowing quantitation of blood flow (*Fig. 1.12*).

Colour Doppler is an extension of these principles, in that blood flowing towards the transducer is coloured red; blood flowing away from the transducer is coloured blue. The colours are superimposed on the cross-sectional image allowing instant assessment of direction of flow. Colour Doppler is particularly useful in echocardiography and for identifying very small

vessels (e.g. calf veins, arcuate arteries in the kidneys). It is also used to confirm blood flow within organs (e.g. testis to exclude torsion) and to assess the vascularity of tumours.

The combination of conventional two-dimensional US imaging with Doppler US is known as Duplex ultrasound (*Fig. 1.13*). As outlined in following chapters, Duplex US is an important technique in the examination of arteries and veins.

2. Intracavitary scanning

An assortment of probes are now available for imaging various body cavities and organs, the most widely used and accepted being transvaginal scanning. This technique allows more accurate assessment of gynaecological problems and of early pregnancy up to about 12 weeks' gestation. Transrectal probes are used to assess the prostate gland. Ultrasound crystals can be attached to endoscopes for assessment of tumours of the upper gastrointestinal tract. To date, this

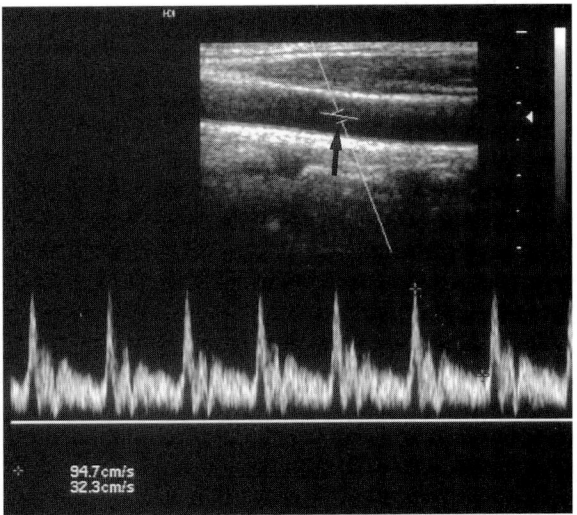

Figure 1.13 *Duplex ultrasound.*
Duplex ultrasound refers to a combination of 2 things: real-time imaging plus pulsed wave Doppler. The area of interest is identified on the real-time image. The Doppler sample gate is set at the appropriate level (arrow). Frequency shifts are displayed as a graph. By knowing the angle between the blood vessel and the ultrasound beam the computer is able to calculate velocities from the frequency shifts so that velocities are directly measured off the graph. In this case peak systolic and end diastolic velocities are displayed.

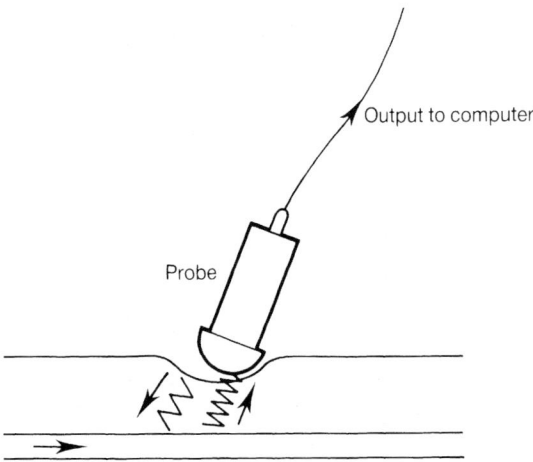

Figure 1.12 *Doppler ultrasound.*
Blood flow is toward the ultrasound probe. As such the returning signal is of higher frequency. The frequency shift is analysed by computer and displayed as a graph.

technique has found greatest application for staging of oesophageal tumours. Echocardiography can also be performed via an endoscopic probe sited in the oesophagus. This removes the problem of overlying ribs and lung which can obscure the heart when performing conventional echocardiography. Tiny ultra-sound probes have also been developed for attach-ment to arterial catheters. These probes provide very accurate cross-sectional images of the arterial wall and, although expensive at present, are under contin-uing development.

3. High frequency scanning

The use of high frequency probes has opened up the area of musculoskeletal ultrasound. This technique has found greatest application in the shoulder joint, specifically in the assessment of the rotator cuff. Most muscles and tendons of the body can also be examined for rupture, inflammation, tumour, etc. In general surgery, high frequency ultrasound has increased the accuracy of small parts imaging, e.g. thyroid, parathyroid. Intra-operative ultrasound also uses high frequency probes directly applied to the organ of interest, e.g. liver, pancreas.

Uses and advantages

The advantages of ultrasound are as follows:

1. Lack of ionising radiation.
2. Relative low cost.
3. Portability of equipment.

Ultrasound scanning is applicable to the solid organs of the body. Initially, studies were directed to the liver, kidneys, spleen, and pancreas and to the pelvic organs. Higher frequency, smaller probes led to the use of ultrasound in diseases of the thyroid, breast, and testes, as well as the musculoskeletal system as above. The lack of ionising radiation is a particular advantage in the assessment of pregnancy and in paediatrics. Used in conjunction with Doppler, ultra-sound is now used in a wide variety of cardiovascular applications including: echocardiography; assessment of carotid, renal, mesenteric, and peripheral arteries for stenosis; assessment of deep veins for thrombosis or incompetence.

Disadvantages and limitations

Ultrasound cannot penetrate gas or bone. Hence lesions lying behind or within gas or bone cannot be visualised. Therefore ultrasound is not used for pulmonary conditions and bowel gas may obscure structures deep in the abdomen (e.g. the pancreas or renal arteries). Bone lesions are not usually amenable to assessment with ultrasound. Similarly, the intra-cranial contents cannot be examined due to the overlying skull vault. The two exceptions to this are:

1. Infants where the fontanelle is still open and provides a 'window'.
2. Intra-operative localisation of brain lesions during craniotomy.

Computed tomography (CT)

Physics and terminology

Computed tomography (CT) is an imaging technique whereby cross-sectional images are obtained with the use of X-rays. The patient passes through a gantry which rotates around at the level of interest. The gantry has an X-ray tube on one side and a set of detectors on the other. Information from the detectors is analysed by computer and displayed as an image (*Fig. 1.14*). Owing to the use of computer analysis, a much greater array of densities can be displayed than on conventional X-ray films. This allows differentiation of solid organs from each other and from pathological processes such as tumour or fluid collections. It also makes CT extremely sensitive to the presence of minute amounts of fat, calcium, or contrast material.

As with plain radiography, high density objects cause more attenuation of the X-ray beam and are therefore displayed as lighter grey than objects of lower density. White and light grey objects are therefore said to be of 'high attenuation'; dark grey and black objects are said to be of 'low attenuation'. Furthermore, the image information can be manipulated by the computer to display the various tissues of the body. This is called 'altering the window settings'. For example, in chest CT where a wide range of tissue densities are present, a good image of the mediastinal structures shows no lung details.

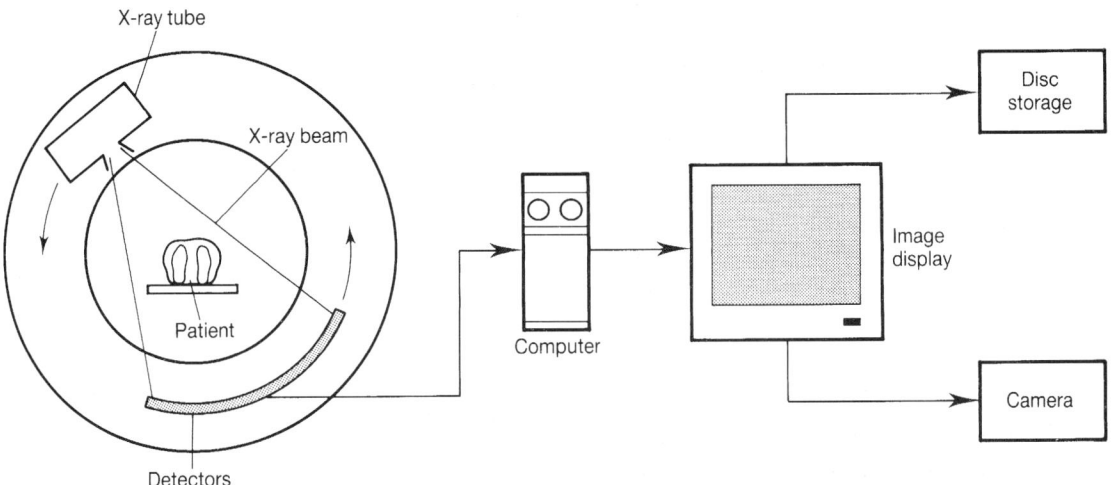

Figure 1.14 *Computed tomography – CT.*

By setting a lung window the lung parenchyma is seen in remarkable detail, though the mediastinal structures are poorly differentiated (*Fig. 1.15*).

This technique can also be used to accentuate a subtle difference in tissue density. For example, the use of 'liver windows' allows greater differentiation of tumours whose tissue density closely approximates that of surrounding normal liver tissue.

Intravenous contrast is used in CT for a number of reasons, as follows:

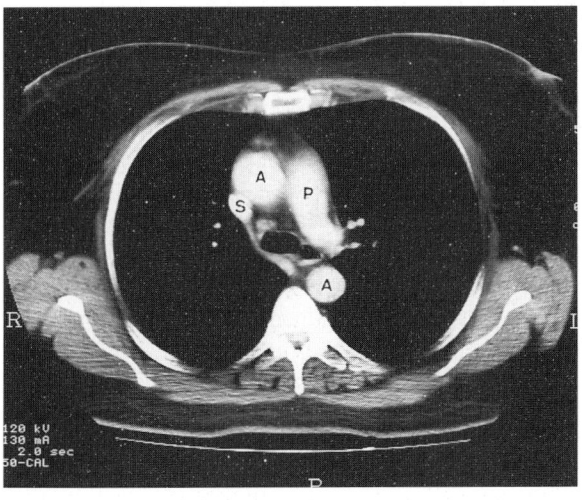

a

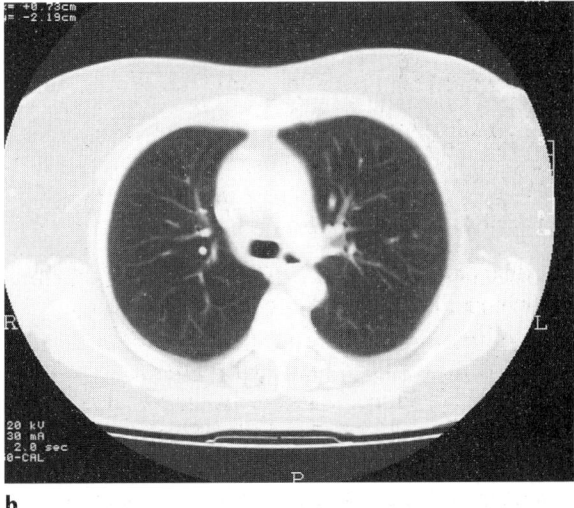

b

Figure 1.15 *CT windows.*
(a) Mediastinal window. Note that mediastinal anatomy is well shown; no lung detail can be seen. Note also the following structures:
- *aorta (A)*
- *SVC (S)*
- *pulmonary artery (P).*
(b) Lung window. Note that the vascular anatomy of the lungs is now well seen.

1. Differentiation of normal blood vessels from abnormal masses, e.g. hilar vessels versus lymph nodes.

2. To make an abnormality more apparent, e.g. liver metastases.

3. To demonstrate the vascular nature of a mass and thus aid in characterisation.

Oral contrast is also used for abdomen CT to allow differentiation of normal enhancing bowel loops from abnormal masses or fluid collections. For detailed examination of the pelvis, rectal contrast and a vaginal tampon will aid in the differentiation of these structures from pathology.

Further developments

Helical (spiral) CT

CT scanners have now been developed which allow continuous acquisition of data as the patient passes through the gantry. These machines differ from conventional scanners in that the tube and detectors rotate without stops as the patient passes through on the scanning table. In this way, a volumetric set of data is obtained which has a helical configuration (*Fig. 1.16*).

This remarkable advance has been due to a number of factors:

1. Better X-ray tube technology.

2. Better detector technology.

3. More sophisticated computer software allowing calculation of the complex data.

4. Development of slip-ring technology. The X-ray tube and detectors rotate on a number of slip-rings; these are metal rings which have three functions:
   (i)   supply of high-voltage electricity to the X-ray tube;
   (ii) supply of low-voltage electricity for various control mechanisms;
   (iii) transfer of digital data from the detectors to the computer.

The major advantages of helical scanning over conventional scanning are:

1. Increased speed of examination.

2. Rapid examination at optimal levels of intravenous contrast concentration.

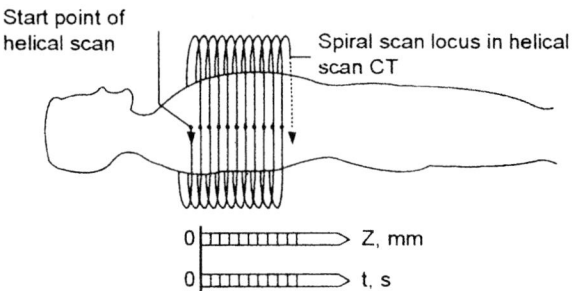

Figure 1.16 *Spiral CT.*
A schematic diagram to show the scanning method of spiral CT. 'Z' represents the Z-plane, i.e. the direction of passage of the patient through the scanner; 't, s' equals time in seconds. Obviously the scanner spins in a circle. The spiral 'shape' of acquired data is due to movement of the patient through the spinning gantry. (Courtesy of GE Medical Systems Australia Pty Ltd.)

3. Images can be retrospectively reconstructed at any desired level.

4. The continuous volumetric nature of data allows accurate high quality 3D reconstruction. This has many applications such as planning of cranial and facial reconstruction surgery; repair of fractures in complex areas, e.g. acetabulum; CT angiography, i.e. display of blood vessels such as the aorta prior to surgery.

Uses and advantages

The first CT scanners developed, due to their small size, were used only for examination of the head and its contents. With the development of larger scanners, CT is now applied to all areas of the body. CT is the modality of choice for the mediastinum and for many pulmonary conditions. It is also the method of choice for examination of the retroperitoneum and for many disorders of the solid abdominal and pelvic organs. It is excellent in the delineation of bony pathology and it has been used extensively for spinal diseases despite some limitations, as outlined below.

Limitations and disadvantages

Disadvantages of CT relate to its use of ionising radiation, hazards of intravenous contrast, lack of portability of equipment, and its relatively high cost.

A number of areas of the body are imaged relatively poorly with CT. These include the pituitary fossa and the posterior intracranial fossa where artefact from adjacent bony structures obscures normal anatomy. Magnetic resonance imaging (MRI) is the modality of choice for these areas. In the spine, despite its excellent soft tissue contrast capabilities, CT is unable to differentiate spine/spinal cord/nerve roots from surrounding cerebrospinal fluid (CSF) (unless the CSF has been opacified by myelography which is obviously invasive). For this reason, MRI is the imaging modality of choice in the spine.

CT imaging is usually limited to the transverse (axial) plane. Exceptions relate to areas of the body that can be tilted in the gantry (e.g. the head or ankles) to give coronal scans. Helical scanning allows reconstructive imaging in the sagittal plane, e.g. for assessment of the spine.

Scintigraphy (nuclear medicine)

Physics and terminology

Scintigraphy refers to the use of gamma radiation to form images following the injection of various radio-pharmaceuticals. The key word to understanding scintigraphy is 'radio-pharmaceutical', where the 'radio' part refers to the emitter of gamma rays (i.e. a radionuclide).

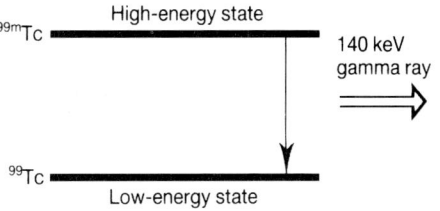

Figure 1.17 *Gamma ray production. The metastable atom ^{99m}Tc in passing from the high-energy state to the lower-energy state releases gamma radiation which has a peak energy of 140 keV. This makes it very suitable for use in imaging. ^{99m}Tc has a half-life of about 6 hours.*

The most commonly used radionuclide in clinical practice is technetium, written in this text as ^{99m}Tc, where 99 is the atomic mass; and the small 'm' stands for 'metastable', the property which causes the material to emit gamma radiation. Metastable means that the technetium atom has two basic energy states: high and low. As the technetium passes from the high-energy state to the low-energy state, it emits a packet of energy in the form of a gamma ray which has an energy of 140 keV (kiloelectron volts) (*Fig. 1.17*). The gamma rays are detected by a gamma camera which converts the absorbed energy of the radiation to an electric signal. This signal is analysed by a computer and displayed as an image (*Fig. 1.18*). Other commonly used radionuclides include gallium citrate (^{67}Ga), thallium (^{201}Tl), indium (^{111}In) and iodine (^{131}I).

'Pharmaceutical' refers to the compound to which the radionuclide is bound. This compound will depend on the area to be examined. For example, sulphur colloid is taken up by the reticulo-endothelial cells of the liver

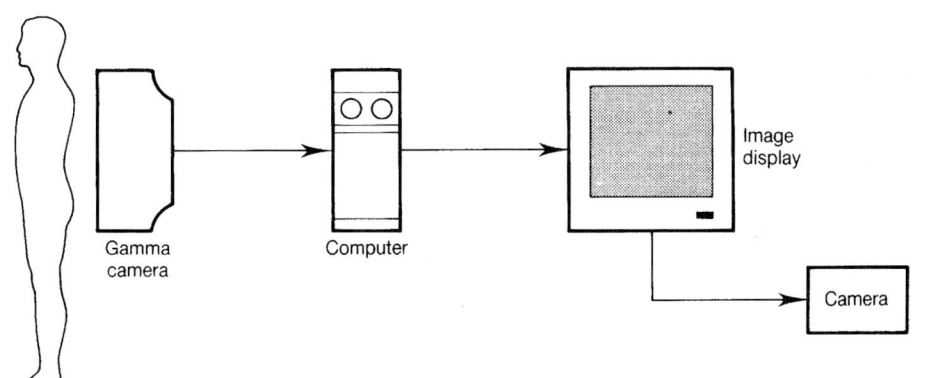

Figure 1.18 *Scintigraphy.*

Table 1.1 *The common radio-pharmaceuticals and their applications*

Organ	Radio-pharmaceutical	Clinical application
Kidneys	99mTc-DTPA 99mTc-MAG3	Renal function, anatomy, drainage of collecting systems
	99mTc-DMSA	Cortical scars in children with urinary tract infection
	99mTc in saline passed into the bladder by catheter	Vesico-ureteric reflux in children with urinary tract infection
Bone	99mTc-MDP	Bone metastases, activity of bone lesions, stress fractures
Lungs	Ventilation: 99mTc-DTPA aerosol Perfusion: 99mTc-MAA	Pulmonary embolism
Liver/spleen	99mTc-colloid	Liver/spleen metastases and other masses
Bile ducts	99mTc-HIDA	Acute cholecystitis, biliary obstruction, biliary atresia, post-liver transplant
Thyroid	99mTc	Thyroid function, thyroiditis, function of thyroid masses, location of aberrant thyroid tissue
Gated cardiac study	Stannous pyrophosphate to reduce Hb then 99mTc which binds reduced Hb and thus red blood cells	Left ventricular ejection fraction, localised wall motion defects
Bleeding studies	99mTc-labelled red blood cells as for gated cardiac study	Acute gastrointestinal bleeding
Myocardium	201Tl	Ischaemic/infarcted myocardium
Parathyroid	99mTc-sestamibi	Hyperparathyroidism
Adrenal medulla	131I-MIBG	Localisation of phaeochromocytoma; staging of neuroblastoma
CSF	111In-DTPA	Differentiation of communicating hydrocephalus from cerebral atrophy

and spleen and is therefore used in imaging these organs. For some applications a pharmaceutical is not required. An example would be the use of free technetium (^{99m}Tc), referred to as pertechnetate, for thyroid scanning.

Areas of high uptake of pharmaceutical and therefore of the radionuclide to which it is bound show resultant high emission of gamma rays. These areas are referred to as 'hot'. Areas of low uptake are referred to as photon-deficient or 'cold'.

Uses and advantages

The main advantages of scintigraphy are:

1. Highly sensitive, e.g. early osteomyelitis may not be visible on plain films for 7–10 days, while scintigraphy will be positive at the time of presentation.

2. Functional information is provided as well as anatomical information, e.g. diethylenetriamine pentaacetic acid (DTPA) renal scans provide information on renal function, as well as renal size and drainage of the collecting systems.

Gallium (^{67}Ga) scanning is used in a number of clinical situations. Gallium is bound to plasma proteins, most strongly to transferrin. It is also taken up by white blood cells. Scanning is performed at 24, 48, and occasionally 72 hours post-injection. The three most common indications for gallium scanning are:

1. To localise occult infection usually in a patient with pyrexia of unknown origin or suspected abdominal abscess not localised by CT or ultrasound.

2. To confirm or deny that an abnormality seen on other studies (e.g. plain films or ^{99m}Tc-MDP bone scan) is infective in nature.

3. In staging and follow-up of Hodgkin's disease, although this role is usually performed by CT.

Limitations and disadvantages

The main disadvantage of scintigraphy is its non-specificity. To take a common example, an isolated 'hot spot' on a bone scan could be due to infection, trauma, or neoplasia and correlation with clinical history and other imaging studies is of paramount importance. On the other hand, multiple 'hot spots' on the bone scan of an elderly man being staged for prostatic carcinoma are easily diagnosed as skeletal metastases. Furthermore, given the high sensitivity of bone scans, a normal study in such a patient virtually excludes skeletal metastatic disease.

Other disadvantages relate to the use of ionising radiation, the cost of equipment, and the extra care required in handling radioactive materials.

Further developments

1. SPECT (single photon emission computed tomography)

This is a technique whereby the computer is programmed to analyse data coming from a single depth within the patient. In this way, cross-sectional scans analogous to plain tomography are obtained. This technique allows greater sensitivity in the detection of subtle lesions overlain by other active structures (e.g. pars interarticularis defects in the lower spine). The main applications of SPECT are in bone scanning, ^{201}Tl cardiac scanning, and in cerebral perfusion studies.

2. PET (positron emission tomography)

This technique uses positron-emitting radionuclides. Research indicates that PET can produce good functional information and may have uses particularly in the brain for assessment of epilepsy, degenerative cerebral conditions, and in various psychiatric conditions. Unfortunately, the radionuclides used for PET are very short lived and must be produced by a cyclotron. As such, PET is yet to find wide acceptance beyond research institutions.

Magnetic resonance imaging (MRI)

Physics and terminology

Over the past 10 years, MRI has become accepted as a powerful imaging tool. It uses the magnetic properties of the hydrogen atom to produce images. The physics of MRI is extremely complex and a full discussion would require a much larger book than this (and another author!). The following is a brief summary of the physical principles behind MRI.

The nucleus of the hydrogen atom is a single proton. Being a spinning, charged particle, it has magnetic properties and, for the sake of discussion, may be thought of as a small bar magnet with North and South poles (*Fig. 1.19*). The first step in MRI is the application of a strong, external magnetic field. For this purpose, the patient is placed within a large

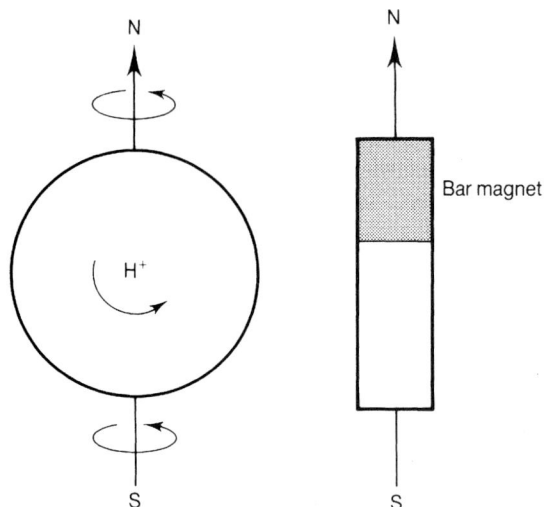

Figure 1.19 *The spinning hydrogen atom.*
The hydrogen atom, being a spinning charged particle,
has a small magnetic field, analogous to a bar magnet.

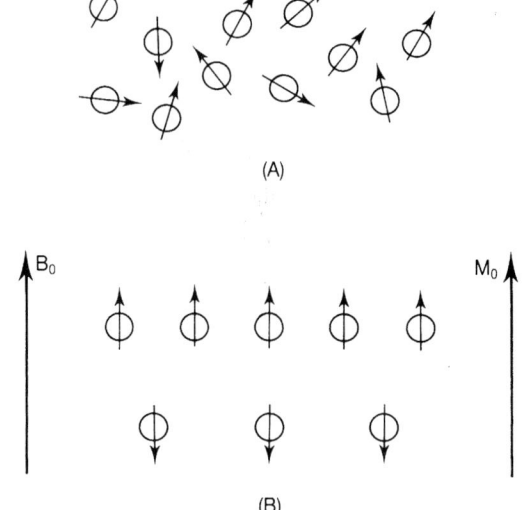

Figure 1.20 *Effect of application of a strong external*
magnetic field. In (A), the hydrogen atoms are randomly
aligned in the normal resting state. In (B), a strong
external magnetic field, B_0, is applied. The atoms align
either parallel or anti-parallel to this field. The majority
align parallel so their net magnetic vector, M_0, is in the
same direction as the external field, B_0.

magnet, either a permanent or superconductive
magnet.

The hydrogen atoms within the patient align in a
direction either parallel or antiparallel to the strong
external field. A greater proportion align in the parallel direction, so that the net vector of their alignment,
and therefore the net magnetic vector, will be in the
direction of the external field (*Fig. 1.20*).

Though aligned in a strong magnetic field, the hydrogen nuclei do not lie motionless. Each nucleus spins
around the line of the field in a motion known as
precession. The frequency of precession is an inherent
property of the hydrogen atom in a given magnetic
field and is known as the *Larmor frequency* (*Fig. 1.21*).
The Larmor frequency therefore changes in proportion
to magnetic field strength. It is of the order of 10 MHz
(megahertz), a frequency in the same part of the
electromagnetic spectrum as radio waves.

A second magnetic field is now applied at right angles
to the original external field. This second magnetic
field is applied at the same frequency as the Larmor
frequency and is known as the *radiofrequency pulse*
(RF pulse). The RF pulse is applied by a second
magnetic coil, the RF coil. The RF pulse causes the net
magnetisation vector of the hydrogen atoms to turn
towards the transverse plane, i.e. a plane at right
angles to the direction of the original, strong external

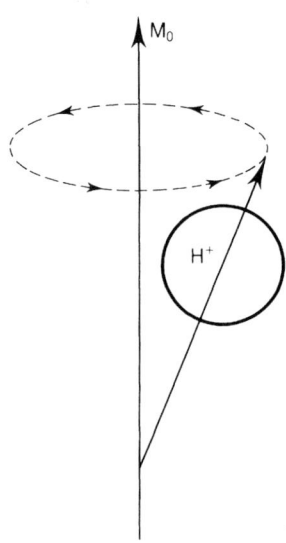

Figure 1.21 *Precession.*
The hydrogen atom spins around the line of the
magnetic field in a motion called precession at a
frequency called the Larmor frequency.

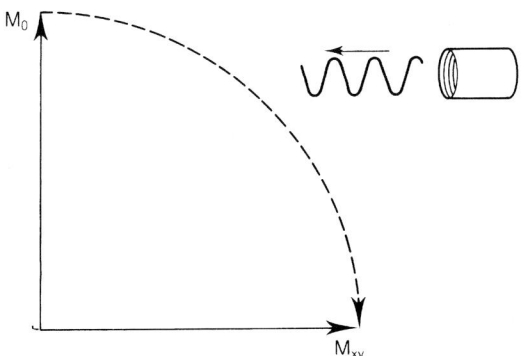

Figure 1.22 *Application of the RF pulse.*
Application of a pulsed magnetic field at 90° to the original field and at the Larmor frequency causes the net magnetic vector of the hydrogen atoms, M_0, to rotate through 90° onto the xy plane.

field. (*Fig. 1.22*). As such, the RF pulse adds energy to the system. Following cessation of the RF pulse, the extra energy is dissipated to the surrounding chemical lattice in a process known as *T1 relaxation*. In addition, the RF pulse brings the precessing protons into phase, i.e. their spins are now in synchrony. The process of dephasing, which occurs due to tiny inhomogeneities in the nuclear magnetic environment, is known as *T2 relaxation*.

The component of the net magnetisation vector in the transverse plane induces a current in magnetic coils

known as *radiofrequency*, or *RF receiver coils*. This current is known as the *MR signal* and is the basis for formation of an image. Note that the MR signal can be produced only when the precession of the spinning protons is in phase. Complex computer analysis of the MR signal from the RF receiver coils is used to produce an *MR image* (*Fig. 1.23*).

Whereas CT depends on tissue density and ultrasound on tissue echogenicity, much of the complexity of MRI arises from the fact that the MR signal depends on many varied properties of substances being examined. These properties include:

- Proton density.

- The chemical environment of the hydrogen atoms (e.g. whether in free water or bound by fat).

- Flow (e.g. in blood or CSF).

- Magnetic susceptibility.

- T1 relaxation time.

- T2 relaxation time.

By altering the duration and amplitude of the RF pulse, as well as the timing and repetition of its application, various sequences have been developed to use and accentuate these various properties. The most common types of images produced have been:

(a) *T1 weighted:* excellent anatomical definition, though with lower sensitivity to pathology.

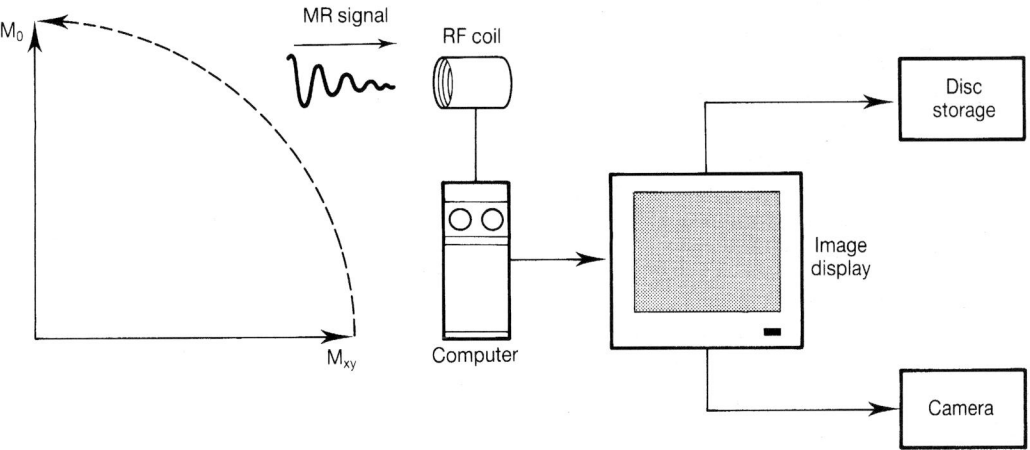

Figure 1.23 *Production of the MR signal.*
When the RF pulse is switched off, the net magnetisation vector returns to its original direction and emits a signal which is received by the RF coil. This signal is analysed by computer to produce an image.

(b) *T2 weighted:* highly sensitive to the presence of pathology.

Numerous other image types are now used. A common example is fat suppression sequences which are excellent for demonstrating pathology in areas containing a lot of fat, e.g. the orbits and bone marrow. Note that in viewing MRI images, white or light grey areas are referred to as 'high signal'; dark grey or black areas are referred to as 'low signal'. On certain sequences flowing blood is seen as a black area referred to as a 'flow void'.

Uses and advantages

The main advantages of MRI are as follows:

1. Excellent soft tissue contrast

- As explained above, MRI uses many varied properties of matter in the generation of an image.

2. Lack of artefact due to adjacent bones

- This makes MRI the imaging modality of choice in areas such as the posterior fossa and pituitary fossa where the quality of CT images is degraded by artefact.

3. Multiplanar capabilities

- MRI is able to obtain images in any plane. The sagittal plane is particularly useful for the spine and this property, combined with the excellent soft tissue contrast, makes MRI the modality of choice for imaging of spinal disorders. Multiple planes are also useful in the musculoskeletal system, e.g. sagittal and coronal planes for the knee, coronal and oblique planes for the shoulder.

4. Lack of ionising radiation

In summary, MRI is the imaging modality of choice for most brain and spine disorders. It has also found wide acceptance in the assessment of musculoskeletal disorders. Although excellent for visualisation of the heart, echocardiography is more widely used as it produces functional as well as anatomical information. MRI has not displaced other modalities, such as CT, ultrasound, and endoscopy, in the imaging of most thoracic and abdominal disorders.

Limitations and disadvantages

1. Cost

- The equipment for MRI is very expensive. Running and maintenance costs are also high. Potential benefits to patient care must be carefully weighed against these costs.

2. Artefacts

- Although free of artefacts from bony structures, a wide variety of artefacts do occur in MRI.

3. Metal foreign objects

- MRI is potentially hazardous for patients with metal foreign bodies in the eyes and for patients with ferromagnetic intracranial aneurysm clips. MRI is contraindicated in patients with cardiac pacemakers and cochlear implants. Also artefacts from even small fragments of metal from orthopaedic surgery cause serious image degradation, though this is minimised with the use of titanium.

4. Reduced sensitivity for certain substances

- MRI is less sensitive than CT in the detection of small amounts of calcification and in the detection of acute haemorrhage. As such, CT is still the imaging modality of choice for the assessment of acute subarachnoid haemorrhage and for acute head injury.

5. Fine bone detail

- MRI is unable to provide the degree of bone detail possible with CT, although it is more sensitive in the detection of infiltrative disorders of bone marrow.

Further developments

1. Contrast material

Although not as widely used as in CT imaging, intravenous contrast is now available for MRI. Gadolinium (Gd) is a paramagnetic substance which causes increased signal on T1-weighted images. Unbound gadolinium is highly toxic. For this reason, binding agents are required for in vivo use. The most common of these is DTPA: Gd-DTPA is non-toxic and used in a dose of 0.1 mmol per kilogram.

The main indications for the use of Gd-DTPA are as follows:

(i) *Brain:*

- Multiple lesions (e.g. metastases, multiple sclerosis).
- Selected tumours (e.g. acoustic neuroma, meningioma).
- Tumour residuum/recurrence following treatment.

(ii) *Spine:*

- Metastases: intraspinal, CSF.
- Tumour recurrence.
- Post-operative to differentiate fibrosis from recurrent disc protrusion.
- Infection.
- Selected tumours, e.g. neurofibroma.

(iii) *Musculoskeletal system:*

- Soft tissue tumours.
- Intra-articular Gd-DTPA in subtle shoulder disorders.

2. Magnetic resonance angiography (MRA)

With varying sequences, flowing blood can be shown as either signal void (i.e. black), or increased signal (i.e. white). Computer reconstruction techniques allow the display of blood vessels in 3D, and allow viewing of the blood vessels from any angle. Indications would include: imaging of the carotid arteries for stroke (transient ischaemic attack (TIA)), aneurysm, AVM, etc.; imaging of the peripheral vessels for claudication.

3. Fast imaging

New, complex sequences are under constant development. Much research is currently directed at very rapid image acquisition.

Further Reading

1. Brink JA. Technical aspects of helical (spiral) CT. *Radiological Clinics of North America* 1995; **33**:825–841.

2. Foley WD, Erickson SJ. Color Doppler flow imaging. *AJR* 1991; **156**:3–13.

3. Kalender WA. Technical foundations of spiral CT. *Seminars in US, CT, and MRI* 1994; **15**:81–89.

4. Villafana T. Fundamental physics of magnetic resonance imaging. *Radiological Clinics of North America* 1988; **26**: 701–715.

5. Weir J, Abrahams PH (eds.). *An Imaging Atlas of Human Anatomy*, 3rd edn. Wolfe Publishing, 1992.

6. Wells PNT. Doppler ultrasound in medical diagnosis. *British Journal of Radiology* 1989; **62**:399–420.

7. Zeman RK, Silverman PM, Vieco PT, Costello P. CT angiography. *AJR* 1995; **165**:1079–1088.

8. Zeman RK, Fox SH, Silverman PM *et al*. Helical (spiral) CT of the abdomen. *AJR* 1993; **160**:719–725.

2 Acute abdomen

In assessing the patient with an acute abdomen the surgeon may complement a full history and examination with other investigations, including laboratory tests (e.g. white cell count, ESR), laparoscopy, and imaging studies. Plain abdominal films remain the first line of imaging investigation for most patients with an acute abdomen, and the most common findings are outlined below. A plain film of the supine abdomen can show abnormal gas patterns (e.g. dilated bowel loops, free gas, gas in the biliary tree), soft tissue masses, foreign bodies, or abnormal calcifications (e.g. renal calculi, pancreatic calcification).

A plain film of the erect chest can show free gas beneath and above the diaphragm, chest conditions which may present as acute abdomen (e.g. basal pneumonia, pulmonary embolus), or chest manifestations of abdominal conditions (e.g. pleural effusion, basal atelectasis).

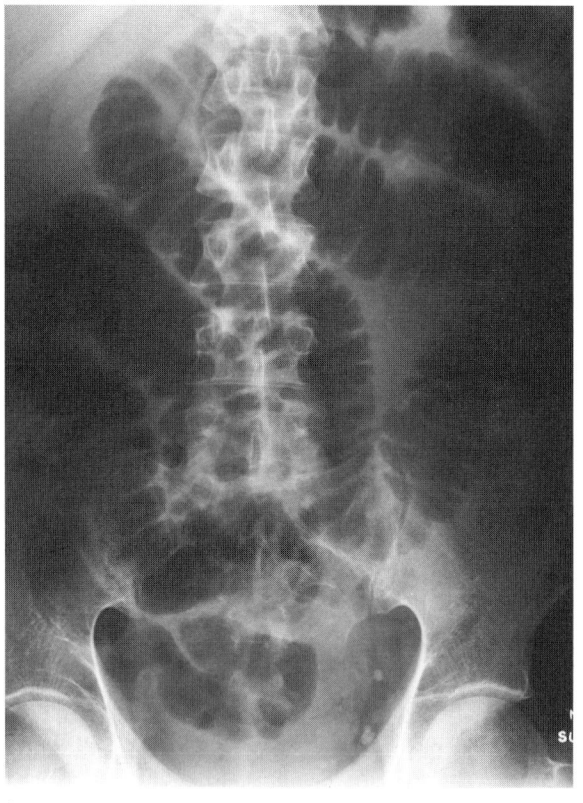

a

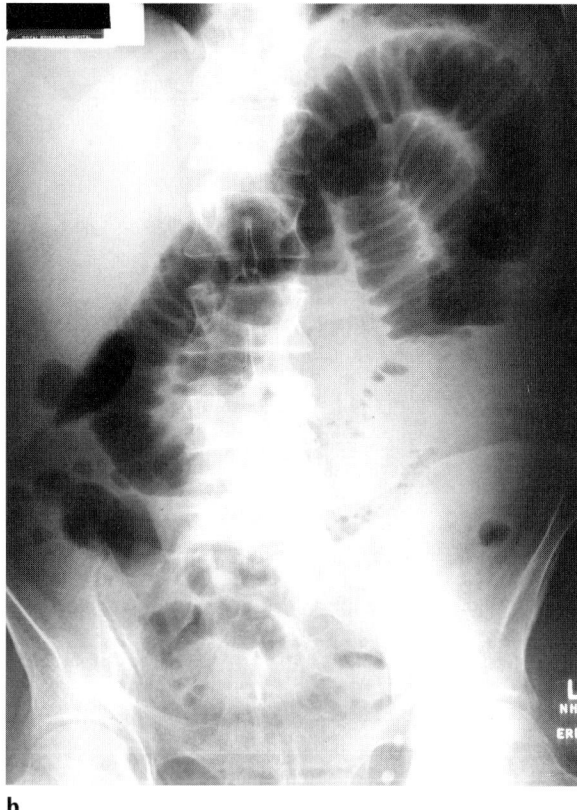

b

Figure 2.1 *Small bowel obstruction.*
(a) Supine film. Note that small bowel loops are mainly central in position; numerous; measure less then 5.0 cm in diameter; have a small radius of curvature; contain valvulae conniventes which pass across the bowel lumen and are thin and close together. (b) Erect film. Note:
- *features of small bowel loops, as above*
- *numerous air–fluid levels.*

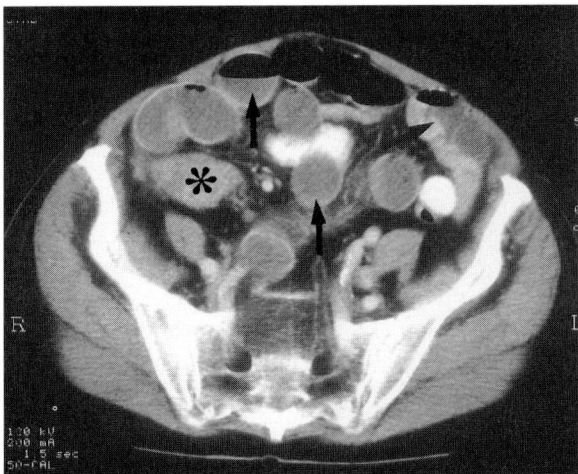

Figure 2.2 *Small bowel obstruction – CT.*
Note:
- *distended small bowel loops some of which contain air–fluid levels (arrows)*
- *soft tissue mass in the distal ileum (*)*
- *the mass was excised and found to be an adenocarcinoma.*

Plain films of the erect abdomen are less frequently used. These should be reserved for cases of suspected intestinal obstruction, or suspected perforation.

Other imaging modalities, i.e. CT, US, and contrast studies are used where appropriate. In particular CT has found an increasing role in the diagnosis of bowel disorders. CT provides excellent delineation of bowel wall thickening, bowel masses, pericolonic inflammation, and sinus and fistula tracts. As will be discussed in this and subsequent chapters CT is useful in the investigation of small bowel obstruction, small bowel neoplasms, inflammatory bowel disease, and lower abdominal pain.

Intestinal obstruction

Small bowel obstruction

- Plain films remain the primary investigation of choice in suspected small bowel obstruction. Plain film signs include:
  (i)   Dilated small bowel loops which tend to be central, numerous, 2.5–5.0 cm diameter, have

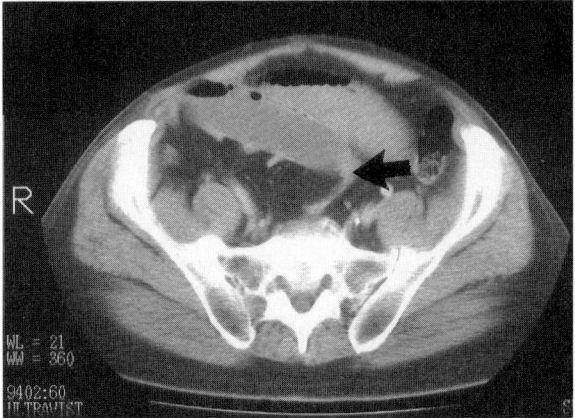

Figure 2.3 *Small bowel obstruction – CT.*
Typical case of small bowel obstruction due to adhesions. Note the dilated small bowel loops with a focal transition zone to distal collapsed bowel (arrow).

a small radius of curvature, have valvulae conniventes which extend right across the bowel, and do not contain solid faeces.
  (ii) Multiple fluid levels on the erect film.
  (iii) 'String of beads' sign on the erect view due to small gas pockets trapped between valvulae conniventes.
  (iv) Absent or little air in the large bowel (*Fig. 2.1*).

- Limitations of plain films include:
  (i)   partial or early obstruction;
  (ii) strangulation;
  (iii) closed-loop obstruction.

- CT is the investigation of choice when clinical and plain film assessment are inconclusive.

- CT is highly accurate for:
  (i)   establishing the diagnosis of small bowel obstruction;
  (ii) location and cause of obstruction (*Fig. 2.2*);
  (iii) associated strangulation.

- CT signs of small bowel obstruction:
  (i)   Small bowel loops measuring > 2.5 cm in diameter.
  (ii) Identifiable focal transition zone from pre-stenotic dilated bowel to post-stenotic collapsed bowel loops (*Fig. 2.3*).

- CT signs of strangulation:
  (i)   Thickening of bowel wall with multiple layers producing a target appearance.

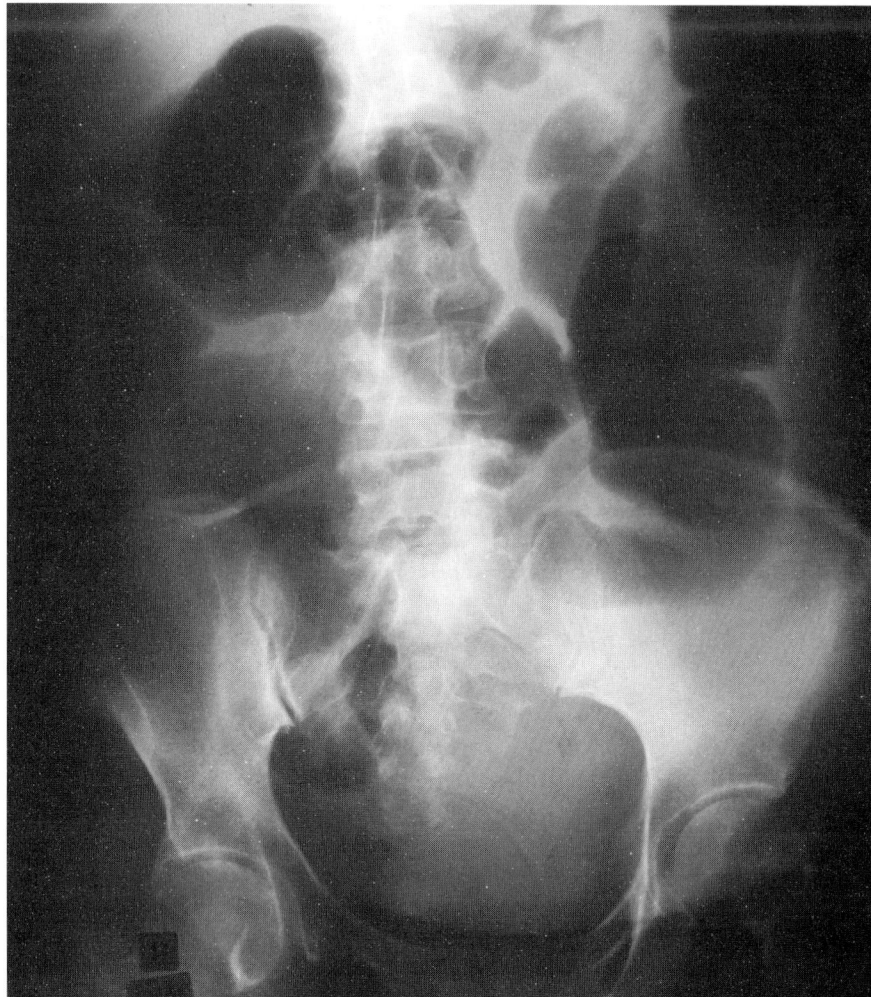

Figure 2.4 *Large bowel obstruction.*
Note the features of large bowel loops:
- *peripheral*
- *few in number*
- *wide radius of curvature*
- *greater than 5.0 cm. in diameter*
- *contain haustra which are thick and widely separated.*

a

(ii)   Gas in the bowel wall.
(iii) Portal vein gas.
(iv)   Streaky soft tissue opacity in mesenteric fat.

- Oral contrast studies (small bowel follow-through) using barium or water soluble contrast are often misleading, i.e. unable to differentiate obstruction from paralytic ileus, and may in fact delay diagnosis.

- Enteroclysis (small bowel enema) remains the investigation of choice for grading severity and location of partial obstruction.

- In summary, the majority of small bowel obstructions are diagnosed with clinical assessment and plain films. CT is the investigation of choice in doubtful cases, with enteroclysis occasionally useful in partial obstruction.

Large bowel obstruction

- Dilated large bowel loops which tend to be peripheral, few in number, large (above 5.0 cm diameter), have a large radius of curvature, have haustra which may or may not extend right across the bowel (distinguished from valvulae conniventes in that they are thick and widely separated), and contain solid faeces (*Fig. 2.4*).

- Caecum may be dilated.

- Small bowel may be dilated.

- Contrast enema may be helpful:
  (i)   to differentiate 'pseudo-obstruction' which occurs most commonly in elderly patients and may be indistinguishable on plain films from mechanical obstruction;

Figure 2.4 continued

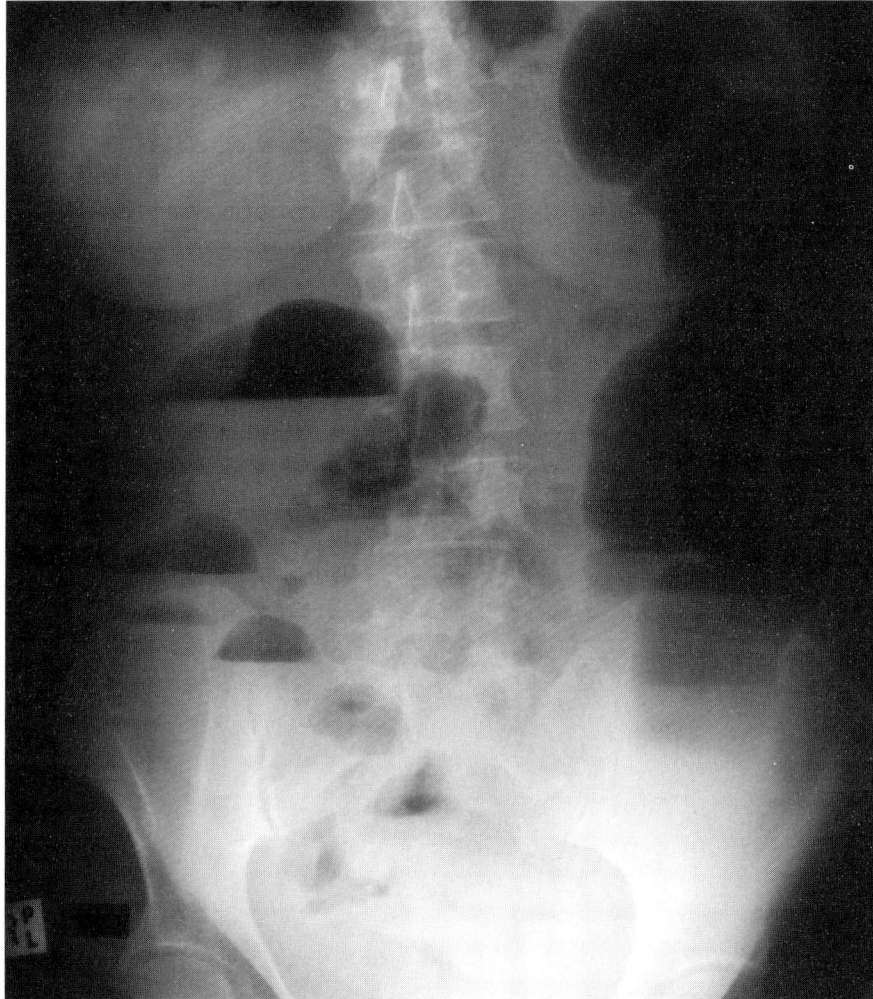

b

(ii) to localise the point of obstruction;
(iii) to diagnose the cause of obstruction, e.g.
      tumour, inflammatory mass;

Paralytic ileus

1. Localised:

Dilated loops of bowel ('sentinel loops'), usually small
bowel, overlying a local inflammation, e.g. right upper
quadrant: acute cholecystitis; left upper quadrant:
acute pancreatitis (*Fig. 2.5*); lower right abdomen:
acute appendicitis.

2. Generalised:

Non-specific dilatation of small and large bowel;

scattered irregular fluid levels on the erect view; may
occur post-operatively or with peritonitis.

Specific causes of intestinal obstruction which may be diagnosed with plain films

Caecal volvulus (*Fig. 2.6*)

- Markedly dilated caecum containing one or two
  haustral markings.

- Caecum may lie in right iliac fossa or left upper
  quadrant.

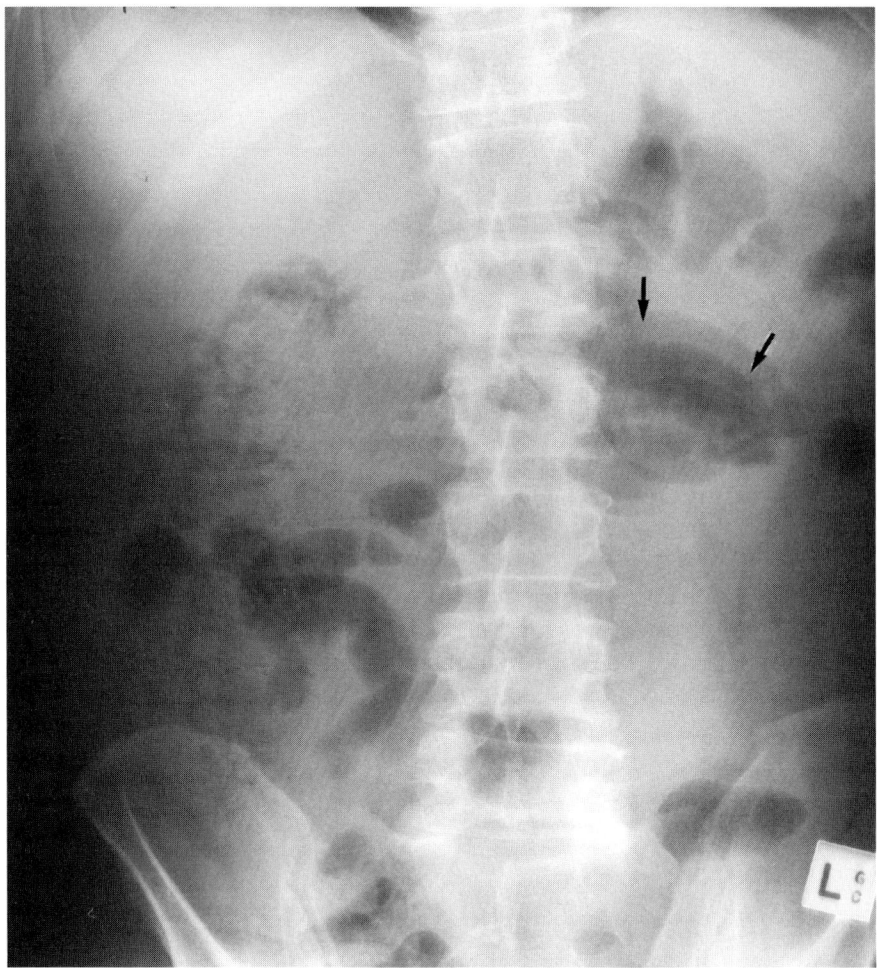

Figure 2.5 *Sentinel loops. Multiple dilated loops of small bowel (arrows) are grouped in the left upper abdomen in a patient with pancreatitis.*

- Attached gas-filled appendix.
- Small bowel dilatation.
- Collapse of left half of colon.

Sigmoid volvulus (*Fig. 2.7*)

- Massively distended sigmoid loop in the shape of an inverted 'U', which can extend above T10 and overlap the lower border of the liver.
- Usually has no haustral markings.
- The outer walls and adjacent inner walls of the U form three white lines which converge towards the left side of the pelvis.

- Overlap of the dilated descending colon, i.e. 'left flank overlap' sign.

Strangulated hernia (*Fig. 2.8*)

- Gas-containing soft tissue mass in the inguinal region.
- May have a fluid level on the erect view.
- Gas in the bowel wall in the presence of infarction.

Gallstone ileus

- Small bowel obstruction.

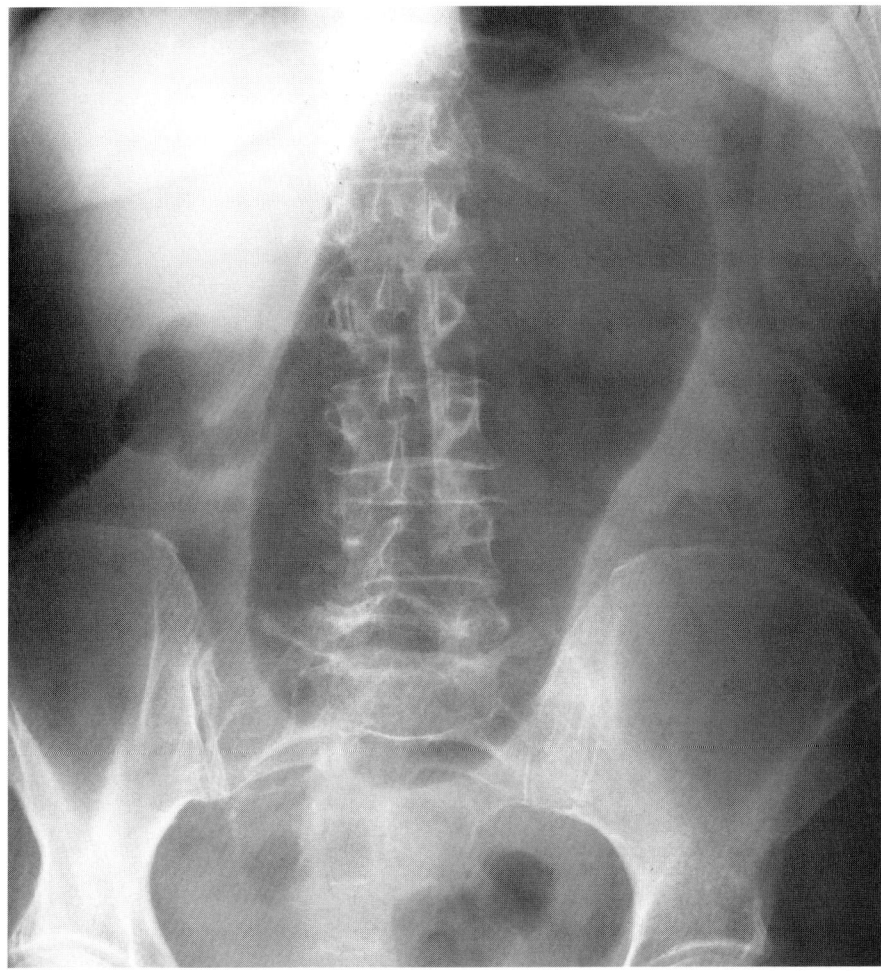

Figure 2.6 *Caecal volvulus. Massively dilated caecum in the central abdomen. Note that the distal large bowel is not dilated.*

- Gas in the biliary tree seen as a branching pattern of gas density in the right upper quadrant.

- Calcified gallstone lying in an abnormal position is occasionally seen.

Intussusception (*see* Chapter 11)

Acute appendicitis

The plain film diagnosis of acute appendicitis is unreliable and some, all, or indeed none of the following signs may be seen:

- Faecolith: calcified opacity usually in the right iliac fossa.

- Distal small bowel obstruction or localised paralytic ileus.

- Blurred right psoas margin and right pro-peritoneal fat stripe.

- Lumbar scoliosis convex to the left.

- Decreased abdominal gas due to vomiting and diarrhoea.

- Gas in the appendix.

- Appendix abscess: soft tissue mass in the right iliac fossa which may separate gas-filled ascending colon from properitoneal fat stripe.

US and CT have an increasing role in the assessment of right lower quadrant pain and are useful for the following:

- Diagnosis of appendicitis.

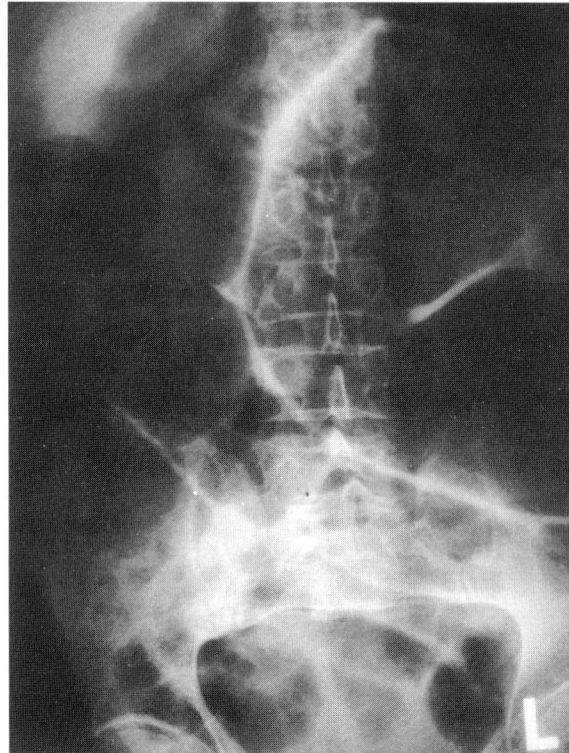

Figure 2.7 *Sigmoid volvulus.*
Massively dilated sigmoid colon arising from the pelvis to the level of the lower thoracic vertebrae. Note:
- *lack of haustral markings*
- *convergence into the pelvis of outer and inner walls of the dilated loop*
- *overlap of dilated descending colon in the left abdomen.*

- Diagnosis of complications of appendicitis, e.g. abscess, mucocele.

- Diagnosis of alternate causes of right lower quadrant pain, e.g. pelvic inflammatory disease.

Choice of modality will depend to some extent on local expertise though CT should be used in obese patients or in severely ill patients in whom complications such as peritonitis or abscess are suspected.

US is highly accurate for appendicitis particularly where compression and colour Doppler imaging (CDI) are used, and where the examination is concentrated to the point of maximal tenderness as indicated by the patient (*Fig. 2.9*).

US signs of appendicitis:

- Non-compressible dilated appendix measuring over 7 mm in diameter (normal appendix 5 mm or less).

- Hyperaemia on CDI.

- Complications:
  (a) Gangrene: avascular area on CDI.
  (b) Phlegmon: echogenic mass.
  (c) Abscess: irregular hypoechoic mass.

CT signs of appendicitis:

- Thickened wall of appendix with or without contrast enhancement.

- Peri-appendiceal/pericaecal inflammation.

- Calcified faecolith.

- Complications:
  (a) Abscess: irregular mass containing fluid/gas.
  (b) Mucocele: thin-walled, well-defined fluid-filled mass (*Fig. 2.10*).

Perforation of the gastrointestinal tract

Signs of free gas

- Erect chest X-ray: gas beneath diaphragm (*Fig. 2.11*).

- Supine abdomen: gas outlines solid organs (liver and spleen) and outlines anatomical structures (e.g. falciform ligament); bowel walls seen as white lines with gas both inside and outside (*Fig. 2.12*).

- Free gas also identified on erect abdomen film: if the patient is too ill to stand then either decubitus or shoot-through lateral films can be performed.

Contrast studies

- Use water soluble contrast as opposed to barium.

- Contrast meal for suspected perforated duodenal or gastric ulcers.

- Contrast enema for suspected perforated colon (*Fig. 2.13*).

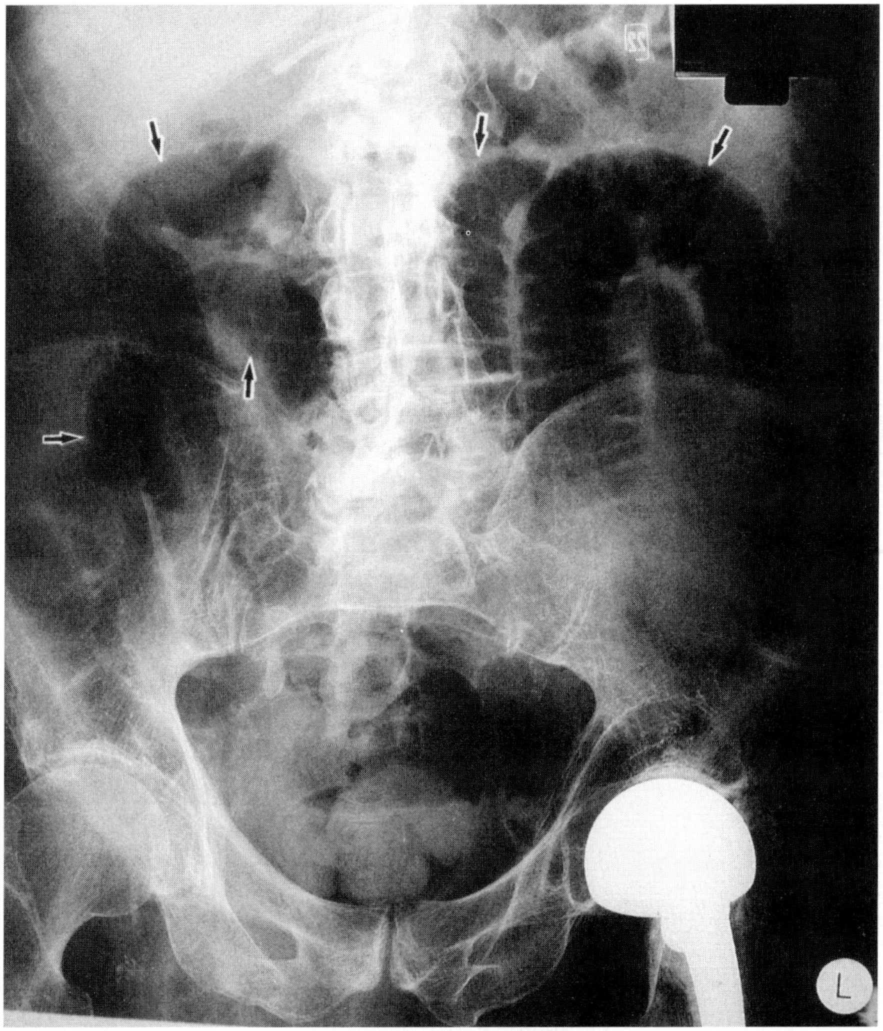

Figure 2.8 *Strangulated inguinal hernia. Distended small bowel loops (arrows). Increased soft tissue density plus gas-containing bowel loops seen below the right inguinal ligament.*

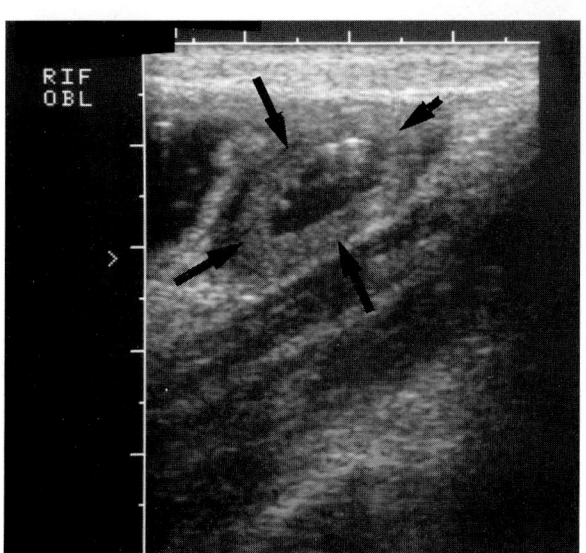

Figure 2.9 *Acute appendicitis – US. The inflamed appendix is well seen (arrows) and has the following features:*
- *distended*
- *thick walled*
- *non-compressible*
- *acutely tender to probe pressure.*

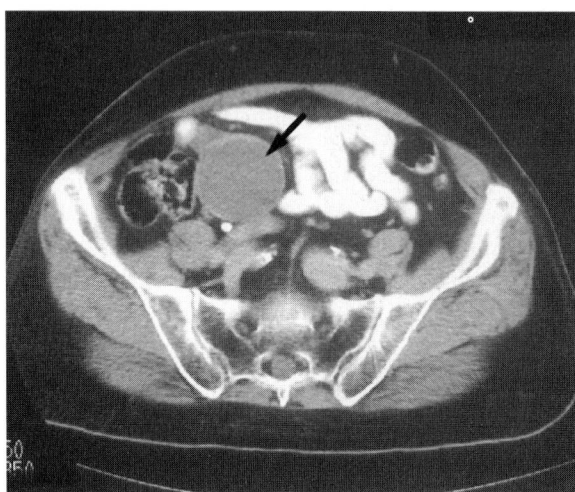

Figure 2.10 *Mucocele of the appendix.*
Thin walled cyst (arrow) with homogeneous low
attenuation fluid contents lying medial to the caecum.

- May also identify sinus and fistula tracts (e.g. colovesical fistula in diverticular disease).

Acute cholecystitis

Ultrasound

US is the investigation of choice for suspected acute cholecystitis. US signs include:

- Gallstones: hyperechoic lesions with acoustic shadowing which are mobile (*Fig. 1.11*).
- Thickening of gallbladder wall (greater than 4 mm) (*Fig. 2.14*).
- Hypoechoic gallbladder wall due to oedema.
- Surrounding fluid or localised fluid collection.
- Distended gallbladder.
- Localised tenderness to direct probe pressure.

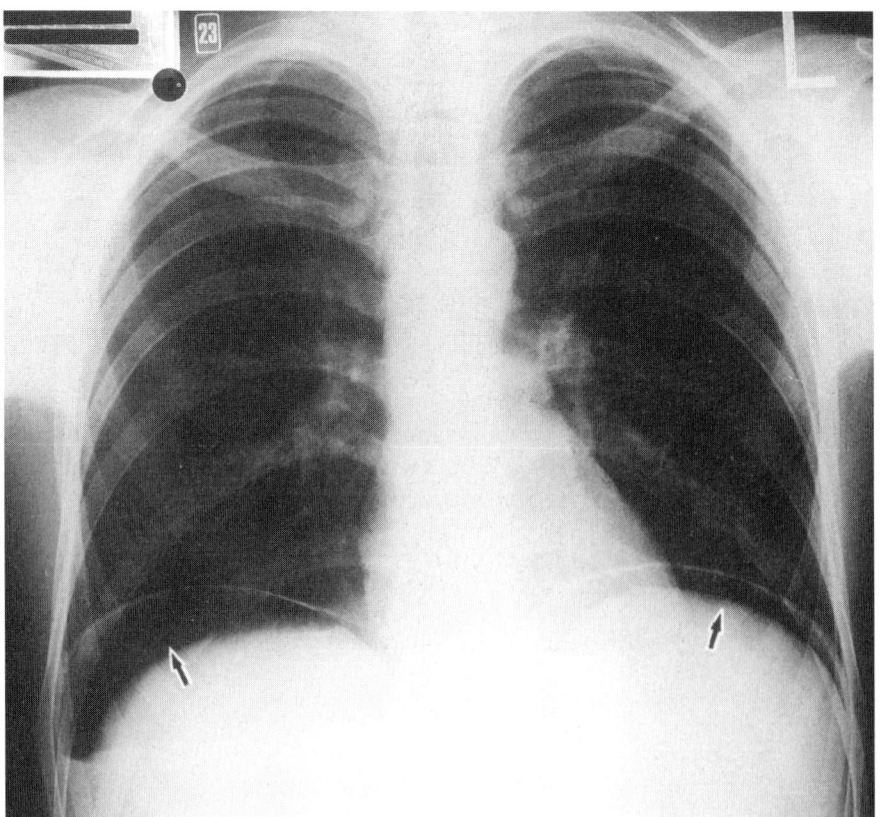

Figure 2.11 *Perforation of the colon.*
Excellent demonstration of free gas beneath the diaphragm (arrows).

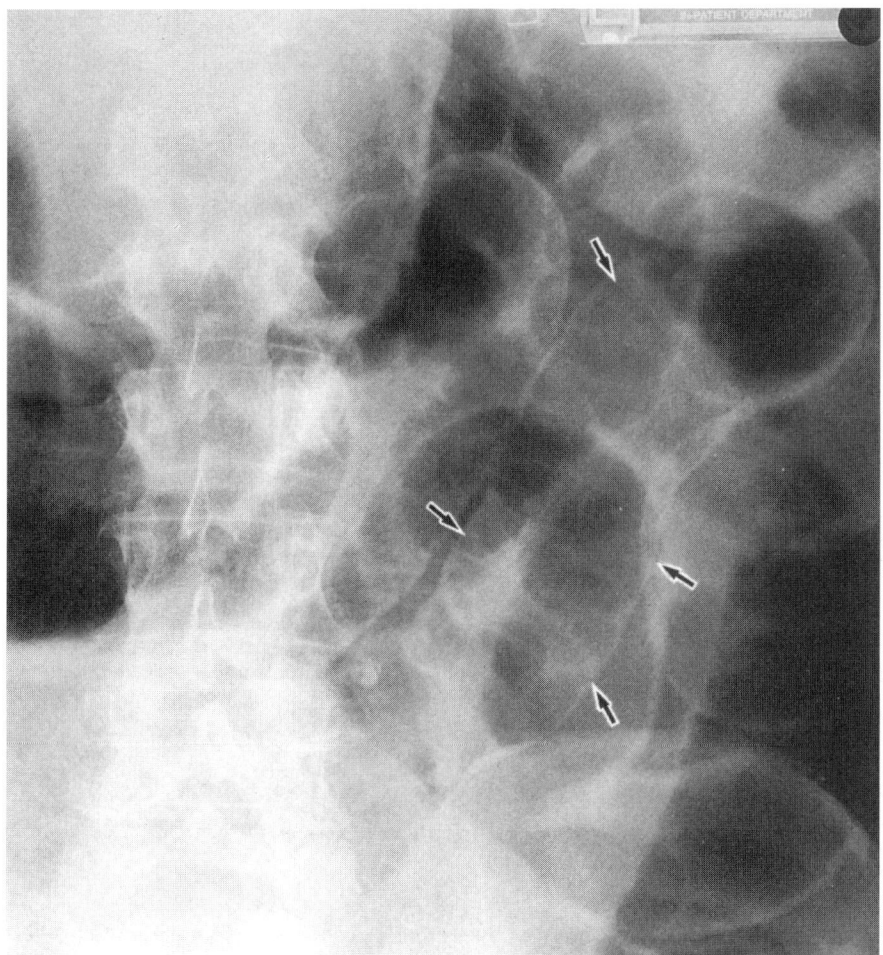

Figure 2.12
Pneumoperitoneum-supine abdomen.
The bowel wall is outlined by gas within the lumen and by free gas outside the bowel within the peritoneal cavity (arrows).

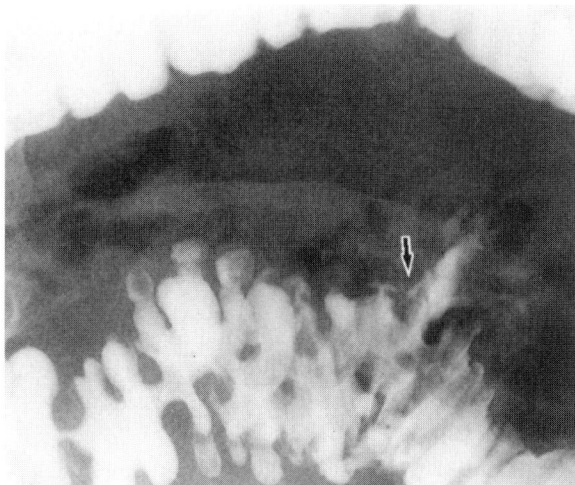

Figure 2.13 *Perforated large bowel.*
Leakage of contrast from large bowel (arrow) due to diverticular disease.

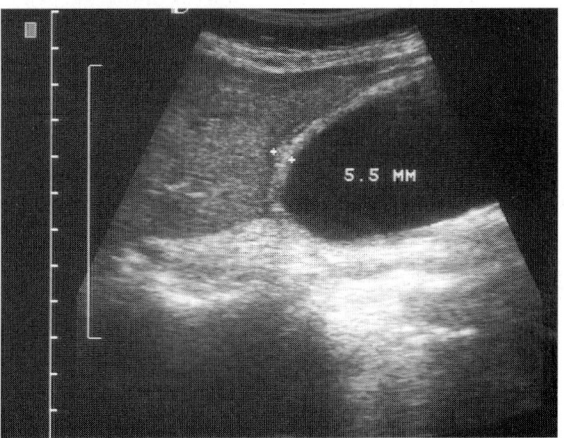

Figure 2.14 *Thickened gallbladder wall – US.*
The gallbladder wall normally measures 3 mm in thickness or less. Thickening of the gallbladder wall is well demonstrated in this case of acalculous cholecystitis.

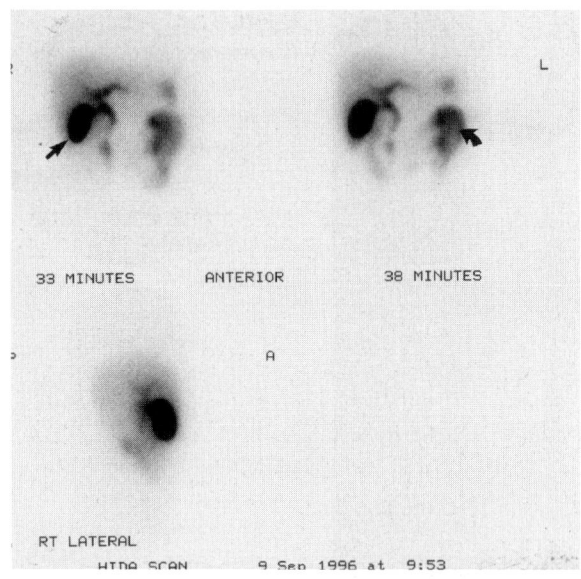
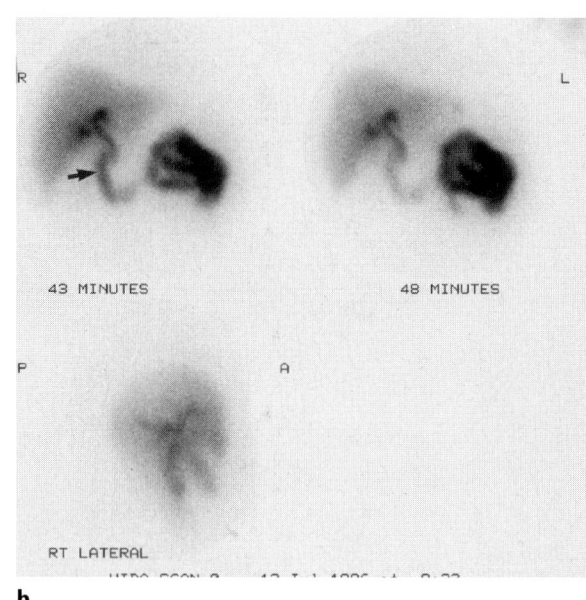

a   b

Figure 2.15 *Acute cholecystitis – HIDA scan.*
(a) Normal HIDA scan. Following normal hepatic uptake there is good filling of the bile ducts and the gallbladder (straight arrow). Note also normal activity in the duodenum and jejunum (curved arrow). (b) Acute cholecystitis. There is normal hepatic uptake of tracer. The bile duct is outlined (arrow) and tracer has entered the bowel. The gallbladder is not seen due to acute cholecystitis. Compare this appearance with (a).

Scintigraphy

Scintigraphy with ^{99m}Tc-labelled iminodiacetic acid (IDA) compounds has a limited role in difficult cases where clinical assessment and ultrasound are doubtful. Acute cholecystitis is indicated by non-visualisation of the gallbladder with good visualisation of the common bile duct and duodenum one hour after injection (*Fig. 2.15*). Visualisation of the gallbladder excludes acute cholecystitis.

Plain films

Plain films are insensitive for acute cholecystitis; signs are usually non-specific and include:

- Gallstones (only seen in 10%).

- Soft tissue mass in the right upper quadrant due to distended gallbladder.

- Paralytic ileus in the right upper quadrant.

Acute pancreatitis

CT

- Investigation of choice:
  (i)   Confirmation of the diagnosis.
  (ii) Identification of necrotic gland tissue.
  (iii) Diagnosis of complications.
  (iv) Guidance of interventional procedures.

- CT signs include:
  (i)   Diffuse or focal gland enlargement with decreased density and indistinct gland margins.
  (ii) Fine sections during infusion of contrast (i.e. dynamic scans) can differentiate necrotic from viable gland tissue as necrotic tissue does not enhance.
  (iii) Thickening of surrounding fascial planes (e.g. left paranephric fascia) (*Fig. 2.16*).
  (iv) Fluid collections most commonly related to the gland, in lesser sac, and in the left pararenal space (*Fig. 2.17*).

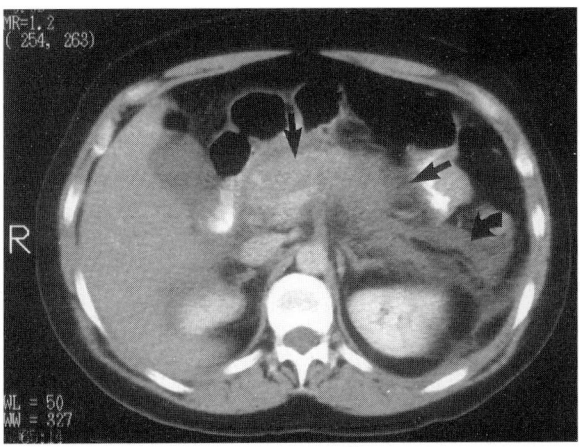

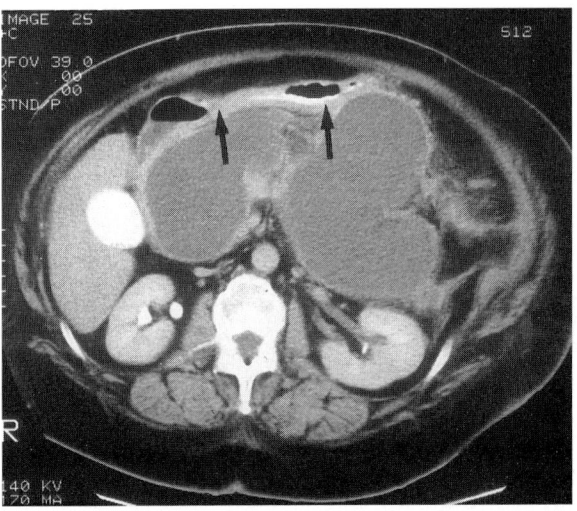

Figure 2.16 *Acute pancreatitis – CT.*
The pancreas is swollen and has indistinct margins due to inflammation of surrounding fat (straight arrows). There is thickening of the left pararenal fascia (curved arrow).

Figure 2.17 *Acute pancreatitis – CT.*
Large fluid collections in the pancreas. The stomach is compressed anteriorly (arrows).

(v) Phlegmon appears as an irregular mass spreading along fascial planes and can be quite extensive.

(vi) Abscess: poorly defined fluid collection; irregular, blurred margin which enhances with contrast; gas, either a large collection or mottled bubbles (*Fig. 2.18*).

(vii) Pseudocyst: either within the gland, adjacent to the gland in the lesser sac or left pararenal space, or less commonly at more distant sites including the mediastinum; uni- or multiloculated fluid collection; contents of water density; well defined wall.

- CT can be used to guide aspiration procedures and placement of drains in abscesses and pseudocysts, and for follow-up either post-operatively or in conservative management.

Ultrasound

- May be difficult in the acute situation owing to overlying dilated bowel loops.

- Pancreas appears enlarged with decreased echogenicity and blurred irregular margins.

- Fluid collections are seen as hypoechoic areas anatomically localised as described for CT.

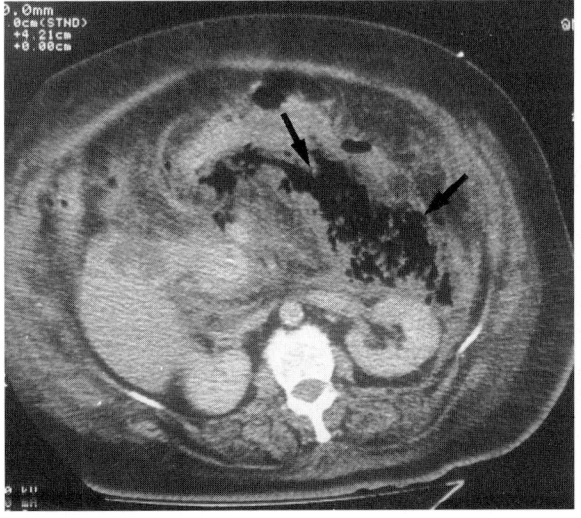

Figure 2.18 *Acute pancreatitis – CT.*
The pancreas is necrotic and largely replaced by abscess formation. Note the presence of gas in the abscess (arrows) as well as inflammatory change in the mesenteric and subcutaneous fat.

- As with CT, US can be used to guide aspiration and drainage procedures, and for follow-up.

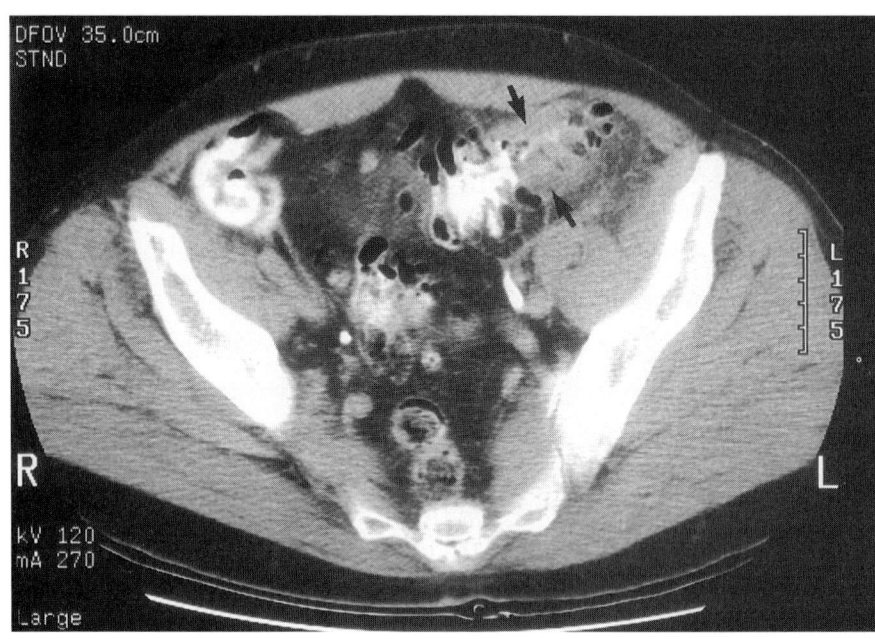

Figure 2.19 *Acute diverticulitis – CT. The wall of the sigmoid colon is thickened with intramural abscess formation (arrows). Note also inflammatory stranding in the pericolonic fat.*

Plain films

- Unreliable: up to two-thirds are normal.
- Plain film signs may include:
  - (i) Paralytic ileus in the left upper quadrant (*Fig. 2.5*).
  - (ii) Generalised ileus.
  - (iii) Loss of left psoas outline.
  - (iv) Separation of greater curve of stomach from transverse colon.
  - (v) Pancreatic calcification with chronic pancreatitis.
- Chest X-ray signs:
  - (i) Left pleural effusion.
  - (ii) Atelectasis of left lower lobe.
  - (iii) Elevated left hemidiaphragm.

Diverticulitis

Diverticulitis refers to diverticular perforation with intramural, pericolonic, or peritoneal inflammation, abscess formation, and sinus/fistula formation. Plain films are usually unhelpful. In the past barium enema has been used to study patients with diverticulitis. Limitations of barium enema include:

- Inability to diagnose pericolonic and peritoneal inflammation.
- Low sensitivity for intramural inflammation.
- Low sensitivity for alternate diagnoses.

CT is now the investigation of choice for assessment of acute left lower quadrant pain:

- Highly accurate for diagnosis of diverticulitis.
- Able to visualise intramural and pericolonic inflammation.
- Where diverticulitis is not present may suggest alternate diagnoses, e.g. small bowel obstruction, pelvic inflammatory disease, pancreatitis, pyelonephritis, etc.

CT signs of diverticulitis (*Fig. 2.19*):

- Localised wall thickening > 5 mm.
- Pericolonic inflammation: soft tissue stranding or haziness in pericolonic fat.
- Abscess/phlegmon: soft tissue mass containing fluid and/or gas.
- Sinus/fistula tracts: linear tracts filled with contrast/gas.
- Contrast/gas in bladder, vagina, or abdominal wall.

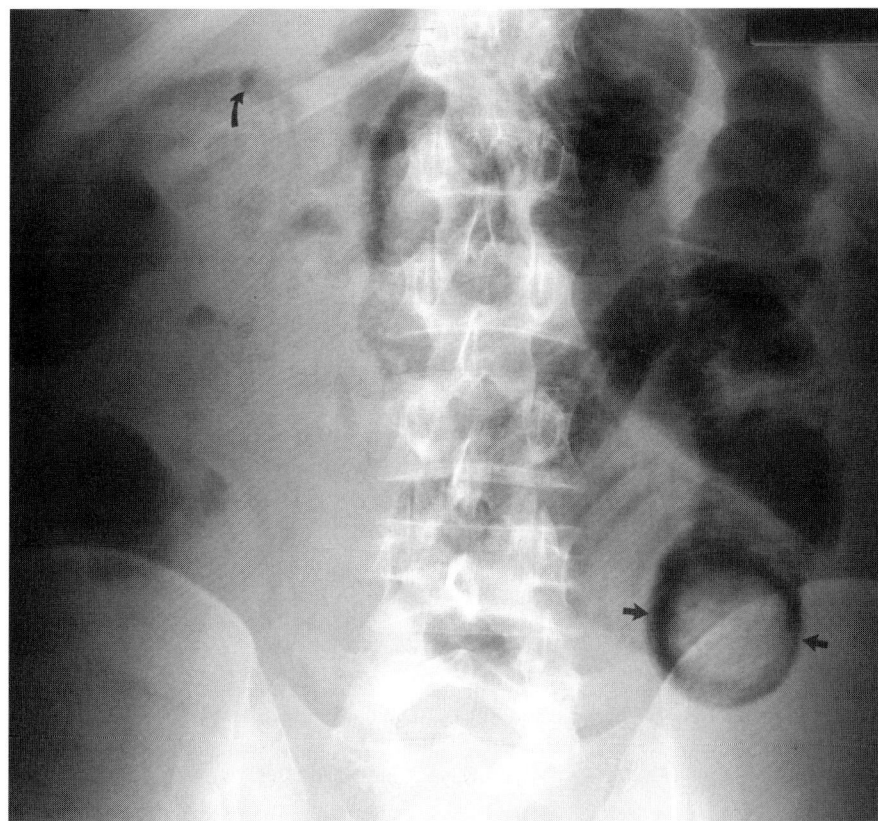

Figure 2.20 *Small bowel infarction.*
There is a large amount of gas in the wall of the small bowel indicating infarction (straight arrows). Note gas in the portal vein (curved arrow).

Acute mesenteric ischaemia (AMI)

AMI is caused by abrupt disruption to blood flow to the bowel. The goal of diagnosis and therapy is prevention or limitation of bowel infarction. Plain films are insensitive for AMI; plain films signs when present usually indicate bowel infarction and include bowel wall thickening, bowel dilatation, gas in the bowel wall and portal vein gas (*Fig. 2.20*).

Early diagnosis requires a high index of suspicion and early angiography in patients with clinical evidence of AMI, i.e. sudden onset of severe abdominal pain and bloody diarrhoea. The most common causes of AMI are superior mesenteric artery (SMA) embolus, SMA thrombosis, and non-occlusive SMA vasospasm. Depending on the cause and clinical situation, particularly the presence or absence of peritoneal signs, treatment will be immediate surgery or interventional radiology.

SMA embolus

• May have a history of cardiac disease, previous embolic event, or simultaneous peripheral artery embolus.

• Angiography: occlusion of SMA usually several centimetres from its origin with a convex filling defect.

• Usually treated with immediate surgery.

SMA thrombosis

• Usually associated with underlying stenotic athero-sclerotic lesion in SMA.

• Onset of pain may be less acute than in SMA embolus.

• Angiography: occlusion of SMA within 1 or 2 cm of its origin; collateral vessels to the more distal SMA.

• Interventional radiology: thrombolytic therapy via a

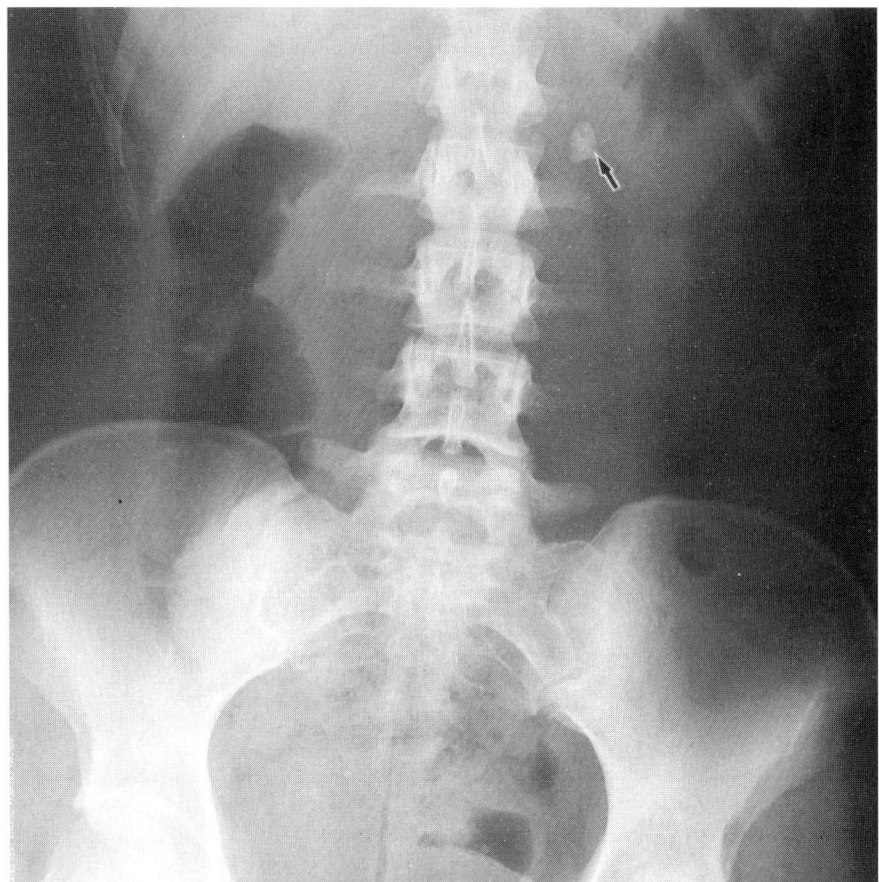

Figure 2.21 *Ureteric calculus.*
Dense opacity on the left at the level of the L1-2 disc (arrow).

catheter placed in the origin of the SMA followed by dilatation of the underlying stenosis by balloon dilatation or stent placement.

Non-occlusive SMA vasospasm

- Mesenteric vasospasm persisting after an episode of severe systemic hypotension.

- Angiography: diffuse arterial narrowing due to vasospasm; poor filling of distal branches; low arterial flow rate; delayed filling of veins.

- Interventional radiology: papaverine bolus and infusion via catheter placed in the SMA.

Renal colic

Common causes of renal colic or renal angle pain:

- Ureteric calculus.

- Renal calculus.

- Pelvi-ureteric junction obstruction.

- Acute pyelonephritis.

- Ureteric stricture.

- Transitional cell carcinoma (TCC) of the ureter causing obstruction.

- TCC of the bladder impinging on the vesico-ureteric junction.

- Clot colic, i.e. colic due to a blood clot complicating haematuria.

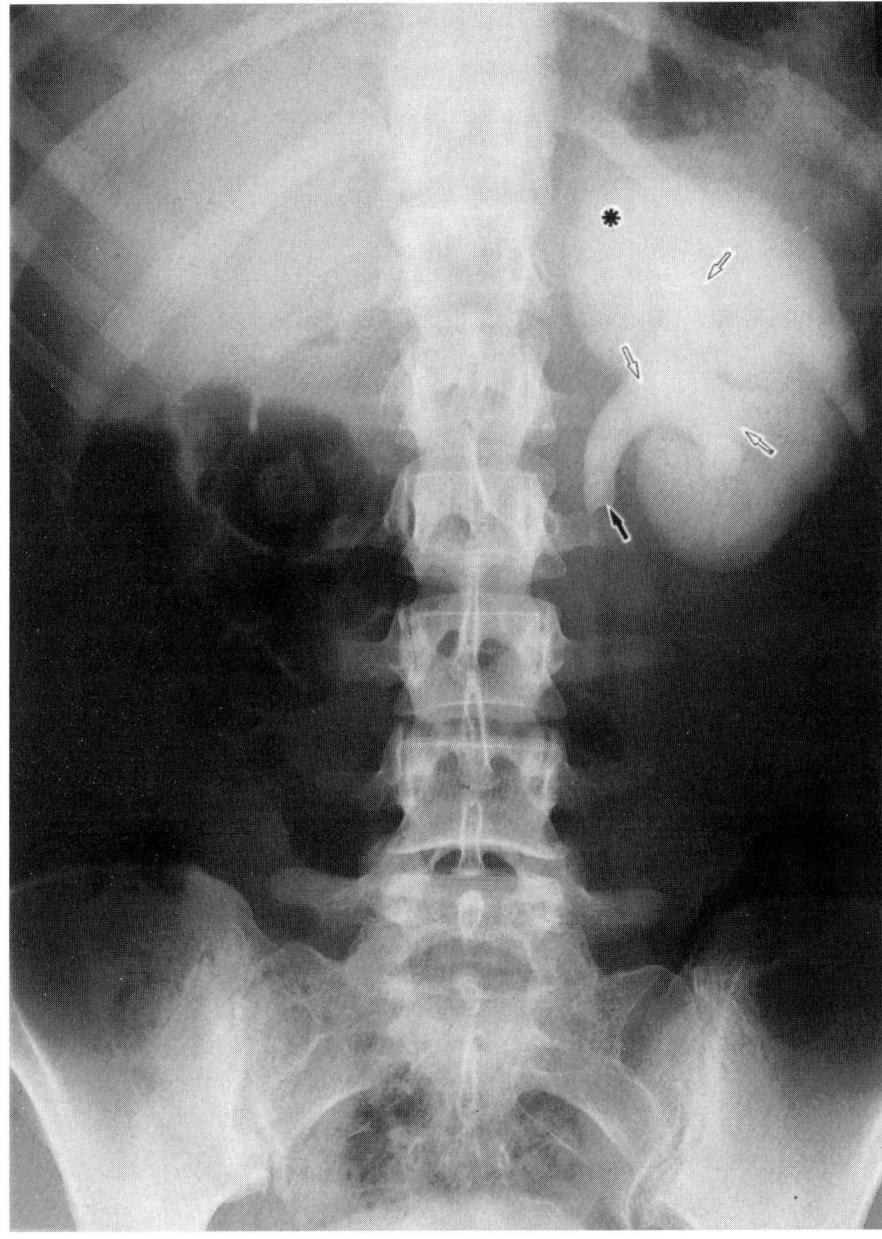

Figure 2.22 *Uteric calculus – IVP.*
A delayed IVP film confirms that the opacity in Figure 2.21 is a calculus in the upper left ureter (black arrow). On this delayed film the signs of obstruction of the left kidney are:
- *dense persistent nephrogram (*)*
- *dilated collecting system above the calculus (white arrows)*
- *no passage of contrast below the calculus.*

Plain films

- 90% of renal calculi contain sufficient calcium to be radio-opaque, i.e. visible on plain films (*Fig. 2.21*).

- Cystine stones (3%) are faintly opaque.

- Urate stones (5%) are lucent.

- Xanthine and matrix stones are rare and lucent.

Note that opacities seen on plain films thought to be renal or ureteric calculi need to be differentiated from other causes of calcification, e.g. arterial calcification, calcified lymph nodes, pelvic phleboliths.

IVP

- Following plain films, IVP is the imaging modality of choice in the assessment of renal colic:

(i)   To prove that an opacity seen on plain films lies within the urinary tract.
(ii) To diagnose lucent calculi not seen on plain films.
(iii) To identify other causes of renal colic, as above, and guide further actions.

- Dilatation of the entire length of the ureter with no apparent obstructing opacity is most commonly due to oedema of the vesico-ureteric junction secondary to recent passage of a calculus.

- An obstructing ureteric calculus shows all or some of the following signs (*Fig. 2.22*):
  (i)   Delayed uptake of contrast by the involved kidney.
  (ii) Persistent contrast outlining the renal cortex, i.e. delayed nephrogram.
  (iii) Delayed appearance of contrast in the collecting system.
  (iv) Dilated collecting system above the calculus.
  (v)   Leakage of contrast with severe obstruction.
  (vi) Increased pain following injection of contrast.

- Renal calculi may be amenable to extracorporeal shock wave lithotripsy (ESWL) which uses highly focused, high intensity ultrasound to shatter calculi into small fragments able to be passed or removed percutaneously.

- Acute pyelonephritis may show no changes on IVP or a focal deformity in the event of inflammatory mass or abscess formation.

- Pelvi-ureteric junction obstruction shows dilatation of the collecting system with marked dilatation of the renal pelvis and failure to opacify the ureter.

- Percutaneous nephrostomy may be required to salvage renal function prior to surgery.

Abdominal abscess

Plain films

Although the following signs may be seen, plain films are unreliable.

- Chest X-ray signs associated with subphrenic abscess:
  (i)   Raised hemidiaphragm.

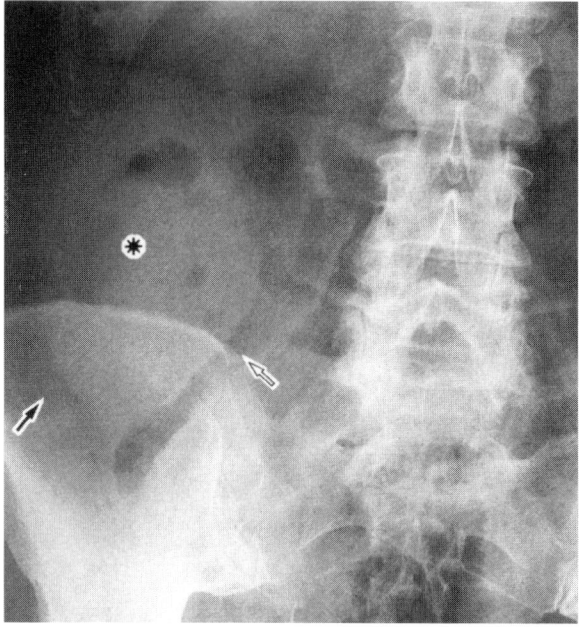

Figure 2.23 *Abscess.*
Mass of mixed soft tissue and gas density (*) lying in the right paracolic gutter separating ascending colon (solid arrow) from pro-peritoneal fat stripe (hollow arrow).

  (ii) Pleural fluid.
  (iii) Lower lobe collapse.
  (iv) Subdiaphragmatic fluid level.

- Abdomen X-ray:
  (i)   Mass, perhaps containing gas or even a fluid level on the erect view (*Fig. 2.23*).
  (ii) Displaced bowel loops.
  (iii) Localised or generalised ileus.
  (iv) Loss of outline of adjacent structures, e.g. psoas muscle.

Ultrasound

- US should be the primary investigation of choice for suspected intra-abdominal abscess. Advantages of US include:
  (i)   Portability.
  (ii) Can differentiate localised fluid collections.
  (iii) Guide needle aspiration and drainage.
  (iv) Especially sensitive for subdiaphragmatic, subhepatic, and pelvic collections (*Fig. 2.24*).

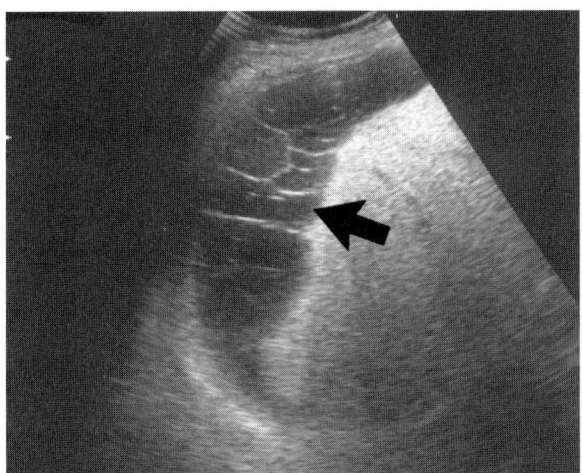

Figure 2.24 *Subphrenic abscess – US.*
A complex fluid collection (arrow) is seen between the right diaphragm and the liver.

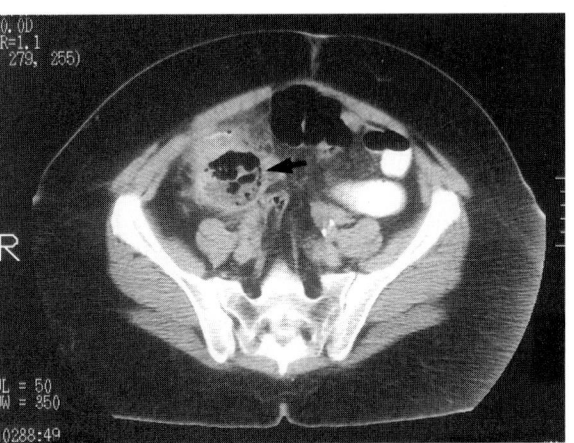

Figure 2.25 *Appendiceal abscess.*
Fluid collection in the right iliac fossa (arrow). Note the presence of gas in the collection as well as inflammatory stranding in the surrounding fat.

- The principal disadvantage of US is that it is less sensitive for central abdominal collections due to overlying intestinal gas.

- US may also be difficult to perform where surgical dressings and drains are present.

CT

- Excellent modality, especially where US is unhelpful.

- Complete bowel opacification with oral and rectal contrast is mandatory as non-opacified bowel loops may mimic fluid collections.

- Guidance of needle aspiration and drain placement.

- CT signs of abscess:
    (i)   low attenuation mass;
    (ii) irregular enhancing wall;
    (iii) may contain gas and fluid levels (*Fig. 2.25*).

Scintigraphy

- Scintigraphy is used to sort out difficult cases where clinical suspicion of an abscess is high but US and CT are negative.

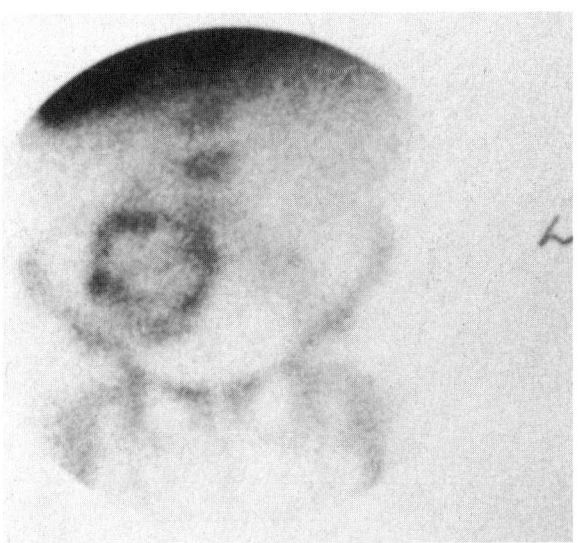

Figure 2.26 *Abscess – scintigraphy.*
Labelled white blood cell scan. There is a ring-shaped area of increased activity in the right iliac fossa indicating uptake of white blood cells in the wall of a large abscess. (Courtesy of Dr W. Lun, Royal Brisbane Hospital.)

- Labelled white cells:
    (i) Indium and more recently, ^{99m}Tc HMPAO (hexamethylpropyleneamineoxime)-labelled white blood cells.

(ii) ^{99m}Tc HMPAO provides better image resolution, lower radiation dose, and easier handling compared with indium.

(iii) More specificity than gallium scanning and results available sooner as imaging performed 3 hours after injection.

(iv) An abscess (or other inflammatory process) shows as an area of focal increased activity (*Fig. 2.26*).

(v) Difficulty of interpretation may occur owing to uptake in the hepatobiliary system, the bowel, and the urinary tract.

• Gallium:
(i) Gallium scanning is extremely sensitive in detecting sites of inflammation.

(ii) Difficulty of interpretation owing to gallium uptake in bowel, liver, and spleen.

(iii) Results not available for up to 48 hours.

Further Reading

1. Balthazar EJ, Birnbaum BA, Yee J et al. Acute appendicitis: CT and US Correlation in 100 patients. *Radiology* 1994; 190:31–35.

2. Cho KC, Morehouse HT, Alterman DD, Thornhill BA. Sigmoid diverticulitis: diagnostic role of CT – Comparison with barium enema studies. *Radiology* 1990; 176:111–115.

3. Frazer D, Medwid SW, Baer JW *et al*. CT of small bowel obstruction: value in establishing the diagnosis and determining the degree and cause. *AJR* 1994; 162:37–41.

4. Paterson-Brown S, Vipond MN. Modern aids to clinical decision making in the acute abdomen. *British Journal of Surgery* 1990; 77:13–18.

5. Sivit CJ. Imaging children with acute right lower quadrant pain. *Pediatric Clinics of North America* 1997; 44:575–589.

6. Young WS. Further radiological observations in cecal volvulus. *Clinical Radiology* 1980; 31:479–483.

3 Miscellaneous gastrointestinal (GIT) conditions

Common GIT radiological procedures

Barium swallow

Indications:

- Dysphagia.
- Swallowing disorders in the elderly, following stroke, or following head injury.
- Suspected gastro-oesophageal reflux.
- Post-oesophageal surgery.

Method:

The patient is asked to swallow contrast material and films taken. Images of the oesophagus are recorded on cine-film, video, or X-ray film. Video is particularly useful in the assessment of swallowing disorders and these studies are often undertaken with the help and cooperation of a speech or swallowing therapist. Barium is usually used though for checking of surgical anastomoses where leakage may occur a water-soluble material such as Gastrografin is preferable. Note that Gastrografin should not be used if pulmonary aspiration is suspected as it is highly osmolar and may induce pulmonary oedema if it enters the lungs.

Barium meal

Indications:

- Dyspepsia.
- Suspected upper GIT bleeding.

- Weight loss/anaemia of unknown cause.
- Assessment of anastomoses post-gastric surgery: use water-soluble contrast (Gastrografin).

Method:

Barium meal is best performed with a 'double contrast' technique. A single contrast study is one where a hollow organ is filled with contrast material such as barium. The outline of the organ can be appreciated though not its mucosal surfaces. If gas is then used to dilate the organ the mucosal surfaces can be seen coated with barium. This is double contrast. The great majority of barium meals and enemas are performed in double contrast as it provides much greater mucosal detail than single contrast. Single contrast studies using barium only may be performed in children, and occasionally in the very elderly.

For a barium meal the patient drinks a small amount of barium followed by gas-forming fluids and films are taken. An antispasmodic is commonly used to halt peristalsis and allow more accurate imaging of the duodenum and stomach. Intravenous hyoscine is used. It rapidly halts peristalsis for 15–20 minutes.

The side effects are rare and due to anticholinergic effects, i.e. dry mouth and blurred vision. Glucagon is used where there is a history of cardiac ischaemia or glaucoma.

Small bowel follow-through

This is a simple screening procedure of limited accuracy used to demonstrate and locate small bowel pathology. The patient drinks a quantity of barium and films are taken until the contrast reaches an obstruction or enters the large bowel.

Enteroclysis (small bowel enema)

Indications:

- Inflammatory bowel disease, especially Crohn's disease.

- Partial small bowel obstruction.

- Suspected small bowel tumour.

- Meckel diverticulum.

- Malabsorption syndromes.

Method:

A nasogastric tube is passed to the stomach and with the aid of a steering wire guided through the duodenum to the duodeno-jejunal flexure. A mixture of barium with either water or methylcellulose is introduced rapidly through the tube into the small bowel producing a double contrast effect. This is usually much more rapid than small bowel follow through and is more accurate owing to better visualisation of mucosal detail. The major disadvantage is the nasogastric tube which is unpleasant for the patient.

Barium enema

Indications:

- Altered bowel habit.

- Non-acute lower GIT bleeding.

- Weight loss/anaemia of unknown cause.

- Failed colonoscopy.

- To outline and define a suspected obstruction.

- Check surgical anastomoses (Gastrografin).

- Suspected perforation.

Method:

Barium is passed into the colon via a rectal cannula followed by air giving a double contrast technique. Single contrast technique may be used in children, in the very elderly, or for suspected obstruction. Transient bacteraemia may occur and patients with artificial heart valves should receive antibiotic cover. Bowel perforation has been reported though is extremely rare.

Dysphagia

Barium swallow

Barium swallow is the simplest and cheapest screening test. For many conditions barium swallow is sufficient for diagnosis; for others it will guide further investigations. The more common surgical conditions encountered on barium swallow are listed below:

Pharyngeal pouch (Zenker's diverticulum) (*Fig. 3.1*):

- Projects posteriorly and to the left above cricopharyngeus through the inferior constrictor muscle.

- May be quite large with a fluid level seen on chest X-ray.

Oesophageal diverticulum (*Fig. 3.2*):

- Most common from the level of the tracheal bifurcation to the diaphragm.

- Project anteriorly and laterally.

- Large diverticulae above the diaphragm may be associated with hiatus hernia.

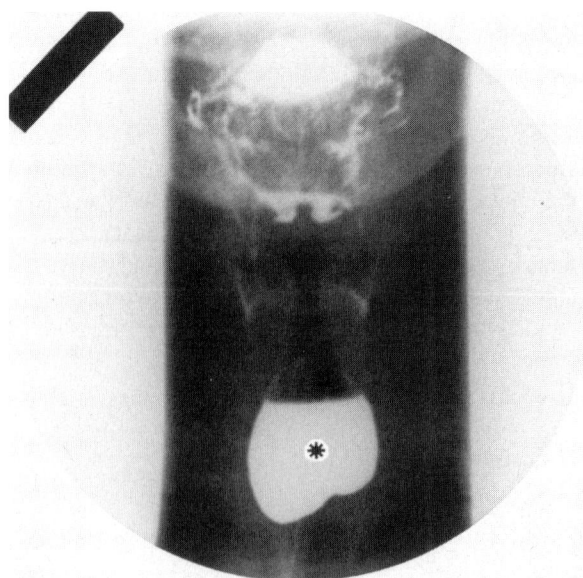

Figure 3.1 *Pharyngeal pouch – barium swallow. Large pharyngeal pouch (*) well outlined with barium.*

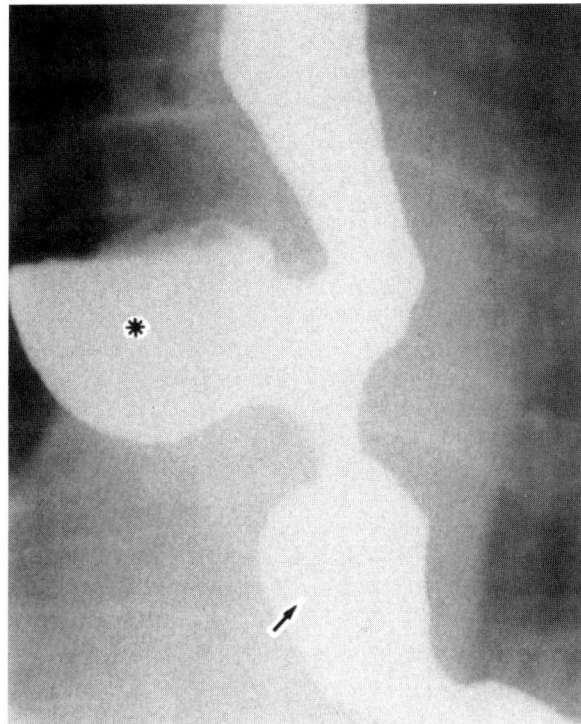

Figure 3.2 *Oesophageal diverticulum.*
This large laterally directed diverticulum (*) of the lower oesophagus is associated with a small hiatus hernia (arrow).

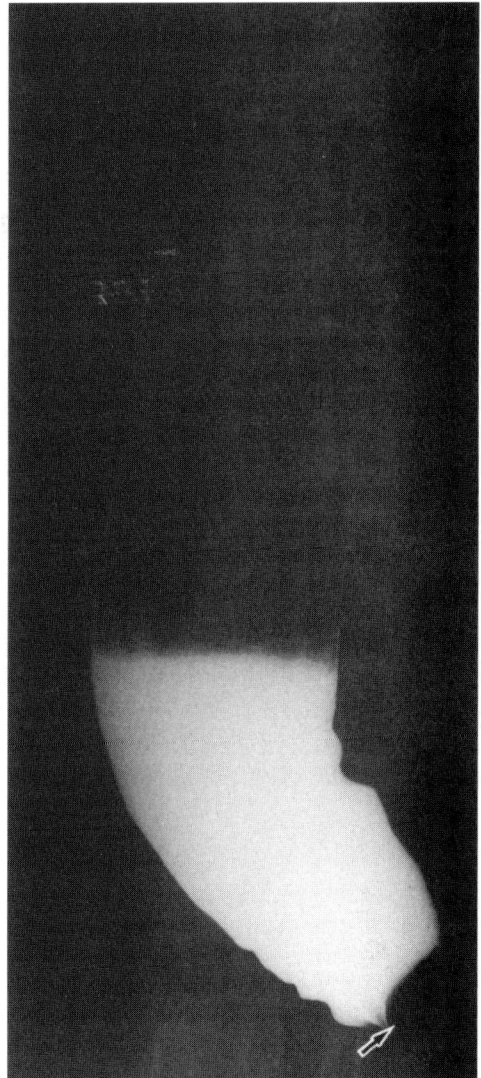

Figure 3.3 *Achalasia – barium swallow.*

Achalasia (*Fig. 3.3*):

- Dilated oesophagus which may also be elongated and tortuous.

- Poor peristalsis.

- Smoothly tapered lower end.

- Chest X-ray may show a mediastinal fluid level, absent gastric air bubble, and evidence of aspiration pneumonia.

Sliding hiatus hernia:

- Range in size from a small clinically insignificant hernia to the entire stomach lying in the thorax (i.e. thoracic stomach) which is at risk of volvulus (*Fig. 3.4*).

- On chest X-ray may show as an apparent mass behind the heart containing a fluid level.

Reflux oesophagitis:

- Erosions give a granular appearance to the mucosa.

- Ulcers seen as larger mucosal defects.

- Chronic reflux may cause a peptic stricture which usually has smooth tapering edges.

Carcinoma of the oesophagus:

- Appearances depend on pattern of tumour growth.

- Early lesions may show only an area of mucosal irregularity and ulceration.

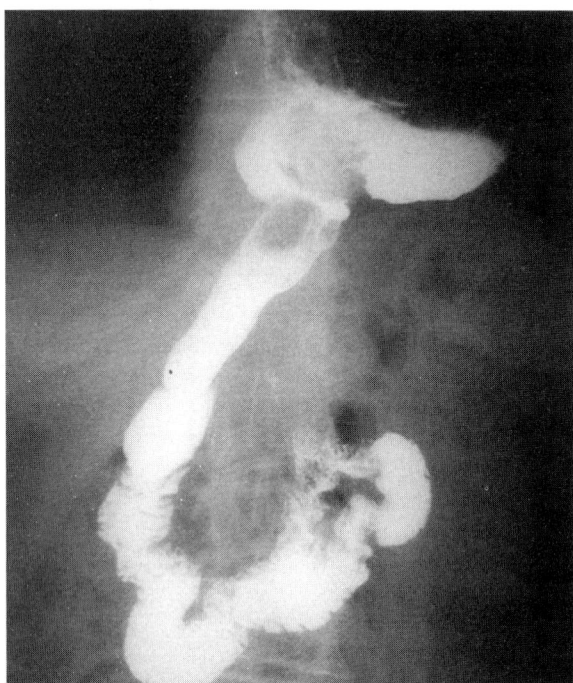

Figure 3.4 *Hiatus hernia.*
Most of the stomach lies within the thoracic cavity. The pylorus is directed vertically downwards into the duodenum.

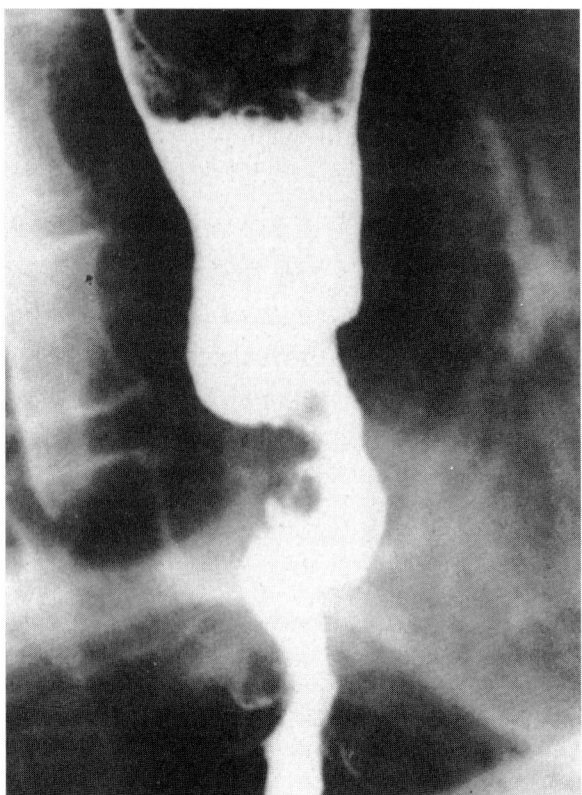

Figure 3.5 *Oesophageal carcinoma – barium swallow. There is a stricture of the lower oesophagus with prominent margins and an intraluminal mass.*

- More advanced lesions present with irregular strictures with elevated margins (*Fig. 3.5*).

- May also present as an irregular intraluminal mass, ulceration, or with sinus/fistula formation.

- For further notes on staging of carcinoma of the oesophagus *see* Chapter 12.

Endoscopy and biopsy

All strictures seen on barium swallow should undergo endoscopic assessment and biopsy as should areas of ulceration and mucosal irregularity.

Peptic ulceration and *Helicobacter pylori*

H. pylori is a Gram-negative bacterium. *H. pylori* infection is the most important cause of gastric and duodenal ulceration, chronic gastritis, and gastric carcinoma. Initial infection causes acute gastritis with parietal cell failure and reduced acid secretion. Chronic infection produces chronic inflammation in the gastric antrum; this chronic superficial gastritis is considered the characteristic pathological lesion produced by *H. pylori*. At this stage acid secretion from parietal cells in the proximal stomach may be normal or raised leading to an increased incidence of peptic ulceration.

The vast majority of gastric and duodenal ulcers are caused by *H. pylori* infection with non-steroidal anti-inflammatory drugs remaining a major causative factor in the stomach. *H. pylori* infection is also associated with an increased incidence of gastric carcinoma. Another type of gastric malignancy associated with *H. pylori* infection is the mucosa-associated lymphoid tissue (MALT) lymphoma; treatment of infection will result in complete or partial regression of this tumour in most patients.

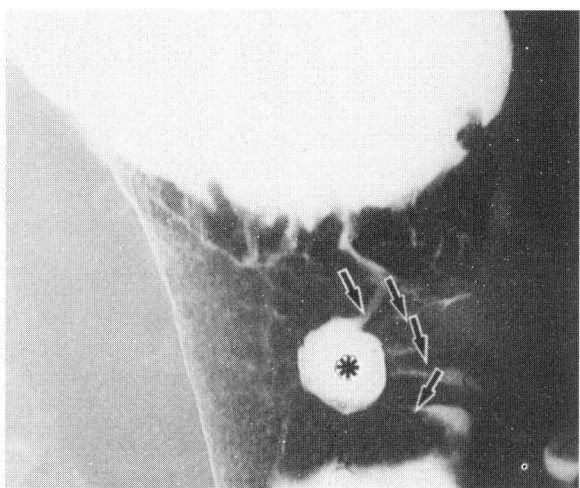

Figure 3.6 *Gastric ulcer.*
Large ulcer crater (*) with radiating mucosal folds (arrows).

Diagnostic tests for *H. pylori* infection include:

- Endoscopic biopsy:
  (i)   histologic examination;
  (ii) culture of biopsy sample.

- Serological tests.

- Urea breath test.

- Double contrast barium meal.

The most characteristic radiological sign of *H. pylori* infection is thickened gastric folds. This fold thickening may be nodular or polypoid and occurs predominantly in the gastric antrum. Other findings may include erosions, ulcers (*Fig. 3.6*), inflammatory polyps, and narrowing of the gastric antrum.

A logical approach to diagnosis and treatment of *H. pylori* would be as follows:

Figure 3.7 *Acute colitis. Featureless loops of large bowel due to acute inflammation of the bowel wall (*). Note faecal shadows throughout the remainder of the colon.*

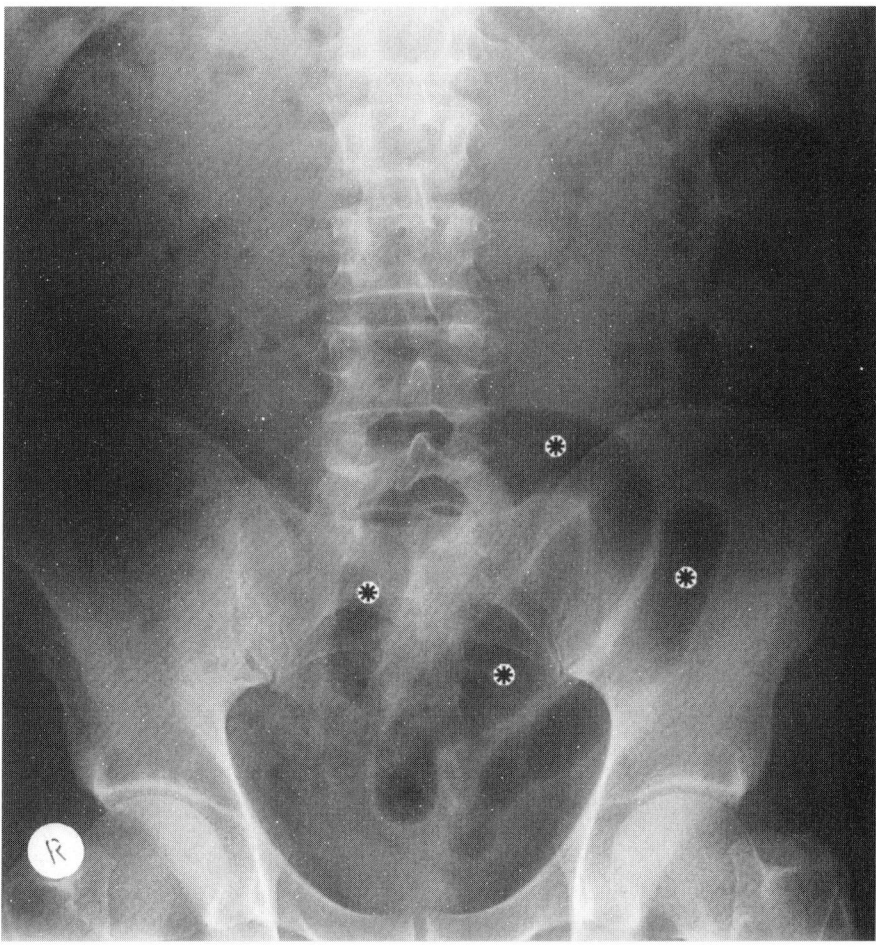

- Young patients, mild symptoms: serological tests or urea breath tests followed by treatment with antimicrobial and antisecretory medications.

- Persistent or severe symptoms: barium meal or endoscopy to exclude ulceration or carcinoma.

Inflammatory bowel disease

Plain films

- Relatively insensitive and non-specific.

- May be useful in acute colitis where barium studies are contraindicated and endoscopy may be difficult and painful.

- Acute colitis: affected bowel shows wall thickening, blurred mucosal margins, absent haustral markings; gasless colon strongly suggests severe disease (*Fig. 3.7*).

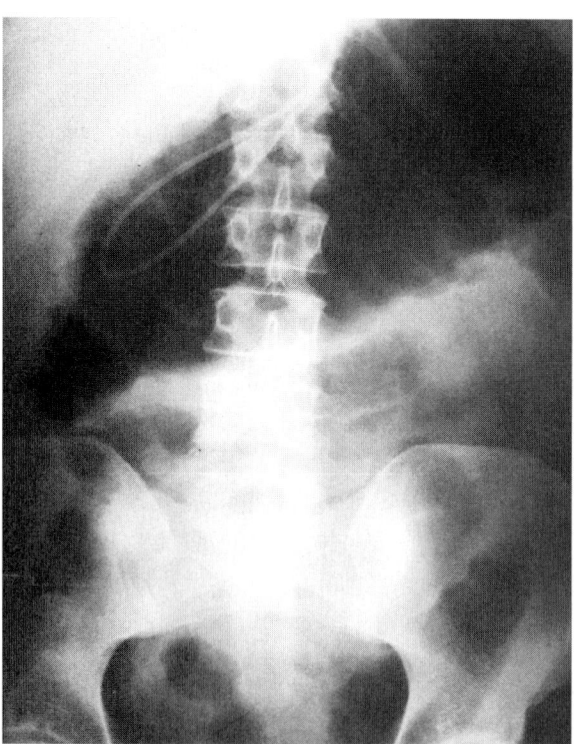

Figure 3.8 *Toxic megacolon.*
Grossly dilated transverse colon. There is also a nasogastric tube lying curled in the stomach.

- Toxic megacolon: marked dilatation, most often of the transverse colon, often greater than 8 cm diameter; may be complicated by perforation and peritonitis (*Fig. 3.8*).

CT

CT is the investigation of choice in the acute situation particularly where barium studies and endoscopy may be difficult or contraindicated. CT is used in inflammatory bowel disease to define:

- Extent and site of bowel involvement.

- Extracolonic inflammation and abscess formation.

- Sinus/fistula formation.

CT signs of Crohn's disease (*Fig. 3.9*):

- Symmetrical thickening of bowel wall up to 3 cm in severe cases.

- Homogeneous enhancement of bowel wall.

- Multiple 'skip' lesions.

- Streaky soft tissue opacification in mesenteric fat.

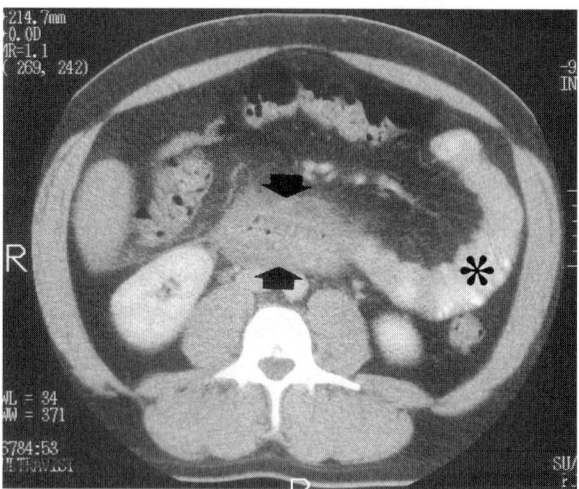

Figure 3.9 *Crohn's disease – CT.*
There is Crohn's disease of the duodenum (arrows).
Note:
- *thickening of the duodenal wall*
- *streaky inflammatory change in fat adjacent to the duodenal wall*
- *normal jejunum (*).*

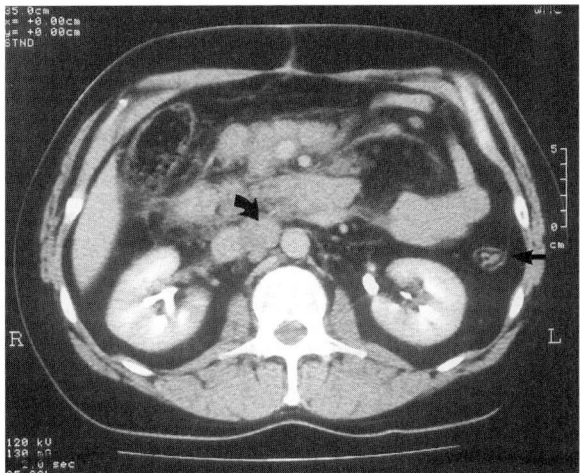

Figure 3.10 *Ulcerative colitis – CT.*
Note that the wall of the descending colon has a target appearance due to submucosal deposition of low attenuation fat (straight arrow). Retroperitoneal lymphadenopathy (curved arrow) is due to secondary spread from a carcinoma of the caecum.

- Pericolonic abscess: low-attenuation mass with irregular enhancing wall.
- Sinus/fistula tracts: contrast/gas-filled tracts; gas in bladder.

CT signs of ulcerative colitis

- Symmetrical bowel wall thickening, usually < 1 cm.
- Inhomogeneous enhancement; alternating layers of oedema, fat, and enhancement in the bowel wall may produce a 'target' appearance (*Fig. 3.10*).
- Diffuse non-segmental distribution from distal to proximal colon.

Barium studies

Barium studies for Crohn's disease

- Small bowel study: best images obtained by entero-clysis (small bowel enema) (*Fig. 3.11*).

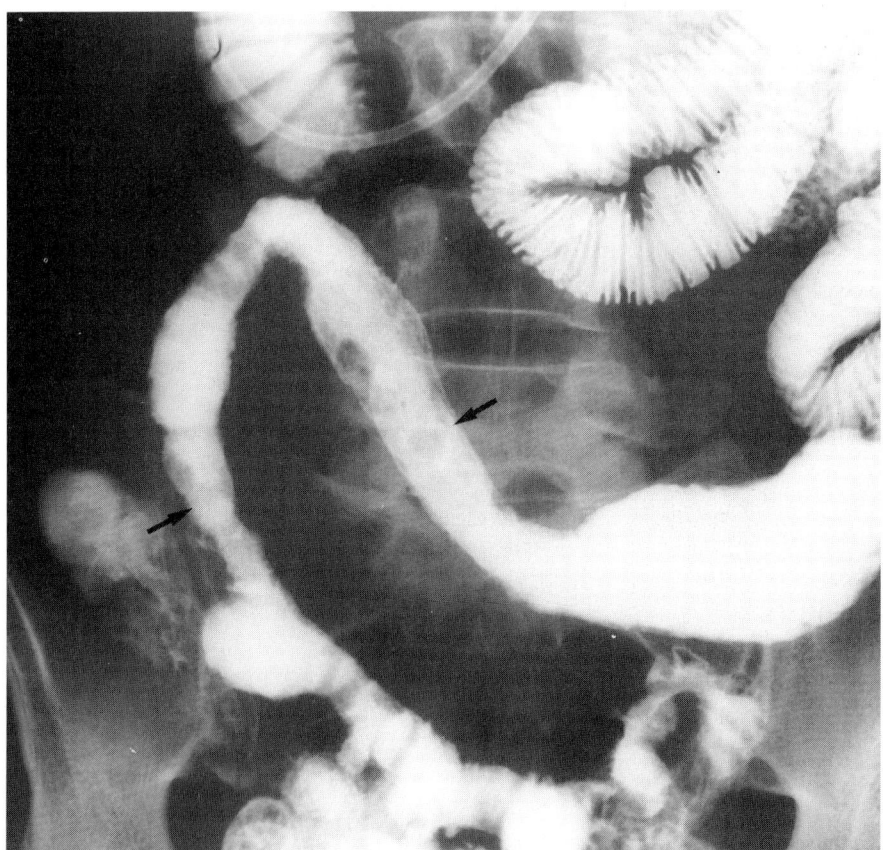

Figure 3.11 *Crohn's disease – enteroclysis.*
The diseased small bowel loop (arrows) shows the following features:
- *thickened bowel wall with loss of normal mucosal pattern*
- *ulceration*
- *'cobblestoning'*
- *separation from adjacent bowel loops due to mesenteric inflammation*
- *note the normal small bowel loops proximal and distal to the diseased segment.*

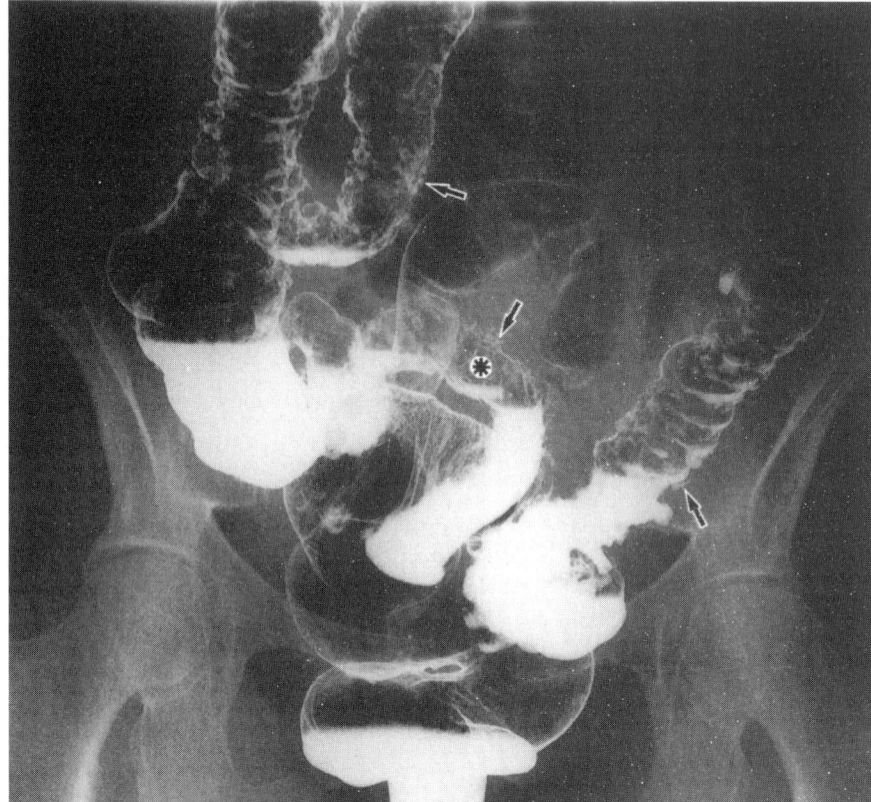

Figure 3.12 *Crohn's disease – barium enema. Numerous 'skip' lesions are seen with loss of mucosal pattern and deep ulceration (arrows). The terminal ileum is also involved (*). The rectum is normal.*

- Barium enema for large bowel involvement (*Fig. 3.12*).

- Signs are numerous and include:
  - (i)   'Skip' lesions (i.e. diseased segments separated by segments of normal bowel).
  - (ii) Ulcers.
  - (iii) Strictures.
  - (iv) 'Cobblestoning' due to fissures separating islands of intact mucosa.
  - (v)   Thickened bowel wall.
  - (vi) Fistulae and sinuses.
  - (vii) Separation of bowel loops due to mesenteric infiltration or abscesses.

Barium studies for ulcerative colitis

- Barium enema is absolutely contraindicated in toxic megacolon.

- Signs:
  - (i)   Rectum involved.
  - (ii) Retrograde involvement of large bowel with no skip lesions.

- (iii) Early there is fine ulceration which later becomes more florid (*Fig. 3.13*).
- (iv) Pseudopolyp formation due to post-inflammatory granulation tissue and fibrosis.
- (v)   Loss of haustral markings.
- (vi) Shortening and narrowing of large bowel.
- (vii) Involvement of distal ileum in total colitis with fine ulceration giving a granular mucosal pattern.

Scintigraphy

- Performed with a variety of techniques (e.g. ^{99m}Tc HMPAO, ^{99m}Tc-labelled sucralfate).

- Affected bowel segments show as areas of increased uptake.

- May be useful in defining anatomical location of disease, to a lesser extent in assessing disease severity, to diagnose relapse in patients with known inflammatory bowel disease, and in acutely ill patients in whom barium studies are contraindicated.

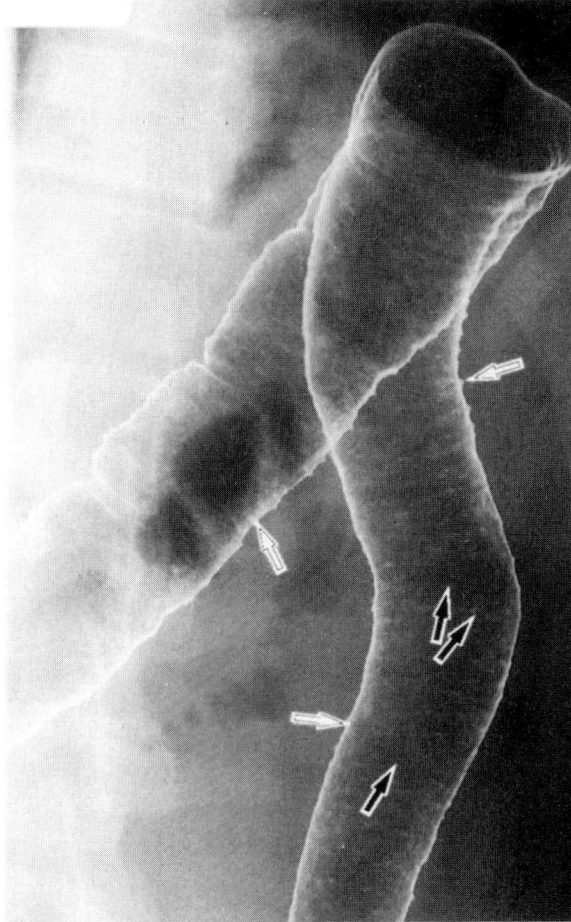

Figure 3.13 *Ulcerative colitis.*
Localised view of the splenic flexure showing the ulcerations. The ulcers are seen as small collections of barium (solid arrows) and as tiny projections beyond the bowel wall (hollow arrows) giving the bowel a rather shaggy outline. (Courtesy of Dr G. McInnes, Aberdeen.)

Gastrointestinal bleeding

Endoscopy is the primary investigation of choice for acute upper and lower GIT bleeding. In a significant proportion of patients however, endoscopy will either fail to find a bleeding point, or fail to achieve haemostasis, and it is in these cases that radiological techniques have an important role.

The goals of diagnosis and treatment of the patient with acute GIT bleeding are:

- Haemodynamic resuscitation.
- Localisation of the source of bleeding.
- Control of blood loss either by surgery, interventional radiology, or a combination of both.

Upper GIT bleeding is excluded by:

- Nasogastric aspirate.
- Upper GIT endoscopy.

Lower GIT bleeding is first investigated by sigmoidoscopy; if this is negative the patient is further assessed by scintigraphy and angiography. Causes of acute lower GIT bleeding include:

- Angiodysplasia.
- Colonic diverticulum: although diverticular disease is most prevalent in the sigmoid colon up to 50% of bleeding from colonic diverticulae occurs in the ascending colon.
- Less common causes: inflammatory bowel disease, colonic carcinoma, solitary rectal ulcer, postpolypectomy.

RBC scintigraphy

- ^{99m}Tc-labelled red blood cells.
- A bleeding point shows as an area of increased uptake outside normal areas of activity, i.e. aorta, IVC, portal vein, renal veins, kidneys and bladder (Fig. 3.14).
- More sensitive than angiography; that is, a lower rate of haemorrhage is required (said to be 0.1–0.2 ml/minute) to produce a positive result.
- Less anatomically specific than angiography; for this reason surgery based on RBC scintigraphy alone is not recommended.
- RBC scintigraphy should be seen as a screening test which will increase the accuracy of subsequent angiography.
- RBC scintigraphy is therefore usually used in a complementary role to establish whether or not acute haemorrhage is occurring prior to angiography.
- A patient with clinical evidence of bleeding and negative scintigraphy should be investigated with elective colonoscopy and barium studies.

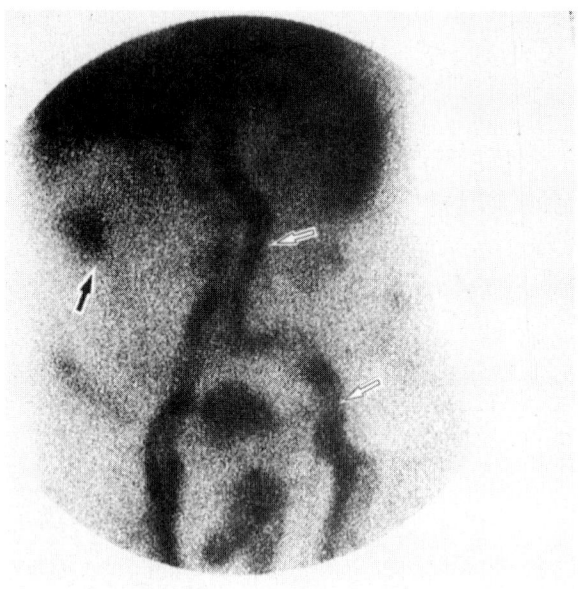 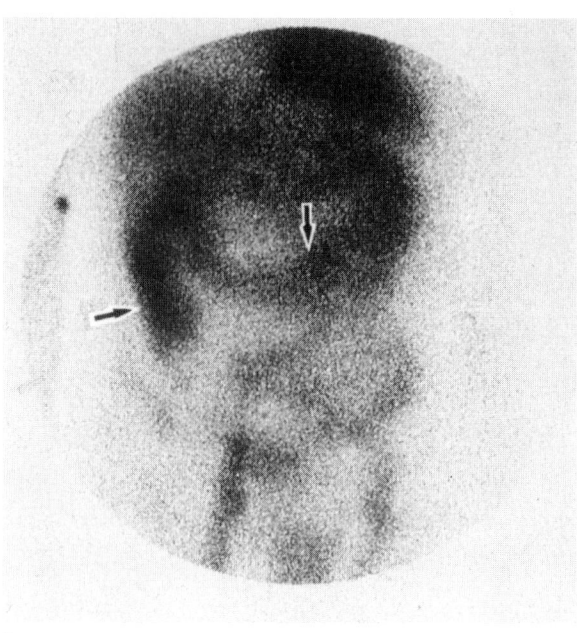

a　　　　　　　　　　　　　　　　　b

Figure 3.14 *Gastrointestinal haemorrhage – scintigraphy.*
(a) ^{99m}Tc-labelled red blood cells. An early scan shows a 'hot' area (solid arrow) on the right side of the abdomen indicating haemorrhage into the upper ascending colon. Note that the aorta and iliac vessels are well outlined (hollow arrows). (b) A later scan shows tracer filling much of the bowel (solid arrows) indicating extensive haemorrhage. (Courtesy of Dr F. Smith, Aberdeen.)

Angiography

- Angiography is performed for two reasons:
  (i)　To locate a bleeding point;
  (ii)　To achieve haemostasis by infusion of vasocon-strictors, or embolisation (*Fig. 3.15*).

- Use selective injection of coeliac axis and superior mesenteric artery for upper bleeds, superior and inferior mesenteric artery for lower bleeds, and in some cases all three vessels where clinical localisation is difficult.

- Active haemorrhage is seen as extravasation of contrast material into the bowel if bleeding of 0.5–1.0 ml/minute is occurring at the time of injection.

- Angiodysplasia is seen as a small nest of irregular vessels with early and persistent filling of a draining vein.

- Interventional radiology:

  (i)　Selective infusion of vasoconstrictors such as vasopressin.
  (ii)　Embolisation of small distal arterial branches following superselective catheterisation.
  (iii)　Most useful where surgery is thought to be too risky or for stabilisation prior to surgery.

Barium studies

In centres where endoscopy services are limited, or where colonoscopy is technically impossible, barium studies of upper and lower gastrointestinal tract have a role in chronic and intermittent bleeding, especially for making certain specific diagnoses such as peptic ulceration, to exclude malignancy of either upper or lower gastrointestinal tract in chronic blood loss, and in the diagnosis of other lesions like polyps
(*Fig. 3.16*), diverticular disease and inflammatory bowel disease. Barium studies have no role in acute bleeding.

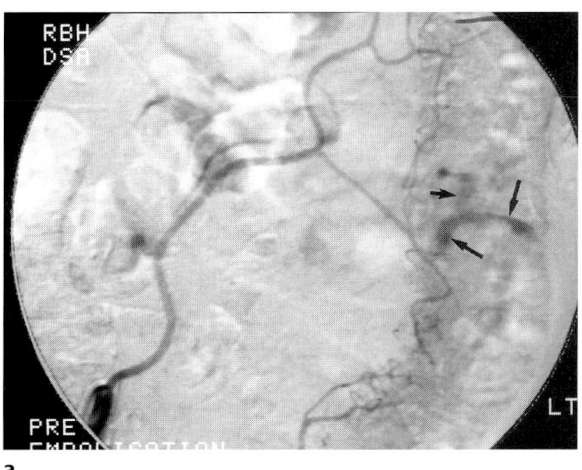

a

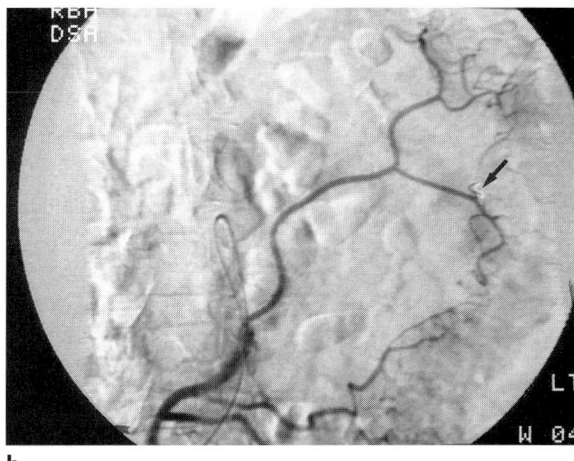

b

Figure 3.15 *Bleeding diverticulum – angiogram.*
(a) Inferior mesenteric angiogram. Selective catheterisation of the inferior mesenteric artery. Acute haemorrhage is seen as a blush of contrast in the bowel arising from a branch of the left colic artery (arrows). (b) Embolisation. Following superselective catheterisation a steel coil is used to occlude the bleeding artery (arrow). Note that leakage of contrast is no longer seen indicating successful embolisation.

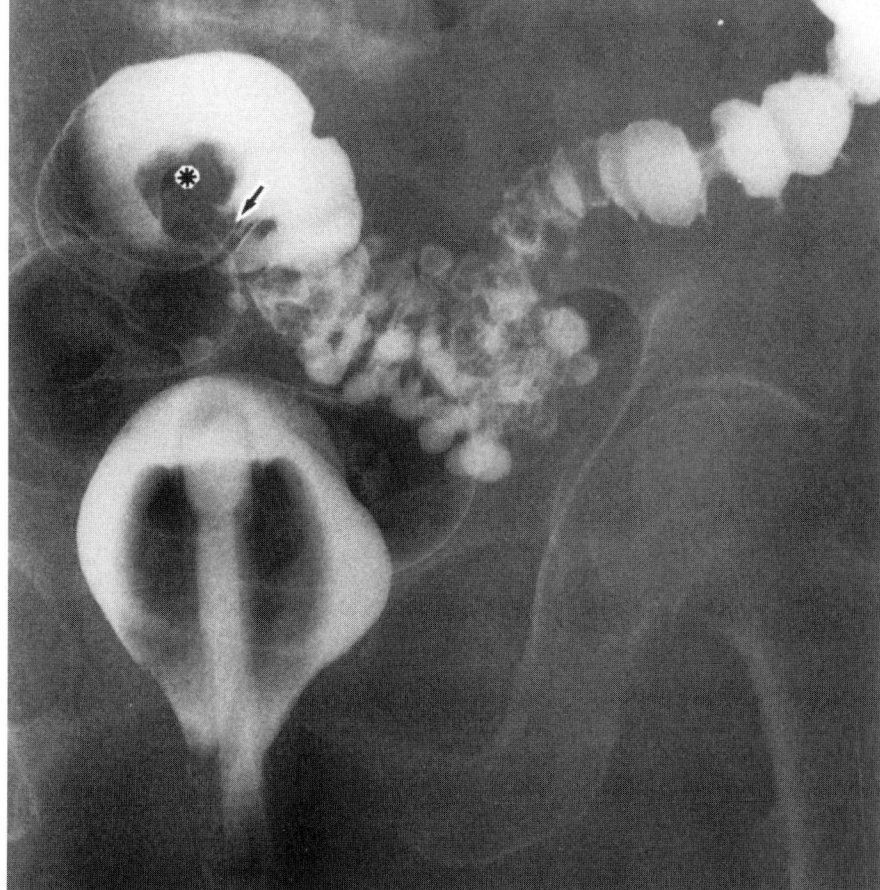

Figure 3.16 *Pedunculated polyp.*
Filling defect in the sigmoid colon (*). Note the stalk of the polyp (arrow).

Meckel diverticulum

Enteroclysis (small bowel enema)

- Most accurate technique and therefore the method of choice where this diagnosis is suspected.

Scintigraphy

- ^{99m}Tc, i.e. free pertechnetate.

- Taken up by gastric mucosa and therefore should be positive in those diverticula which contain ectopic gastric mucosa (*Fig. 3.17*).

- Reduced sensitivity in adults as those patients who remain asymptomatic through childhood are less likely to have a diverticulum containing ectopic gastric mucosa.

- A positive test shows as a small area of increased uptake in the lower abdomen.

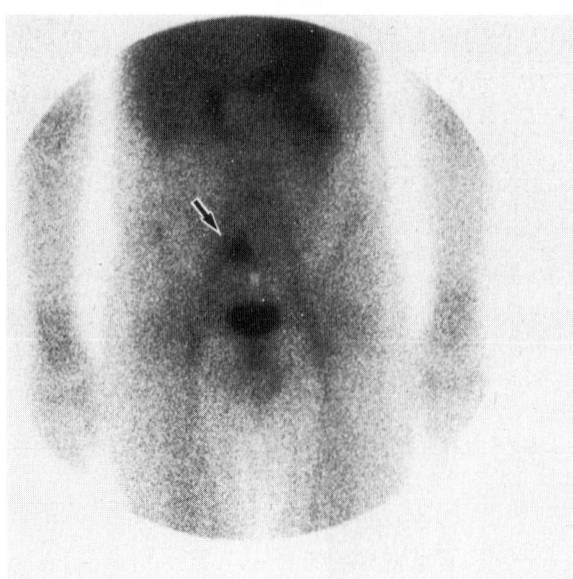

Figure 3.17 *Meckel diverticulum – scintigraphy.* ^{99m}*Tc-pertechnetate. A well defined area of increased uptake (arrow) is seen in the central abdomen above the bladder.*

Angiography

- Best used in acute bleeding.

- Signs:
  (i) Leakage of contrast.
  (ii) Visualisation of an abnormal tortuous group of embryonic vessels as well as the vitelline artery.

Small bowel neoplasms

Small bowel neoplasms may present in a variety of ways and are often very difficult to diagnose. The patient may present with a quite specific clinical picture such as carcinoid syndrome or intussusception, or with less specific signs such as anaemia, weight loss, or frank bleeding. The two principal imaging investigations are barium studies and CT. These studies are complementary in that barium studies show intra-luminal and mucosal tumours whilst CT will image intramural tumours and extra-intestinal spread.

CT will also show lymphadenopathy, liver metastases, and tumour complications such as invasion of adjacent structures, fistula formation, and intussusception.

The primary sign of a small bowel neoplasm on CT is asymmetric thickening of the bowel wall, usually > 1.5 cm. This is compared with bowel wall thickening in benign processes such as Crohn's disease or ischaemia; such thickening is usually concentric, symmetrical, and may show the 'target' sign.

CT is highly accurate for presence, site, and size of tumour, as well as the presence of metastases. CT is less accurate at predicting histology. The exception is lipoma where the fat content is well seen; carcinoid tumour may also have a fairly specific appearance.

Benign tumours

- Lipoma: Characteristic fat content well seen on CT.

- Adenoma/leiomyoma: Well-defined soft tissue masses.

- Benign tumours commonly present as the lead point in an intussusception. Intussusception

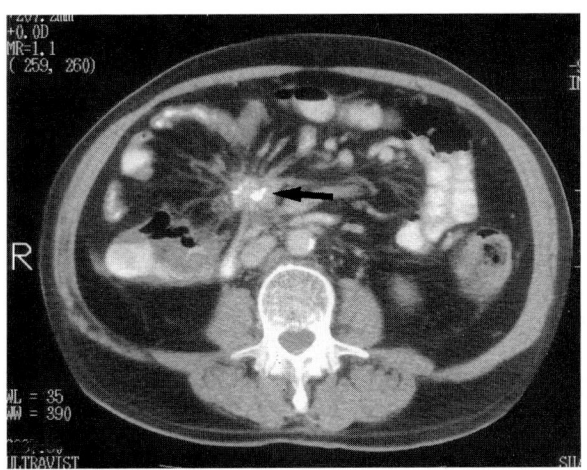

Figure 3.18 *Carcinoid tumour – CT.*
A calcified mesenteric mass (arrow) is surrounded by radiating soft tissue strands due to desmoplastic reaction.

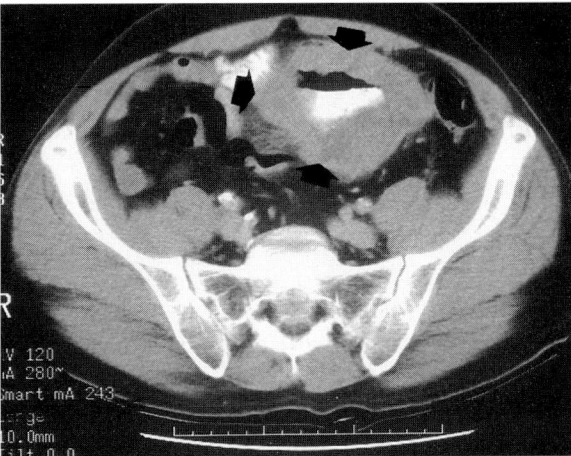

Figure 3.19 *Adenocarcinoma of the jejenum – CT.*
There is a large ulcerative mass arising in the jejunum. Note thickened irregular walls (arrows) with central contrast and air.

appears on CT as a soft tissue mass containing multiple layers giving a target-like appearance.

Carcinoid tumour

- Majority occur in the ileum.

- Often involves the mesentery inciting a desmoplastic reaction.

- CT: soft tissue mass which may be heavily calcified.

- Mesenteric infiltration seen as strands of soft tissue radiating from the mass; adjacent small bowel loops tend to be separated and may be kinked and angular in appearance (*Fig. 3.18*).

- Patients with clinical evidence of carcinoid syndrome will usually also have hepatic metastases.

Adenocarcinoma

- Localised mass or focal area of asymmetric bowel wall thickening (*Fig. 3.19*).

Non-Hodgkin's lymphoma

- Tends to involve a longer segment of bowel than adenocarcinoma.

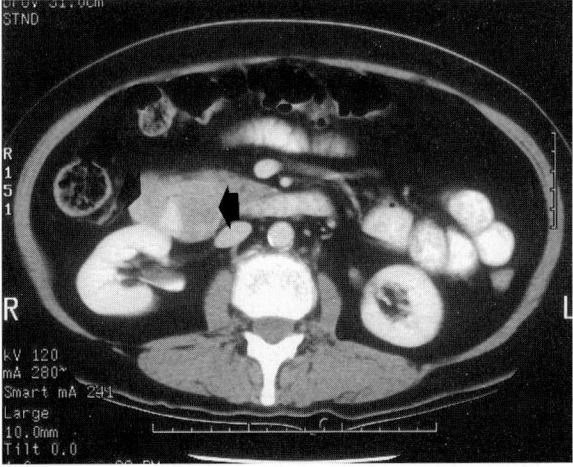

Figure 3.20 *Metastatic melanoma of the duodenum – CT.*
Asymmetric thickening of the distal second part of duodenum (arrow) due to metastatic melanoma.

- Usually a well-defined mass with concentric bowel wall thickening.

- Most commonly involves the ileocaecal region.

- With involvement of mesenteric lymph nodes may see large masses which encase the mesenteric vessels and displace bowel loops.

- In children may present as a lead point in intussusception.

- May also see other CT signs such as lymphadenopathy and splenomegaly.

Leiomyosarcoma

- Bulky mass with central necrosis and ulceration.

Metastases

- Most common primary sites are melanoma (*Fig. 3.20*), lung, breast, and ovary.

- Direct invasion of the small bowel may also occur from the large bowel and pancreas.

Chronic mesenteric ischaemia (CMI)

CMI occurs secondary to atheromatous narrowing of the mesenteric arteries. It is a rare entity owing to the rich mesenteric collateral supply. Symptoms of CMI usually do not occur unless all three major vessels, i.e. coeliac, superior mesenteric and inferior mesenteric arteries are significantly narrowed. These symptoms include pain with eating leading to food avoidance and progressive weight loss.

Doppler US

- Doppler US is an accurate screening test which may be used prior to angiography.

- Direct demonstration of stenoses with colour Doppler.

- Velocity criteria suggestive of stenosis greater than 70%:
  - (i) Coeliac artery: > 200 cm/sec.
  - (ii) Superior mesenteric artery: > 275 cm/sec.

Angiography

- Lateral view of the aorta is the most useful to demonstrate the origins of the three major vessels.

Interventional radiology

- Percutaneous transluminal angioplasty (PTA)/stents for stenoses.

- Arterial occlusions best treated with surgery.

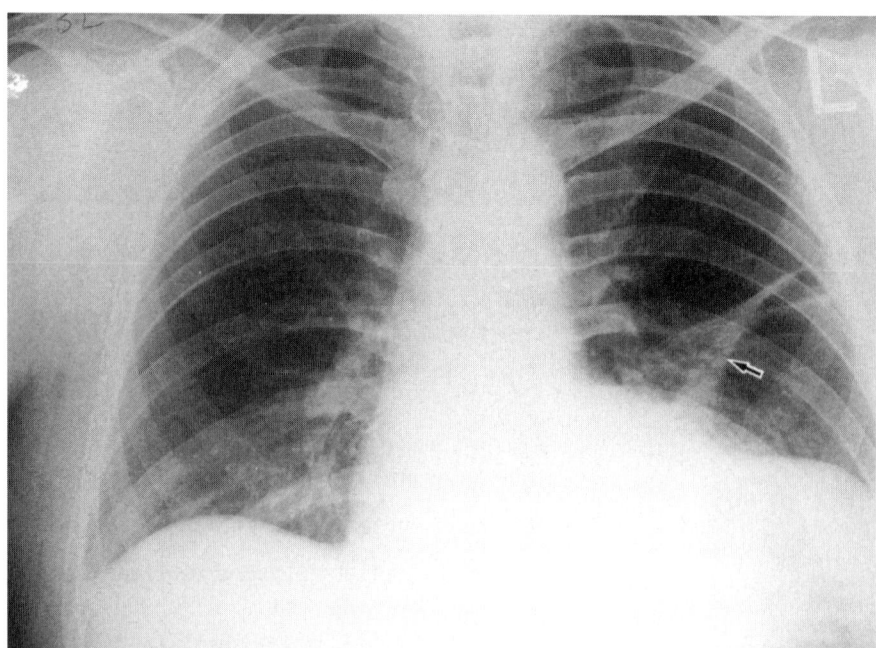

Figure 3.21 *Post-operative atelectasis. Partial collapse of the left lower lobe following laparotomy. Note:*
- *elevation of the left hemidiaphragm with loss of definition of its medial part due to non-aerated lung lying against it*
- *areas of wedge-shaped collapse (arrow).*

CXR changes and complications following abdominal surgery

Atelectasis

- Caused by peripheral mucous plugs in small bronchi and by splinting from abdominal incisions.

- Usually small to large areas of linear atelectasis seen as linear opacities with minimal loss of lung volume (*Fig. 3.21*).

- In more severe cases may see lower lobe collapse.

- Signs of right lower lobe collapse (*Fig. 3.22*):
    (i) decreased volume of right lung;
    (ii) triangular opacity at the right base medially;
    (iii) loss of definition of right diaphragm;
    (iv) heart border not obscured;
    (v) elevation of right diaphragm;
    (vi) depression of right hilum;
    (vii) non-visualisation of right lower lobe artery.

- Signs of right middle lobe collapse (*Fig. 3.23*):

    increased density in the right mid zone with loss of definition of the right heart border.

- Signs of left lower lobe collapse (*Fig. 3.24*):
    (i) decreased volume of left lung;
    (ii) triangular opacity behind the heart;
    (iii) loss of definition of the left diaphragm;
    (iv) left heart border not obscured unless the lingula is also collapsed;
    (v) elevation of the left diaphragm;
    (vi) depression of the left hilum;
    (vii) non-visualisation of the left lower lobe artery.

Pleural fluid

- May be seen following upper abdominal surgery.

- Frequently accompanies lower lobe collapse.

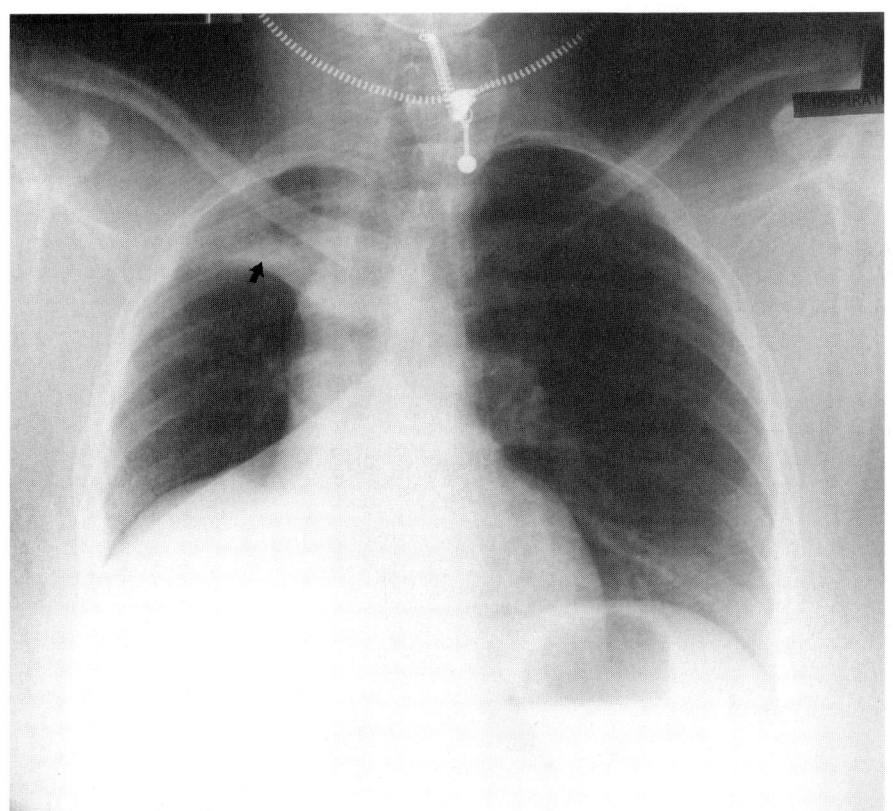

Figure 3.22 *Right lower lobe collapse.*
Note the following signs of right lower lobe collapse:
- *loss of volume of the right lung*
- *triangular opacity at the right base*
- *loss of definition of the right diaphragm.*
There is also collapse of the right upper lobe (arrow):
- *elevation of the horizontal fissure*
- *opacity abutting the right mediastinum*
- *tracheal deviation to the right.*

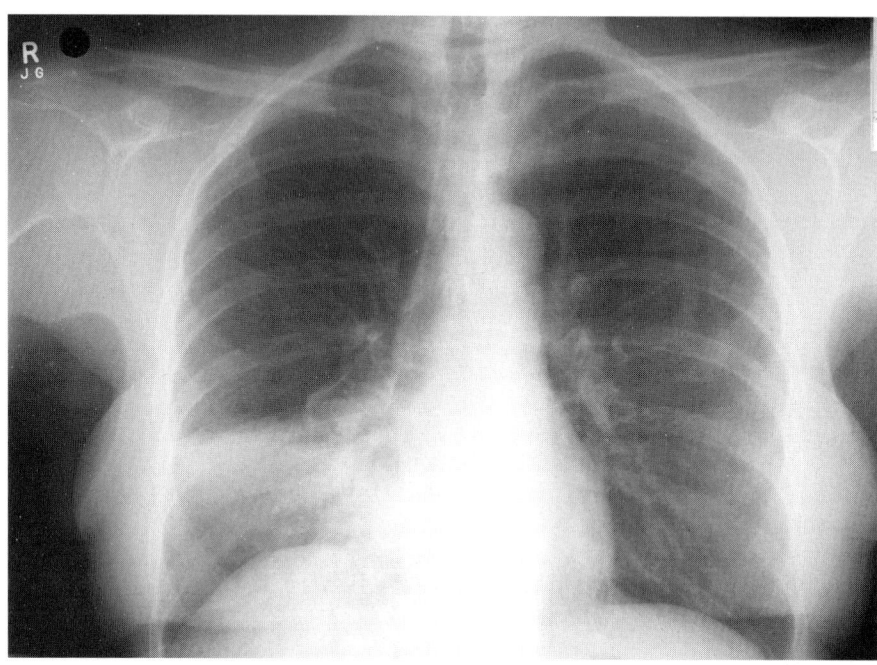

a

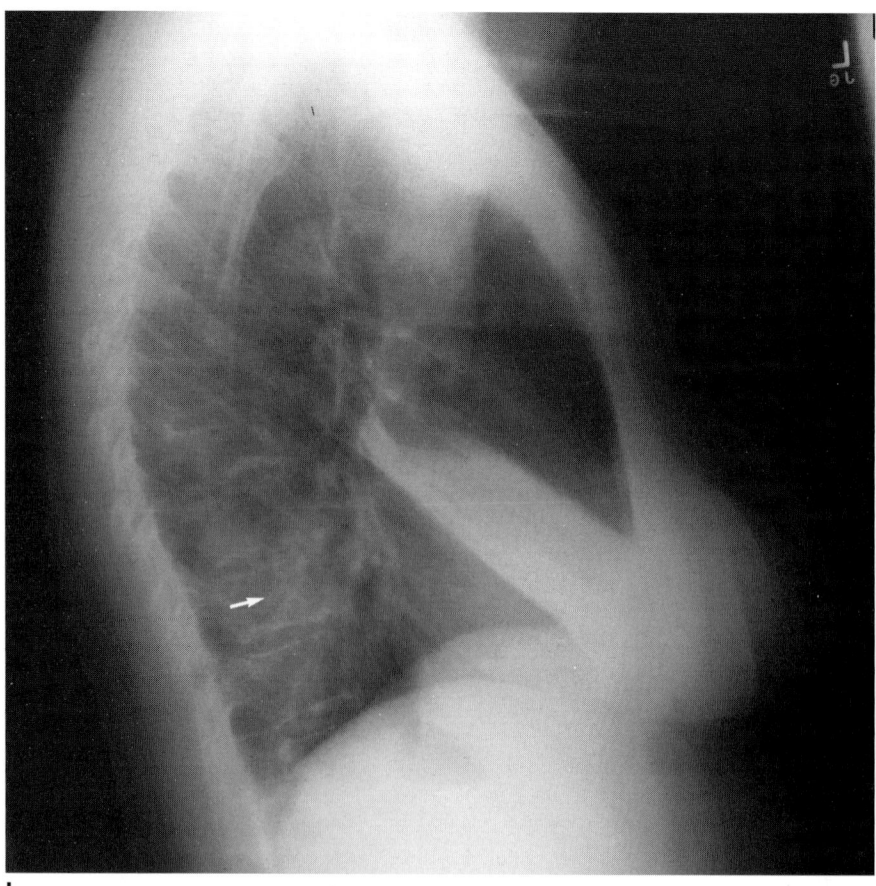

b

Figure 3.23 *Right middle lobe collapse.*
(a) PA film. Note:
- *opacity in right mid- to lower lung*
- *blurring of right heart border (compare with well-defined left heart border).*

(b) Lateral film. Note:
- *dense opacity projected over the heart*
- *well-defined margins due to horizontal fissure anteriorly and oblique fissure posteriorly*
- *consolidation is also seen posteriorly in the right lower lobe (arrow).*

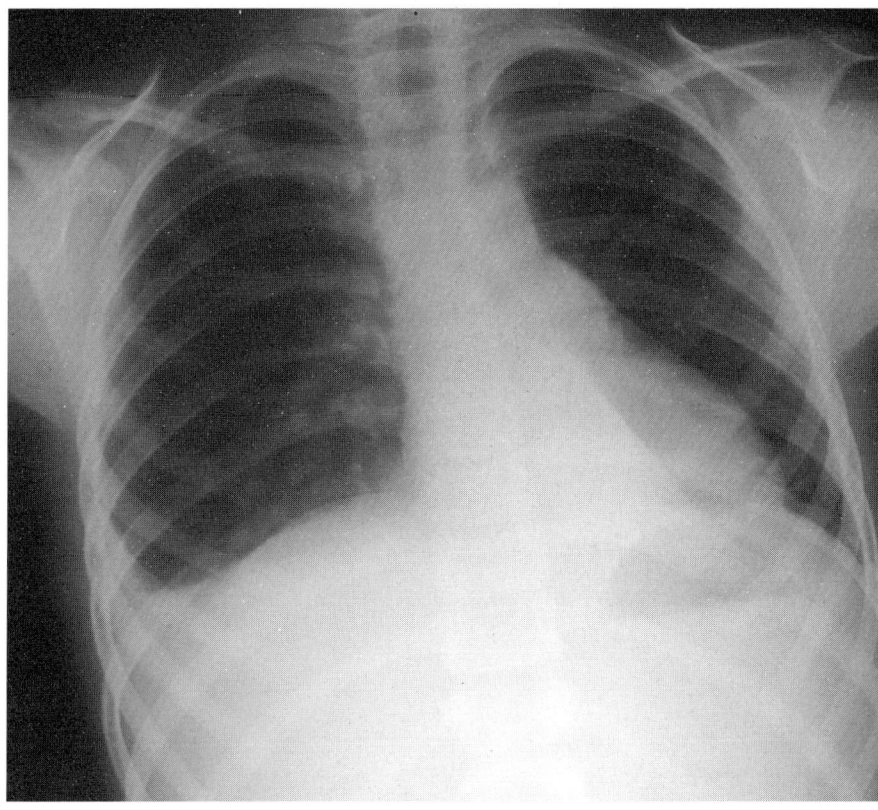

Figure 3.24 *Left lower lobe collapse.*
Note the following signs of left lower lobe collapse:
- *loss of volume of the left lung*
- *triangular opacity behind the heart*
- *loss of definition of the left diaphragm medially*
- *depression of left hilum*
- *non-visualization of the left lower lobe artery.*

- Signs of pleural fluid on supine CXR:
  - (i) opacity over lung apex (pleural cap);
  - (ii) increased opacity of hemithorax;
  - (iii) blunting of costophrenic angle.

Pneumonia

- Localised area of consolidation (*Fig. 3.25*).

- Air bronchograms: air filled bronchi are able to be seen as they are outlined by surrounding consolidated lung.

Pneumothorax

- Usually due to pleural trauma complicating upper abdominal surgery, especially renal surgery.

- Easily diagnosed on an erect CXR.

- Signs of tension:
  - (i) distortion of the shape of the collapsed lung;
  - (ii) increased volume of hemithorax;
  - (iii) contralateral displacement of the mediastinum;
  - (iv) depressed diaphragm;
  - (v) increased space between ribs (*Fig. 3.26*).

- Signs of pneumothorax on supine CXR:
  - (i) important to recognise as a supine pneumothorax may be easily missed in critically ill patients in whom erect CXR cannot be performed;
  - (ii) deep lateral costophrenic angle;
  - (iii) mediastinal structures sharply outlined by adjacent free air;
  - (iv) upper abdomen appears lucent due to overlying air (*Fig. 3.27*).

Adult respiratory distress syndrome

- Bilateral widespread alveolar consolidation.

- Commonly complicated by left lower lobe collapse.

- Beware supine pneumothorax especially in ventilated patients and following insertion of central venous lines.

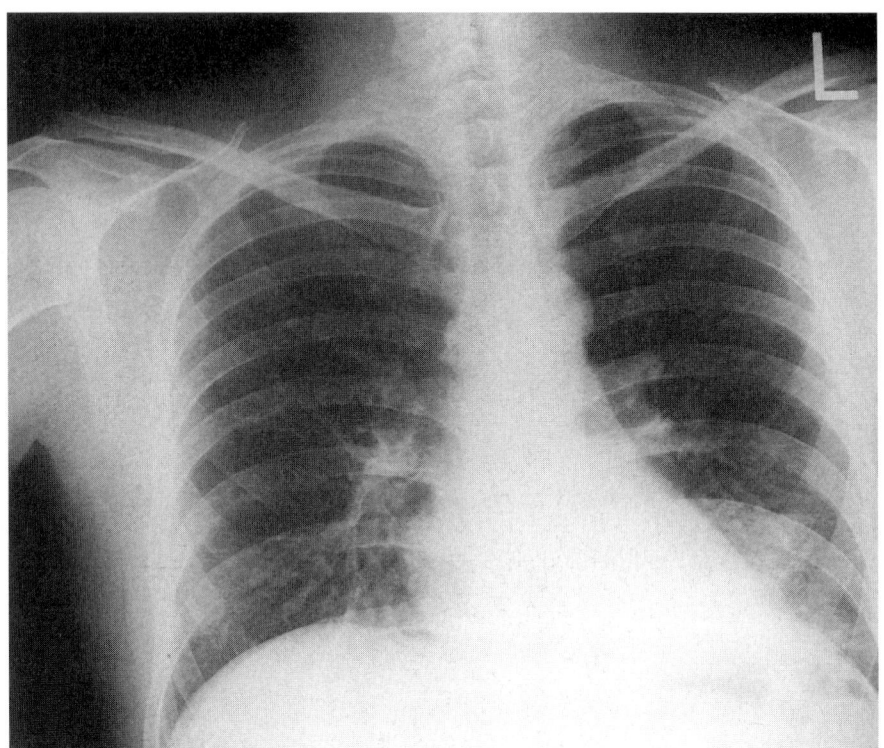

a

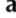

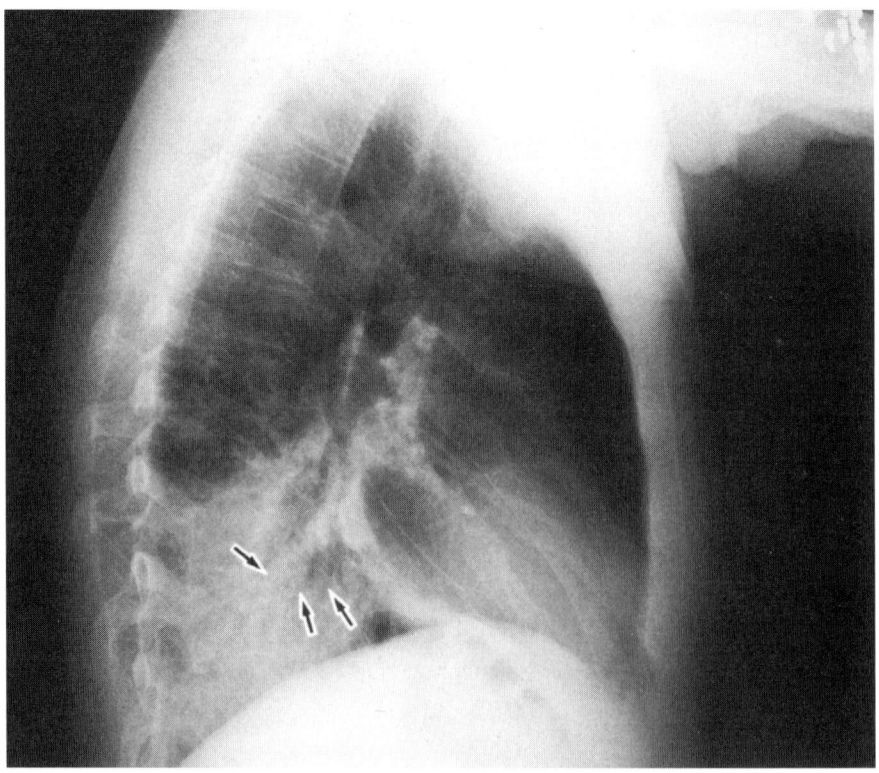

b

Figure 3.25 *Left lower lobe pneumonia.*
(a) PA film. Increased density of left lower hemithorax. Loss of definition of left diaphragm.
(b) Lateral film. Increased density of lower thoracic vertebral bodies. Loss of definition of left diaphragm posteriorly. Air bronchograms (arrows).

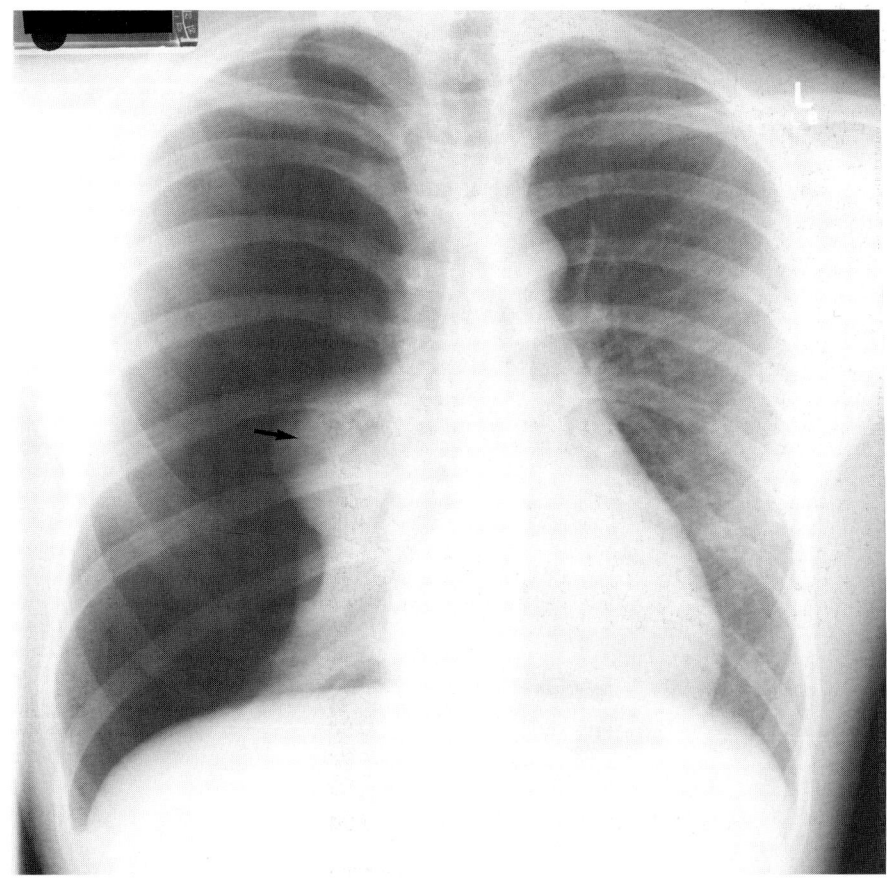

Figure 3.26 *Tension pneumothorax.*
Signs of tension pneumothorax as demonstrated in this case are as follows:
- *total collapse of right lung (arrow)*
- *increased size of right hemithorax*
- *increased space between right ribs*
- *shift of the mediastinum to the left.*

Pulmonary embolism

- CXR signs are non-specific and may include pleural effusion, atelectasis, and focal infiltrates.

- A normal CXR certainly does not exclude pulmonary embolism.

- For notes on the investigation of deep venous thrombosis and pulmonary embolism, *see* Chapter 8.

Summary of interventional radiology of the GIT

Oesophageal stricture dilatation

- Balloon dilatation.

- Rarely may be complicated by perforation.

Oesophageal stent placement

- Palliation of malignant dysphagia.

Percutaneous gastrostomy

- Enteral feeding.

- Fluoroscopic: puncture stomach, pass wire into stomach, dilators over wire to establish track, gastrostomy tube positioned over wire.

- Endoscopic: puncture stomach, pass wire into stomach, wire grasped with endoscope, gastrostomy tube attached to wire and pulled into position.

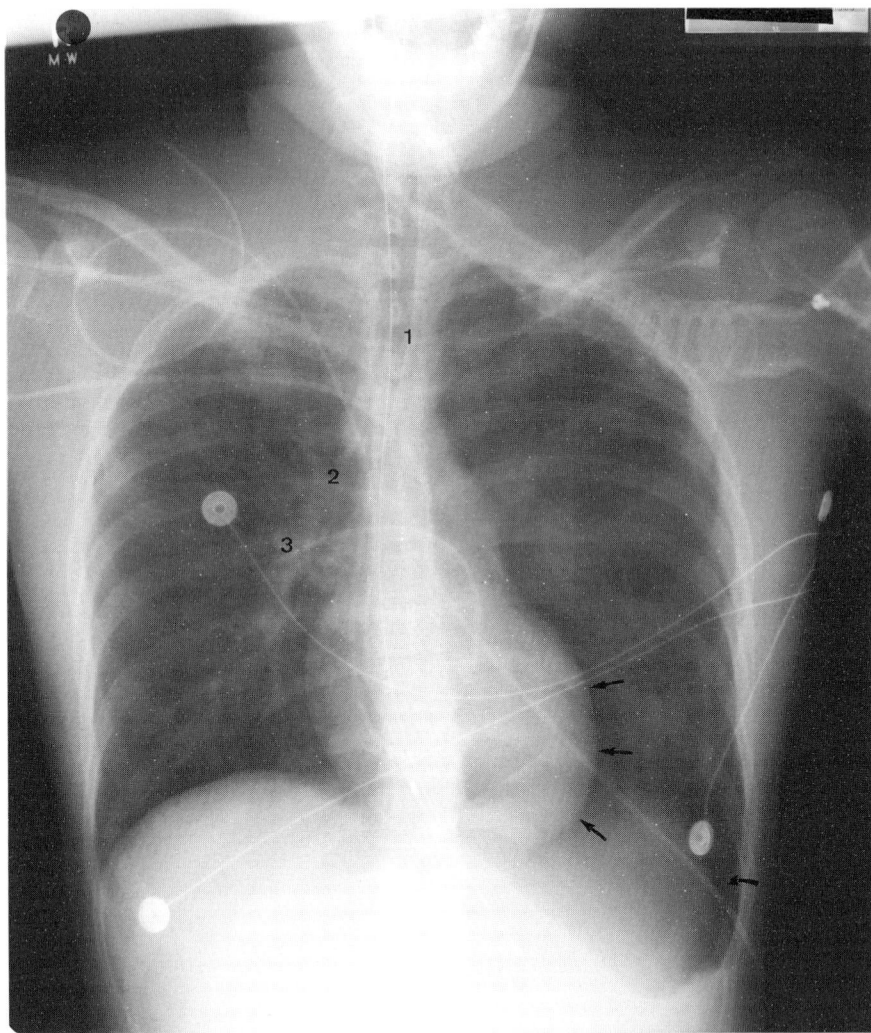

Figure 3.27 *Pneumothorax in a supine patient.*
Note:
- *deep left costo-phrenic angle due to air beneath the lung (curved arrow)*
- *sharp definition of the left cardiac border due to air located anteriorly (straight arrows)*
- *endotracheal tube (1), with tip just above the carina*
- *central venous catheter tip in SVC (2)*
- *Swann–Ganz catheter tip in right pulmonary artery (3).*

Transjugular intrahepatic portosystemic stent shunting (TIPSS)

- Portal hypertension and chronic, recurrent variceal haemorrhage not amenable to sclerotherapy.

- Patient imaged with Doppler US prior to procedure to exclude malignancy and confirm patency of portal vein.

- Technique: Jugular vein puncture, often under US control; wire passed into IVC and hepatic vein catheterised; puncture device passed through catheter; using US to select the most direct route the portal vein is punctured and a wire passed;

tract from hepatic vein to portal vein dilated; stent inserted, usually a metallic prosthesis expanded by balloon (*Fig. 3.28*).

Selective and superselective angiographic procedures

- Vasopressin infusion for GIT bleeding (*see* above).

- Embolisation for GIT bleeding (*see* above).

- Thrombolysis for AMI (*see* Chapter 1).

- Angioplasty for AMI and CMI (*see* Chapter 1 and above).

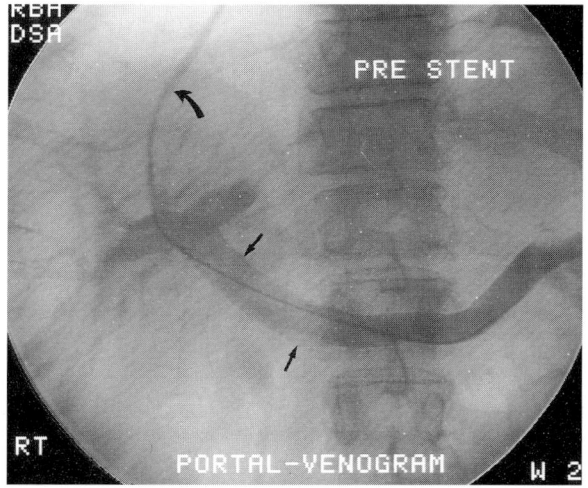

a

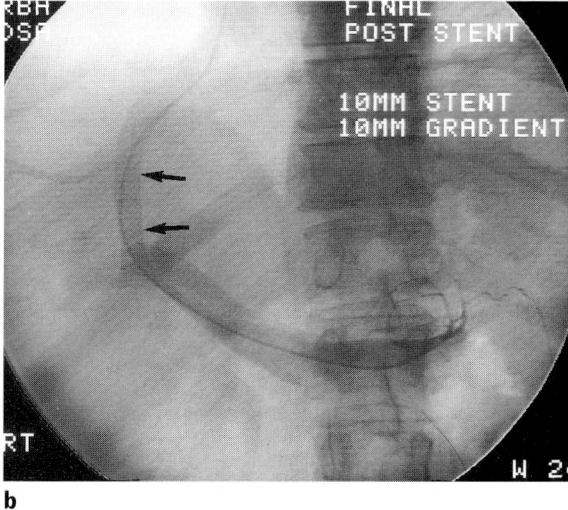

b

c

Figure 3.28 *TIPSS procedure.*
(a). Pre-stent. A guiding catheter is inserted via the right internal jugular vein. Its tip lies in the right hepatic vein (curved arrow). A puncture into the portal vein is then performed via the guiding catheter establishing communication between the portal and systemic venous systems. A fine catheter is passed through the puncture; its tip lies in the splenic vein. Contrast is injected with good opacification of the portal vein (straight arrows). (b) Post-stent. A self-expanding stent is deployed to maintain communication between the portal and systemic venous systems (arrows). (c) Post-stent. A subtraction film shows contrast outlining the portal vein (straight arrow), the shunt (open arrow) and the right hepatic vein (curved arrow).

Further Reading

1. Dixon PM, Nolan DJ. The diagnosis of Meckel's diverticulum: a continuing challenge. *Clinical Radiology* 1987; **38**:615–619.

2. Editorial. Endoscopic ultrasound in oesophageal cancer: the way forward. *Clinical Radiology* 1990; **42**:149–151.

3. Levine MS, Rubesin SE. Radiological investigation of dysphagia. *AJR* 1990; **154**:1157–1163.

4. Levine MS, Rubesin SE. The *Helicobacter pylori* revolution: radiological perspective. *Radiology* 1996; **195**:593–596.

5. Margulis AR, Burhenne HJ. *Practical Alimentary Tract Radiology*. Mosby Year Book, 1993.

6. Mendelson RM. The role of endoscopic ultrasonography in the upper gastrointestinal tract. *Australasian Radiology* 1993; **37**:349–359.

7. Ott DJ, Pikna LA. Clinical and videofluoroscopic evaluation of swallowing disorders. *AJR* 1993; **161**:507–513.

8. Raymond HW, Zwiebel WJ, Swartz JD (eds.). *Seminars in US, CT, and MRI* 1995; **16**(2).

9. Zuckerman DA, Bocchini TP, Birnbaum EH. Massive hemorrhage in the lower gastrointestinal tract in adults: diagnostic imaging and intervention. *AJR* 1993; **161**:703–711.

4   Imaging of trauma

Abdominal trauma

As with the acute abdomen discussed in Chapter 2, the patient with abdominal trauma can be assessed by many aids that supplement the clinical history and examination. These aids to diagnosis include peritoneal lavage, laparoscopy, 'mini-lap', and laparotomy.

Imaging plays an important role and the more common findings in each of the modalities will be outlined below. It should be emphasised that haemodynamically unstable patients should undergo immediate surgery. Contrast enhanced CT is the investigation of choice for suspected abdominal injuries in haemodynamically stable patients. US is used in some centres, particularly in children; it is less sensitive than CT. With CT now widely available plain films are performed less often in the setting of trauma. They are however used to assess spinal and pelvic fractures and it is therefore important to also recognise signs of abdominal trauma.

CT

- Usually following i.v. contrast and oral contrast; oral contrast may need to be administered by nasogastric tube.

- Excellent anatomical definition of intra-abdominal fluid collections and solid organ damage.

- Intraperitoneal and retroperitoneal gas also seen, and may show haematoma in the wall of traumatised gut.

- Blood appears as hypodense material in more dependent parts of the peritoneal cavity, i.e. pelvis (*Fig. 4.1*), hepatorenal pouch, paracolic gutters.

- Splenic trauma:
  (i)   Non-homogeneous density.
  (ii) Altered organ contour.
  (iii) Lacerations appear as hypodense lines separating more dense splenic fragments (*Fig. 4.2*).

- Hepatic trauma:
  (i)   Accurate localisation of haematoma.

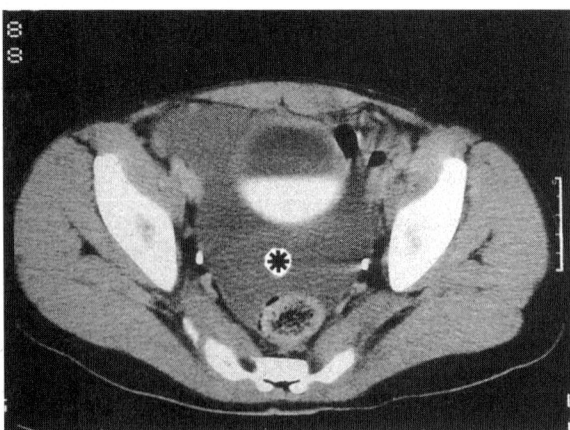

Figure 4.1 *Peritoneal blood – CT.*
Blood in the peritoneal cavity due to traumatic splenic rupture. Blood is seen as low attenuation material (*) separating the bladder from the rectum.

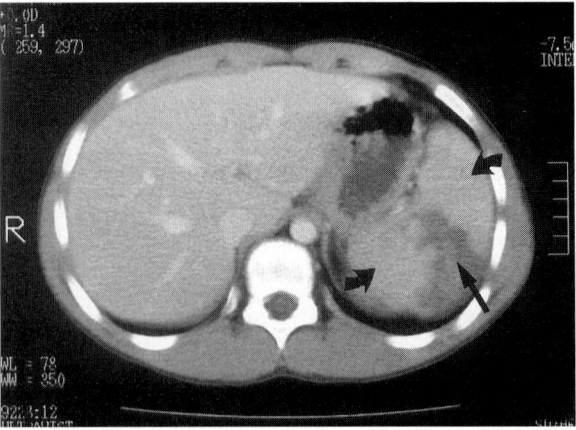

Figure 4.2 *Splenic rupture – CT.*
A large laceration of the spleen is seen as an irregular low attenuation area (straight arrow) separating high attenuation splenic fragments (curved arrows).

(ii)   Intrahepatic haematoma may be of increased or decreased attenuation.

(iii) Lacerations appear as hypodense lines in the liver substance (*Fig. 4.3*).

- Pancreatic trauma:
  (i)   Laceration through the pancreas seen as a low attenuation cleft.
  (ii) May go on to develop acute pancreatitis followed by pseudocyst formation with CT signs as described in Chapter 2.

- Bowel trauma (including duodenum):
  (i)   Pneumoperitoneum: occurs in only 60% of cases of traumatic bowel perforation.
  (ii)   Free retroperitoneal gas may be seen with duodenal rupture (*Fig. 4.4*).
  (iii) Free fluid: low attenuation fluid lying between bowel loops; fluid may be of high attenuation if it contains leaked oral contrast material.
  (iv)   Intramural haematoma: localised bowel wall thickening or intramural mass.
  (v)   Intense contrast enhancement of the bowel wall.
  (vi)   Associated injuries in over 50%, e.g. solid organ damage, Chance fracture, etc.

- Other signs:
  (i)   Sentinel clot sign: high attenuation blood immediately adjacent to the site of injury.
  (ii) Collapsed IVC and renal veins in severe shock.

Ultrasound

- May be difficult in the traumatised patient owing to distended bowel loops, dressings, chest tubes, etc.

- Blood in the peritoneum appears as anechoic fluid, sometimes with septations, separating bowel loops and surrounding solid organs.

- Splenic trauma:
  (i)   Splenomegaly.
  (ii)   Altered organ contour.
  (iii) Non-homogeneous echogenicity.
  (iv)   Intrasplenic haematoma usually anechoic, though may show as an irregular area of increased echogenicity.
  (v)   Subcapsular haematoma shows as an anechoic collection conforming to the shape of the gland.

- Hepatic trauma:
  (i)   Haematomas usually hypoechoic, though acutely they may be hyperechoic with poorly defined margins.
  (ii)   Lacerations appear as hypoechoic lines separating fragments of liver tissue.
  (iii) Subcapsular haematomas conform to the margin of the gland and have a lenticular or biconvex outline.

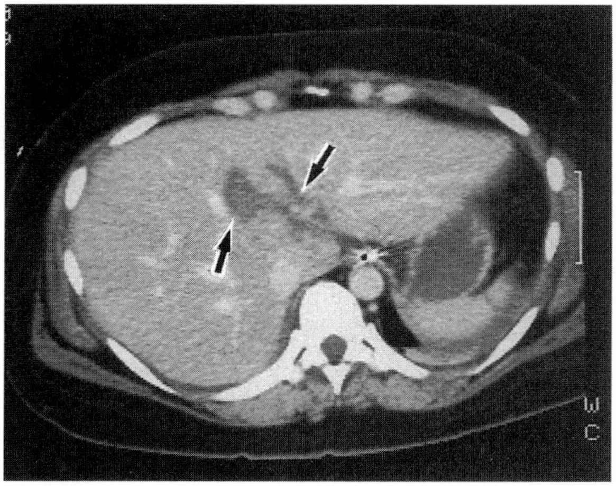

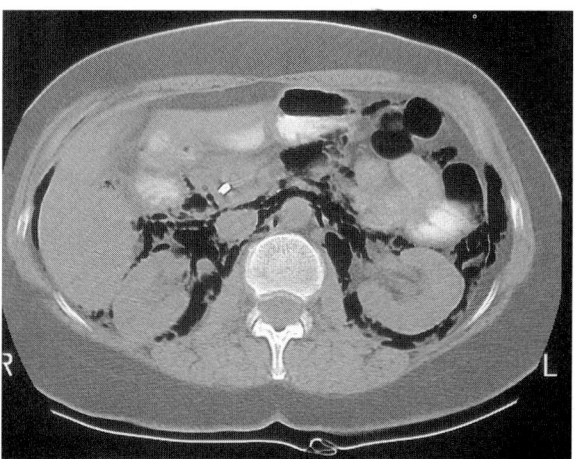

Figure 4.3 *Hepatic trauma.*
Lacerations of the liver are seen as areas of low attenuations within the hepatic parenchyma (arrows).

Figure 4.4 *Duodenal rupture – CT.*
There is extensive free gas in the retroperitoneum following laceration of the duodenal wall. Gas is seen surrounding the kidneys, aorta and IVC.

- Ultrasound is a good technique for follow-up of patients who have been conservatively managed.

- Parenchymal haematomas show decreasing echogenicity and formation of an anechoic cyst prior to resolution.

Plain films: AXR

(a) Intraperitoneal gas:
   - The traumatised patient may not be able to stand, so decubitus or shoot-through lateral views may be required.
(b) Retroperitoneal gas:
   - Streaky gas densities outlining the retroperitoneal structures, e.g. psoas margin.
(c) Intraperitoneal fluid:
   - General 'greyness' of the abdomen.
   - Soft tissue density in the paracolic gutter separating the lateral bowel wall from the properitoneal fat stripe.
   - Displacement of bowel loops by localised haematoma, e.g. downward displacement of hepatic flexure in liver trauma.
(d) Retroperitoneal fluid:
   - Loss of retroperitoneal fat planes, e.g. psoas margins, kidney outlines.
(e) Bone lesions:
   - Fractured lower ribs.
   - Spinal fractures including fractured transverse processes.

CXR changes associated with abdominal trauma

- Pleural effusion.

- Lower lobe collapse.

- Ruptured diaphragm (*Fig. 4.5*).

- Rib fractures.

Angiography

- Limited role in abdominal trauma.

- Used to localise bleeding where other imaging techniques have failed to do so, often as a precursor to embolisation.

Trauma to kidneys and ureters

Imaging is for two purposes: (i) to delineate the nature of injuries; and (ii) to detect pre-existing abnormalities, seen in up to 50% of traumatised kidneys.

CT

- CT with intravenous contrast is the investigation of choice for imaging of renal trauma.

- Good definition of haematoma, lacerations, urinoma (*Fig. 4.6*).

- Functional information when contrast is used.

- Other organs assessed.

Ultrasound

- Intrarenal haematoma: Usually a hyperechoic area, though may be hypoechoic if large.

- Lacerations: Linear defect in the kidney.

- Perinephric haematoma: Hyper- or hypoechoic mass surrounding the kidney.

- Urinoma: Anechoic mass.

- Other organs (spleen, liver) are also assessed.

- No information on renal function.

Plain films

- Signs suggestive of renal trauma include:
   (i) loss of fat planes around the kidney and psoas muscle;
   (ii) fractures of the lower three ribs;
   (iii) fractures of lumbar transverse processes;
   (iv) overlying dilated loops of bowel;
   (v) pleural effusion.

IVP

(a) Non-functioning kidney due to:

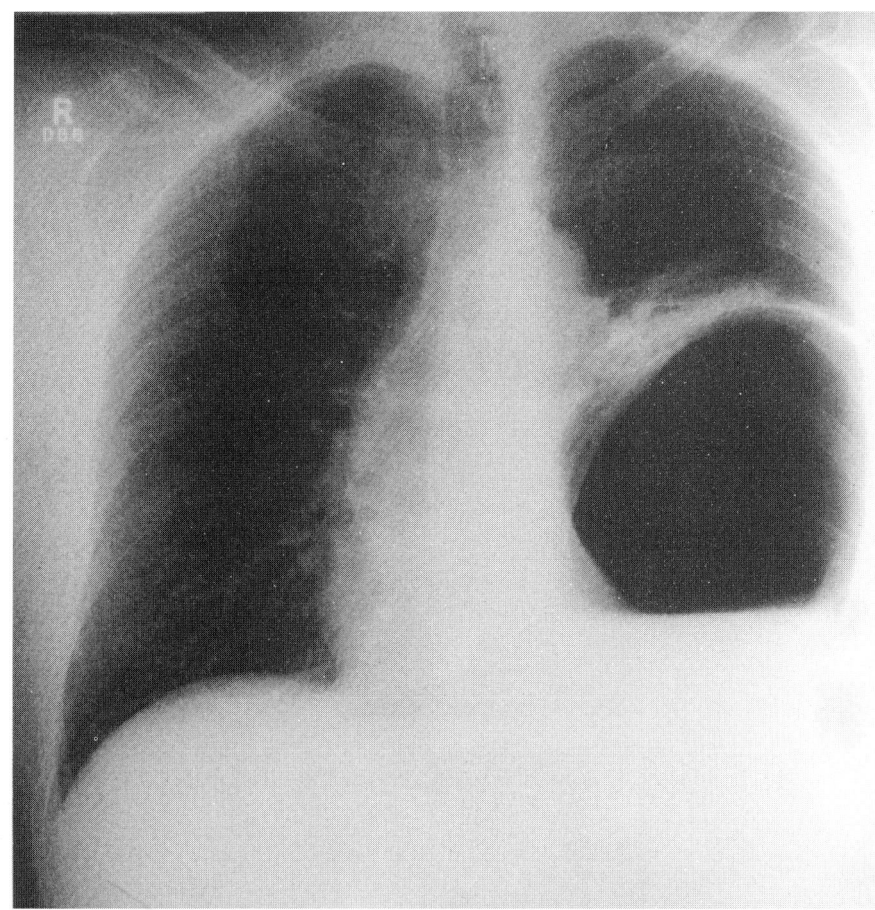

Figure 4.5 *Ruptured left diaphragm.*
The stomach has entered the left thoracic cavity and is dilated. Note:
* *collapse at the base of the left lung*
* *displacement of the heart to the right.*

* Massive parenchymal damage.
* Vascular pedicle injury.
* Obstructed collecting system due to blood clot.

(b) Intrarenal haematoma:
  * Localised filling defect.
  * Displacement of calyces.
(c) Laceration:
  * Well-defined defect.
  * Leakage of contrast if collecting system or ureter involved (*Fig. 4.7*).
(d) Limitations of IVP:
  * Imprecise information on perirenal tissues.
  * Other organs not assessed.

Scintigraphy

* Used in some centres in preference to IVP to provide information on renal function.

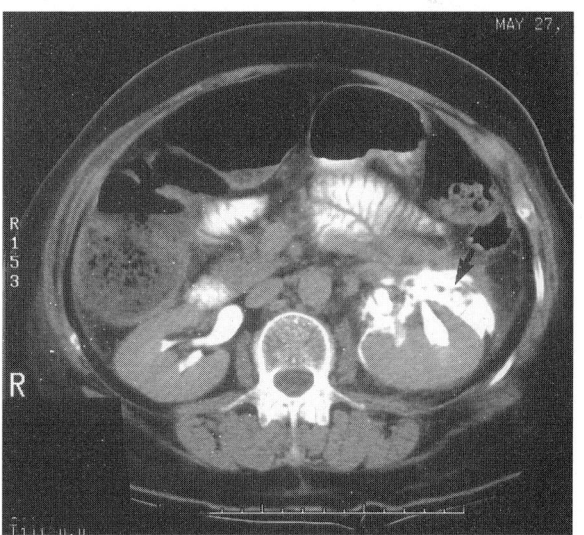

Figure 4.6 *Renal trauma – CT.*
There is leakage of contrast around the left kidney (arrow) indicating laceration of the collecting system.

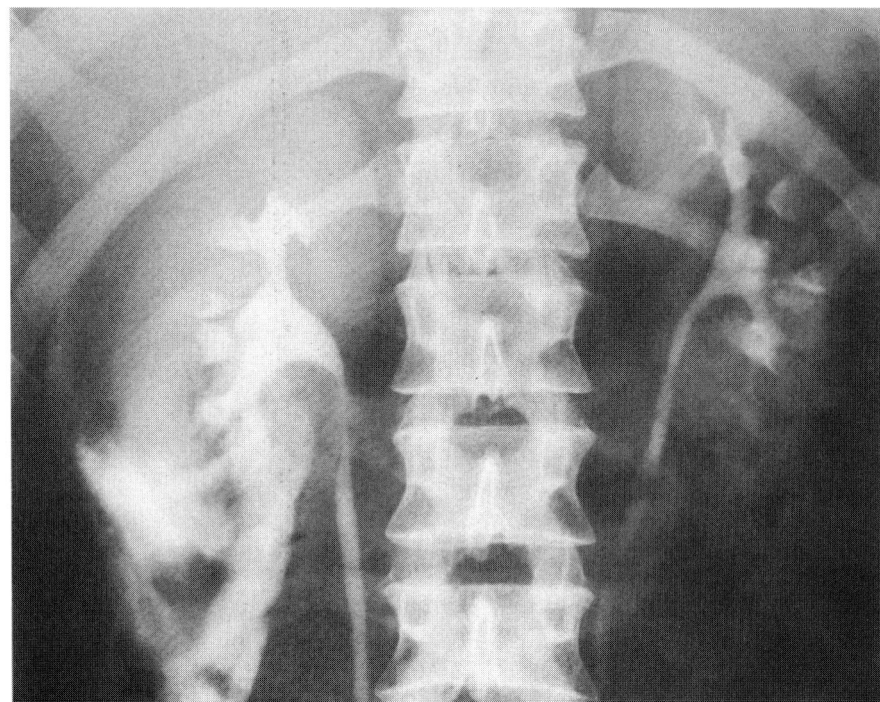

Figure 4.7 *Renal laceration – IVP.*
Leakage of contrast from the lower pole of the right kidney due to a laceration involving the collecting system.

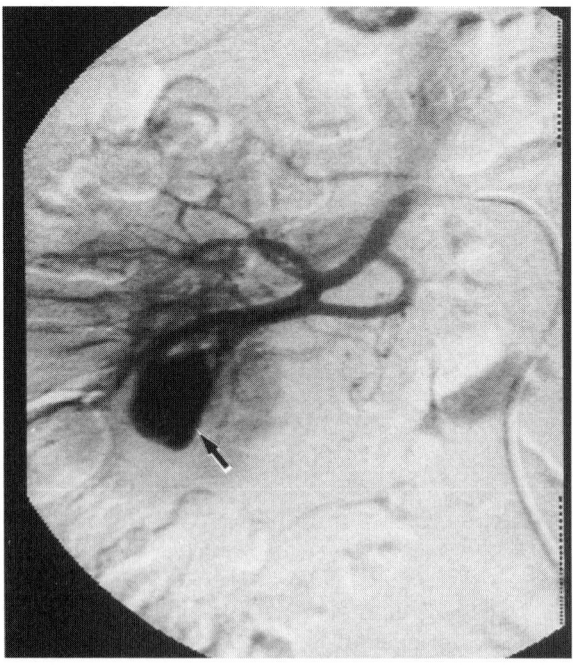

a

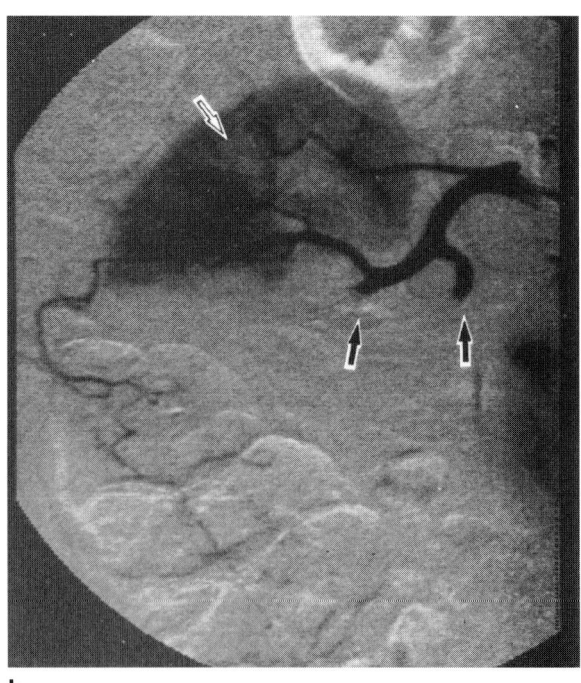

b

Figure 4.8 *Traumatic false aneurysm.*
(a) Pre-embolisation. The patient presented with post-traumatic haematuria. Angiography shows a false aneurysm in the right kidney (arrow). (b) Post-embolisation. Following embolisation the 2 main arteries to the lower pole are occluded (black arrows). This resulted in resolution of haematuria. Note that the upper pole of the right kidney is still well perfused (white arrow).

- Non-function: as above, i.e. massive parenchymal damage, vascular pedicle injury, obstructed collecting system.

- Laceration: leakage of radionuclide.

- Intrarenal haematoma: focal defect.

Angiography

- May be used in selected cases, for example where marked haematuria is not explained by findings of other imaging modalities, or following percutaneous procedures (biopsy, nephrostomy, percutaneous stone removal).

- In these cases, angiography is used to define a bleeding point, arteriovenous fistula, false aneurysm, etc. which may then be embolised or undergo surgery (*Fig. 4.8*).

Trauma to bladder and urethra

Plain films

- Fracture/dislocation of the pelvis (*Fig. 4.9*).

- Soft tissue mass with obliteration of normal fat planes due to leakage of urine.

- Air may be seen in the bladder following penetrating injury.

Urethrogram

- Prior to performing a cystogram for suspected bladder damage, the urethra must be examined.

- Urethral catheterisation should not be attempted prior to urethrogram in any patient with an anterior pelvic fracture/dislocation, or with blood at the urethral meatus following trauma.

- Urethrogram is a simple procedure which can be performed quickly in the emergency room (*Fig. 4.10*).

Cystogram

- If the urethra is normal on urethrogram, a catheter can be passed into the bladder and a cystogram performed.

- Bladder deformity may be seen (*Fig. 4.11*).

- Leakage of contrast may be intraperitoneal,

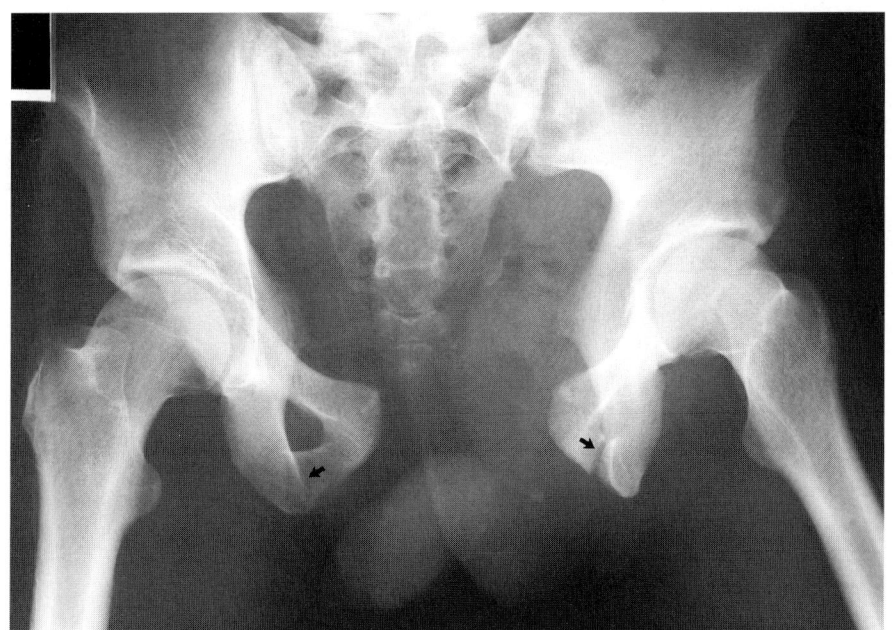

Figure 4.9 *Pelvic trauma. Note:*
- *separation of the pubic symphysis*
- *widening of the left sacroiliac joint*
- *fractures of the inferior ischiopubic rami (arrows)*
- *soft tissue mass on the left due to haematoma.*
Injuries such as this have a high incidence of associated urinary tract damage.

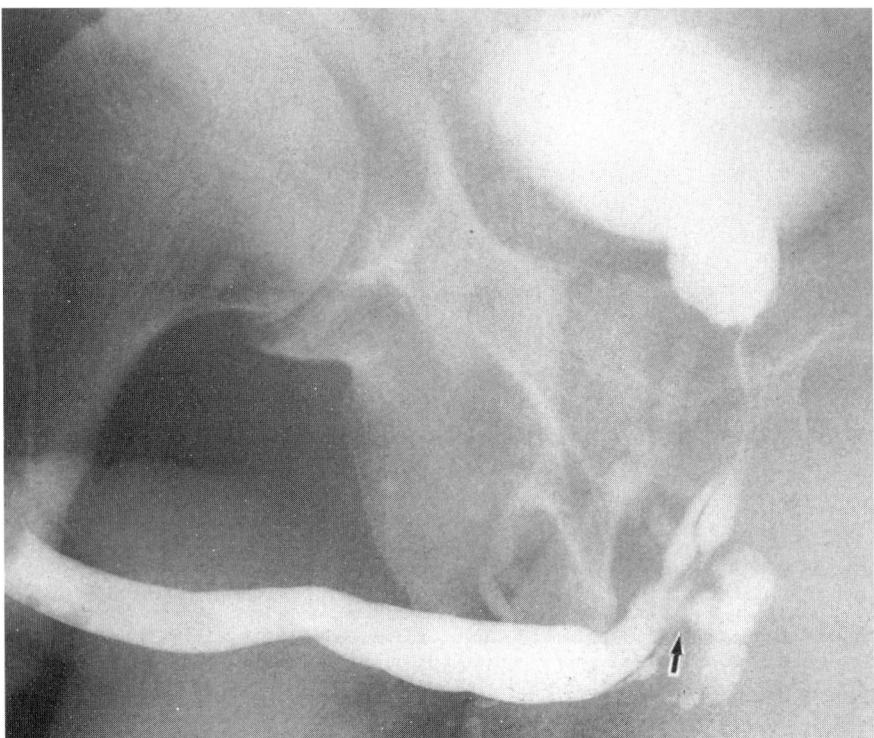

Figure 4.10 *Ruptured urethra – urethrogram. Leakage of contrast from the posterior urethra (arrow).*

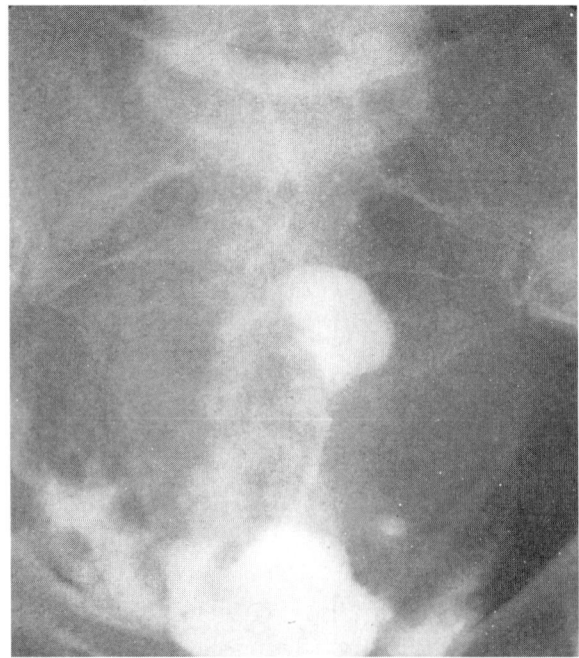

Figure 4.11 *Ruptured bladder. Extensive leakage of contrast from the bladder. The bladder outline is distorted by surrounding haematoma and urine.*

intrapelvic or extrapelvic (contrast streaks along soft tissue planes, sometimes into the thighs).

CT and ultrasound

* Examination of the pelvis should be performed as part of an abdominal trauma scan.

* Both modalities will show:
  (i)   bladder deformity;
  (ii) surrounding fluid: blood and/or urine;
  (iii) air in the bladder from penetrating injury.

Chest trauma

If possible an erect chest X-ray should be performed and perused in the following logical fashion:

1. Thoracic cage.

2. Diaphragm.

3. Pleura.

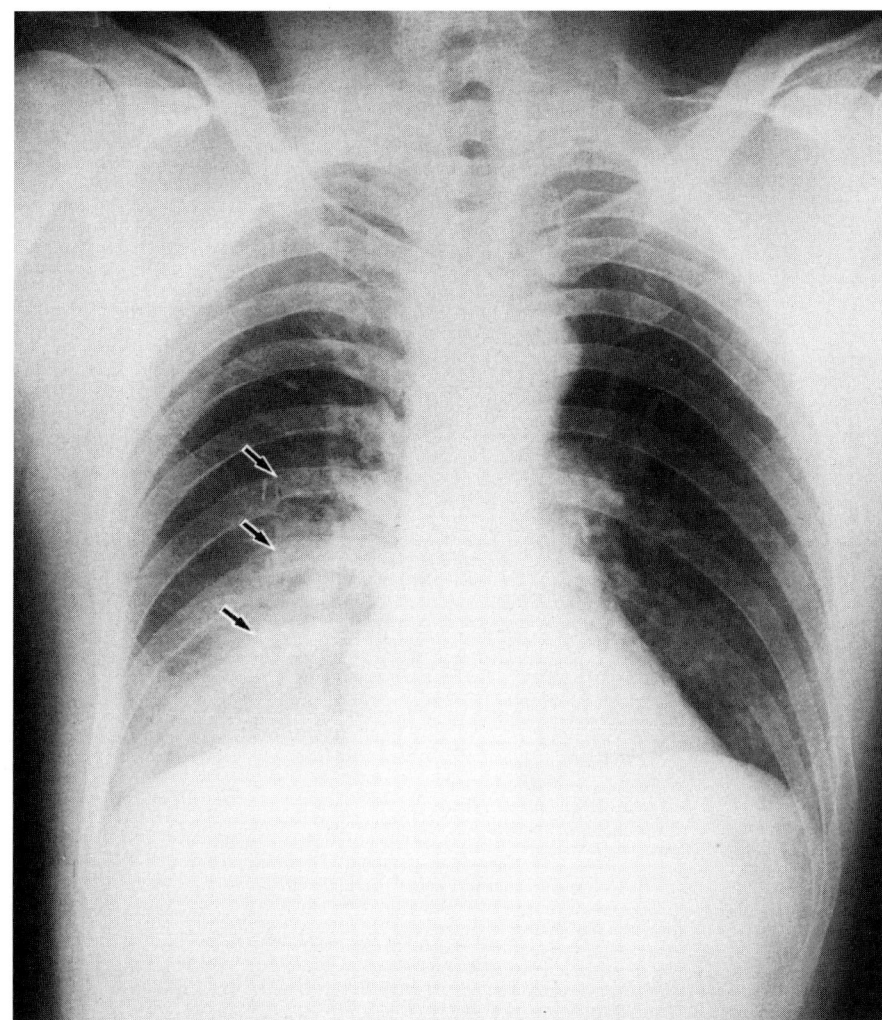

Figure 4.12 *Pulmonary contusion.*
Large contusion in the right lower lobe seen as an area of air-space shadowing. Note posterior rib fractures (arrows).

4. Lungs.

5. Mediastinum and airways.

Rib fractures

- Extensive views looking for subtle rib fractures are not advised in the acute situation; more important are associated injuries.

- Fractured upper three ribs: suspect great vessel damage.

- Fractured lower three ribs: suspect upper abdominal injury (liver, spleen, kidney).

- Complications: flail segment, i.e. segmental fractures of three or more ribs, pneumothorax, subcutaneous emphysema, haemothorax.

Other fractures

- Sternum
  (i)   Lateral view.
  (ii) Fractures usually involve the body of the sternum.
  (iii) High association with myocardial/pulmonary contusion and airway rupture.
  (iv) Fractures of the manubrium are very rare.

- Thoracic spine: penetrated and lateral views, CT.

- Clavicle/scapula/humerus.

Ruptured diaphragm (*Fig. 4.5*)

- Herniation of abdominal structures into the chest.

- Contralateral mediastinal shift.

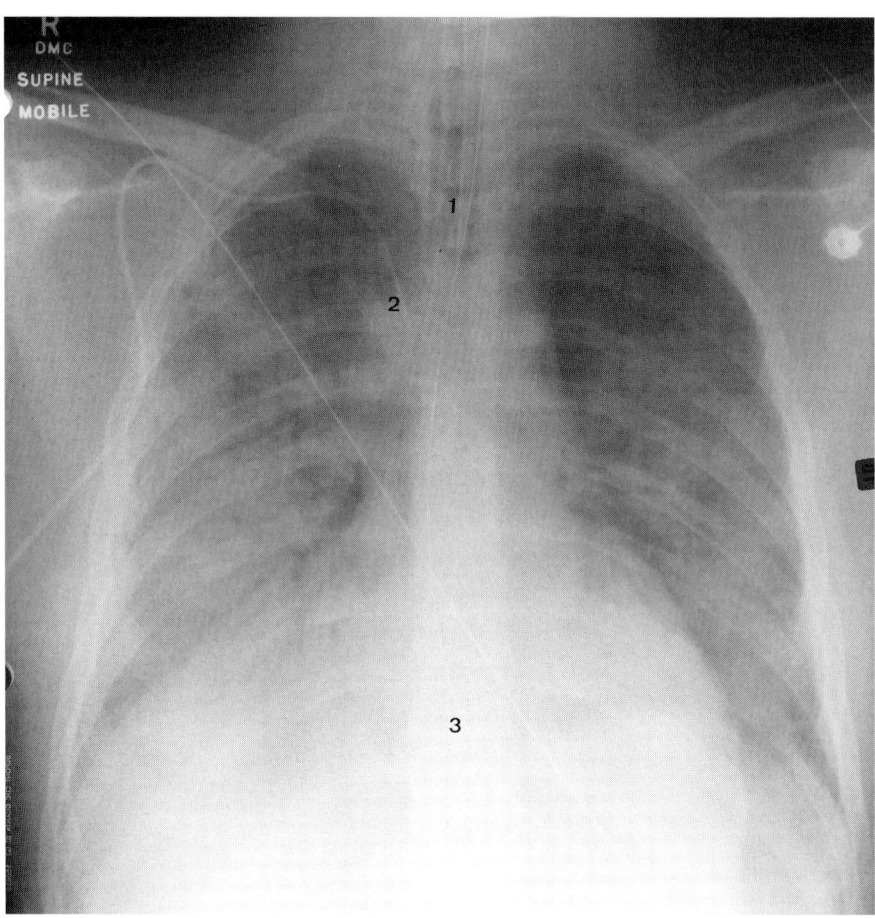

Figure 4.13 *Adult respiratory distress syndrome.*
Air-filled bronchi are seen outlined by surrounding fluid-filled alveoli. Note:
- *endotracheal tube (1)*
- *central venous catheter (2)*
- *nasogastric tube (3)*
- *cardiac monitoring leads.*

- May occur months to years after trauma.

Pneumothorax (*Figs 3.26* and *3.27*)

- Tension indicated by depression of the diaphragm and contralateral mediastinal shift.

- Haemopneumothorax shows as a fluid level.

Lungs

- Pulmonary contusion:
  - (i)   Solitary or multiple.
  - (ii) Patchy consolidation which appears within hours of the trauma and usually clears after 4 days (*Fig. 4.12*).
  - (iii) Usually, though not always, associated with rib fractures.

- Adult respiratory distress syndrome (ARDS): widespread alveolar consolidation with air bronchograms (*Fig. 4.13*).

- Fat embolism (associated with multiple fractures): poorly defined widespread opacities.

Pneumomediastinum

- Vertical lucencies in the paratracheal tissues.

- Air may outline the mediastinal pleura, especially on the left.

- Associated with subcutaneous emphysema, especially in the neck.

- Often complicated by pneumothorax.

Ruptured major airway

- Severe pneumomediastinum.

- Pneumothorax.

Aortic rupture

- Full thickness aortic rupture is usually fatal.

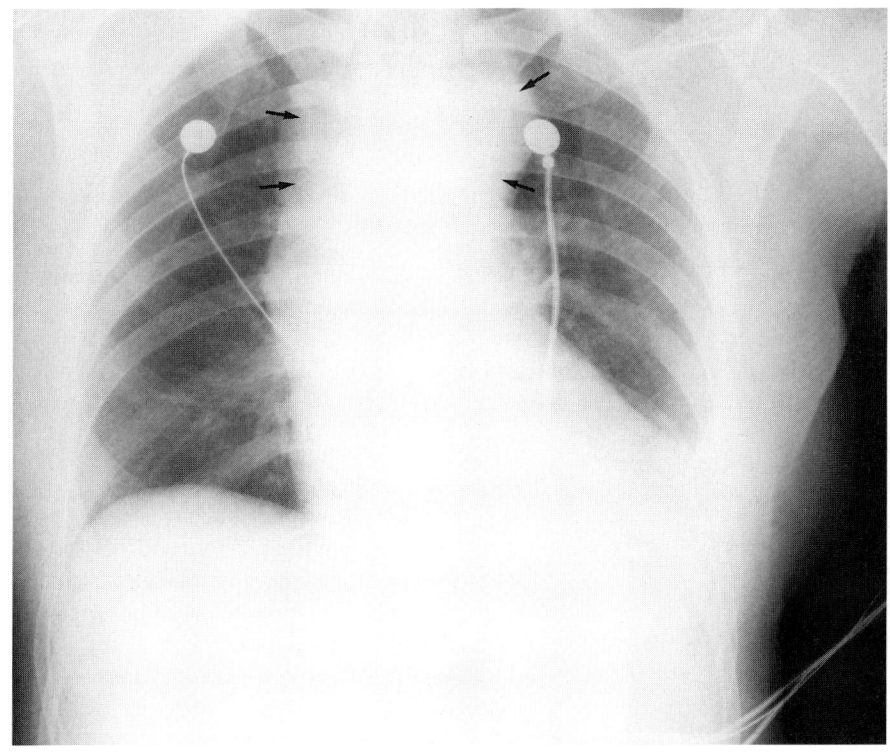

Figure 4.14 *Aortic rupture. Note:*

- *mediastinal widening (arrows) with non-visualisation of normal mediastinal structures due to haemotoma*
- *non-visualisation of the left hemidiaphragm due to haemothorax.*

- Approximately 20% of aortic ruptures are not full thickness, i.e. the adventitia is intact.

- Untreated, there is a high mortality rate with delayed complete rupture occurring up to 4 months following trauma.

- Only around 5% of incomplete ruptures develop a false aneurysm associated with a normal life span.

- It is important to recognise patients with incomplete rupture of the aorta; it is therefore important to recognise signs of mediastinal haematoma on CXR and CT.

- 20% of patients with mediastinal haematoma on CXR/CT will have a positive aortogram; absence of mediastinal haematoma is a reliable predictor of a negative aortogram.

- Note that incomplete aortic rupture implies an intact adventitia; therefore mediastinal haematoma arises in these cases from other vessels, i.e. intercostal, internal mammary etc.

- Incomplete rupture of the aorta is confirmed by aortogram or transoesophageal echocardiogram (TEE).

- Most tears occur at the aortic isthmus, i.e. just distal to the left subclavian artery.

CXR signs of aortic rupture

- Widened mediastinum which may be difficult to assess on a supine film.

- Supine CXR:
    (i) Mediastinal widening is normal and need not imply mediastinal haematoma.
    (ii) The film must be well penetrated and normal mediastinal structures should be well seen: aortic arch, descending aorta, right paratracheal stripe, azygos vein, SVC.

- Signs of mediastinal haematoma (*Fig. 4.14*):
    (i) Obscured aortic knuckle and other mediastinal structures.
    (ii) Displacement of trachea and nasogastric tube to the right.
    (iii) Depression of left main bronchus.

- Left haemothorax giving pleural opacification, including depression of the apex of the left lung.

- Associated fractures of the upper three ribs: not reliable.

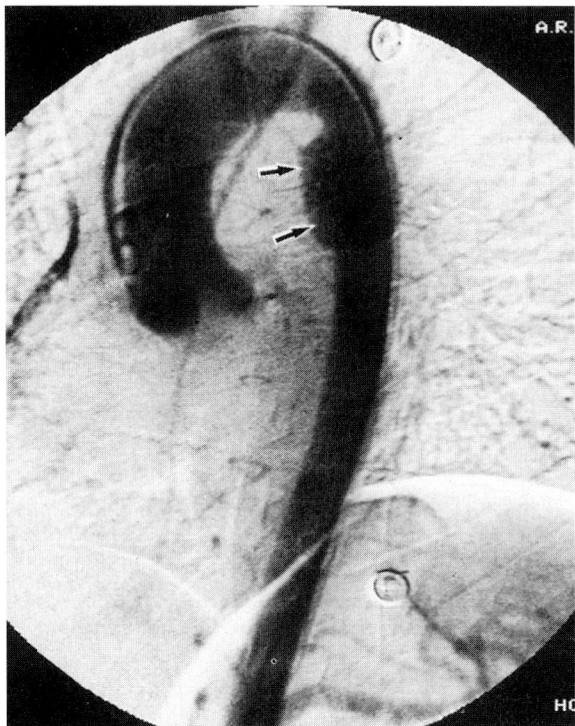

Figure 4.15 *Aortic rupture – aortogram.*
Disruption of the aorta at the isthmus (arrows) i.e.
distal to the origin of the left subclavian artery. This is
the most common site of a traumatic aortic rupture.

Further investigations for aortic rupture

- Where definite signs of mediastinal haematoma are present, aortogram or TEE should be performed (*Fig. 4.15*).

- Where the CXR is equivocal chest CT should be performed; if this is negative no further investigations are required; if positive perform aortogram or TEE.

- MRI:
  (i)   Some centres use MRI as the investigation for suspected aortic injury.
  (ii) The obvious advantage is rapid availability of sagittal images which show the change in calibre of the aortic lumen at the rupture site as well as mediastinal haematoma and haemothorax.

Head trauma

CT

- CT is the investigation of choice for the patient with head trauma.

- CT has replaced skull X-ray in the initial imaging assessment of all significant head trauma.

Indications:

  (i)   Fractured skull.
  (ii)   Confusion/impaired consciousness.
  (iii) Focal neurological signs or fits.
  (iv)   Coma, with or without fracture.
  (v)   Deterioration in level of consciousness or development of further neurological signs.
  (vi)   Confusion or other neurological disturbance for more than 6–8 hours.
  (vii) Compound/depressed vault fracture.
  (viii) Signs of fractured base of skull, i.e. discharge of blood/CSF from nose/ear.

Common CT findings

Acute intracranial haematoma

- Acute intracranial haematoma is of high attenuation (white).

- Over 7–10 days the attenuation gradually decreases to approximately that of adjacent brain tissue; a subdural haematoma of this age may therefore be difficult to see.

- Over the ensuing couple of weeks the attenuation decreases further to approximately that of CSF (black).

Extradural haematoma

- High-attenuation peripheral lesion.

- Convex inner margin (*Fig. 4.16*).

Subdural haematoma

- High-attenuation peripheral lesion often spreading over much of the cerebral hemisphere.

- Concave inner margin.

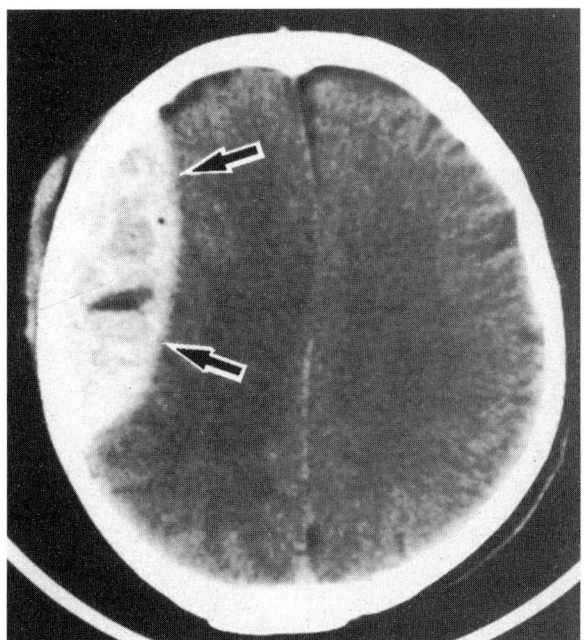

Figure 4.16 *Acute extradural haematoma.*
Peripheral collection of high attenuation. Convex inner margin (arrows) implies that the collection is extradural.

- Usually has severe associated mass effect due to swelling of the underlying damaged brain.

- Decreases in density, so that after 2–3 weeks is of lower attenuation than underlying brain (*Fig. 4.17*).

Subarachnoid haemorrhage

- High-attenuation material in the basal cisterns, Sylvian fissures, cerebral sulci, and ventricles.

Intracerebral haematoma

- High-attenuation area in the brain tissue, usually with a low-attenuation surrounding rim of oedema.

- Decreases in density with resolution to be of lower attenuation than surrounding brain after about 4 weeks.

Other CT signs of brain damage

- Cerebral oedema: low-attenuation areas which may be focal, multifocal, or diffuse; associated mass effect with compression and distortion of ventricles and basal cisterns.

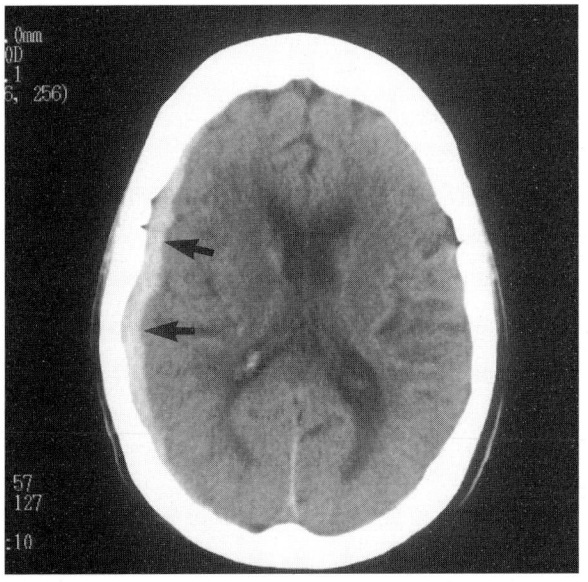

a

b

Figure 4.17 *Subdural haematoma – CT.*
(a) Acute subdural haematoma. Peripheral collection of high attenuation indicating fresh blood. Concave inner margin (arrows) indicates that the collection is subdural. (b) Chronic subdural haematoma. After one month the collection is of low attenuation (arrows), similar in density to CSF.

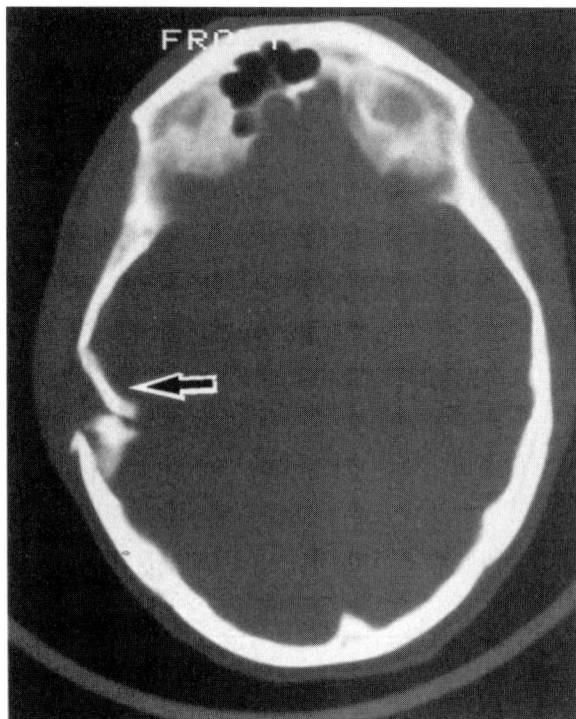

Figure 4.18 *Depressed skull fracture – CT.*
Depressed fragments of bone well demonstrated in cross-section (arrow).

- Cerebral contusion: areas of mixed high and low attenuation which may be focal or multifocal; with time the haemorrhagic component resolves leaving irregular areas of low attenuation; variable associated oedema and mass effect.

- Diffuse axonal (shearing) injuries: small haemorrhagic areas at grey-white matter junction, brainstem, and corpus callosum.

Other CT signs of trauma

- Fractures: CT is especially useful for defining base of skull fractures and all traumatic scans must be perused on bone windows (*Fig. 4.18*).

- Scalp swelling.

- Pneumocephalus: subdural, subarachnoid, intraventricular.

- Opacification and/or fluid levels in sinuses.

- Foreign bodies.

Skull X-ray (SXR)

Indications:

- In view of the wide availability of CT the indications for SXR in a setting of trauma are limited to the following:
  (i) Penetrating injuries.
  (ii) Foreign bodies.
  (iii) Clinical suspicion of a depressed fracture.

- Clinically suspected non-depressed skull fractures with or without neurological signs should be immediately assessed with CT.

Skull fractures:

(a) Fractures need to be differentiated from normal lucent linear markings in the skull, i.e. sutures and vascular markings.

(b) Sutures:

- Position more reliable than appearance; sutures tend to be constant in position so this is the more important parameter.

(c) Lateral film:

- Coronal suture between frontal and parietal bones.

- Lambdoid suture between parietal and occipital bones.

- May also see temporo-parietal and temporo-occipital sutures.

(d) AP film:

- Sagittal suture between parietal bones.

- Lambdoid suture.

(e) Towne's view:

- Lambdoid suture.

(f) Sutures may appear as straight or zigzag lines, or a combination of both.

(g) Vascular markings:

- Appearance more reliable than position; vascular markings are quite variable in position and as such their appearance is the most important parameter.

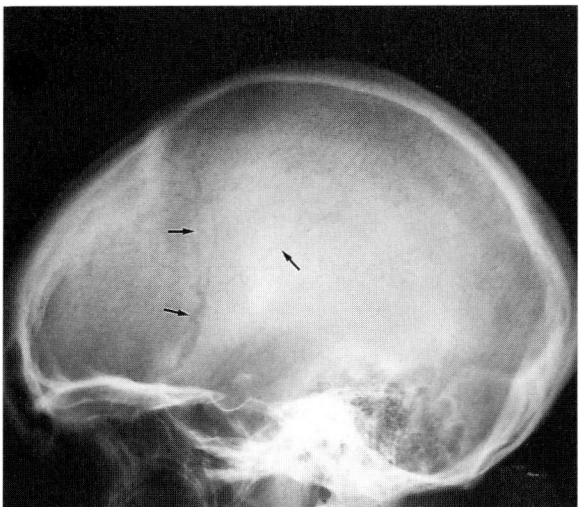

Figure 4.19 *Normal skull – vascular markings.*
The grooves formed by the middle meningeal vessels are
well demonstrated (arrows). Note the typical features of
vascular markings:
- *tortuosity*
- *branching pattern*
- *distal tapering.*

- Vascular markings are tortuous and branching, have well defined corticated (white) margins, become smaller as they pass upwards, and may cross sutures (*Fig. 4.19*).

(h) Fractures have the following features:

- Usually linear and well defined (*Fig. 4.20*).

- Non-corticated margins.

- May occasionally branch.

- May rarely cross a suture; a linear fracture extending to a suture is more often associated with separation of the suture.

- In children isolated separation of a suture may occur without an associated fracture; this most commonly involves the lambdoid and coronal sutures.

(i) Depressed fracture may show as a sharply defined area of high density due to overlapping of bone fragments; depressed fragment seen on tangential views (*Fig. 4.21*).

(j) Other signs of trauma on SXR:

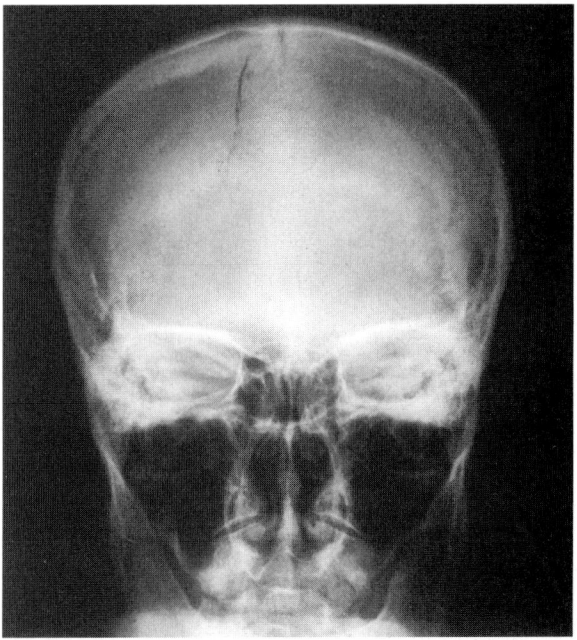

Figure 4.20 *Skull fracture.*
Linear fracture of the left frontal bone.

- Air in the cranial vault indicating penetration or base of skull/sinus fracture (*Fig. 4.22*).

- Air in the ventricles and subarachnoid spaces.

- Air collection (aerocele) anterior to the frontal lobes.

- Opaque sinus or fluid levels in sinuses.

- Opaque middle ear cavities.

- Shift of pineal calcification (an extremely unreliable sign).

MRI

- Owing to relatively poor visualisation of acute haemorrhage, time of examination, and logistical problems with monitoring equipment, MRI has not been recommended for initial screening of acute head trauma.

- MRI is however useful in the non-acute situation of an otherwise stable patient with an ongoing neurological deficit. In particular MRI is highly sensitive for the detection of diffuse axonal injury and 'old' blood products.

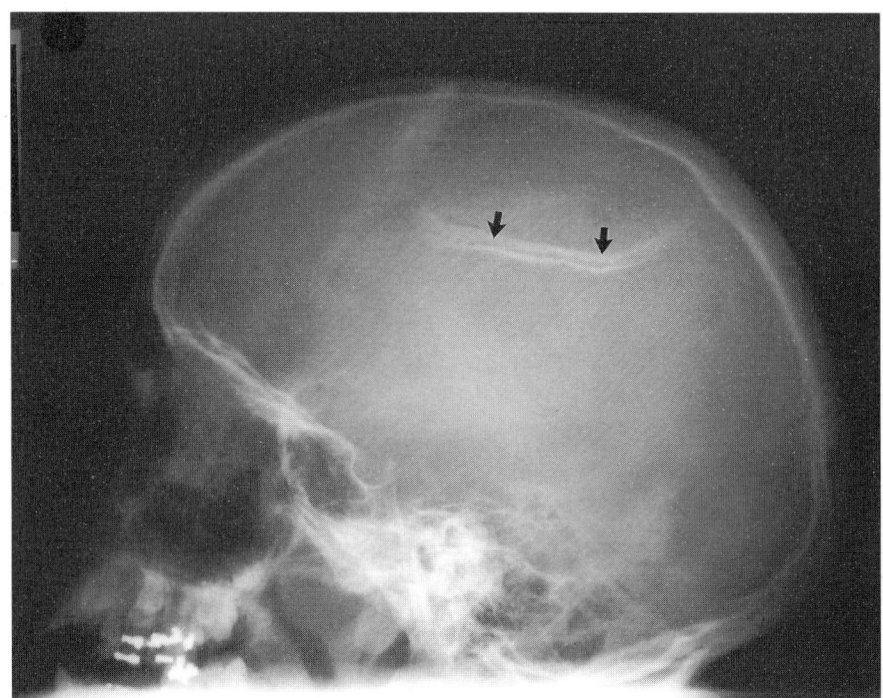

a

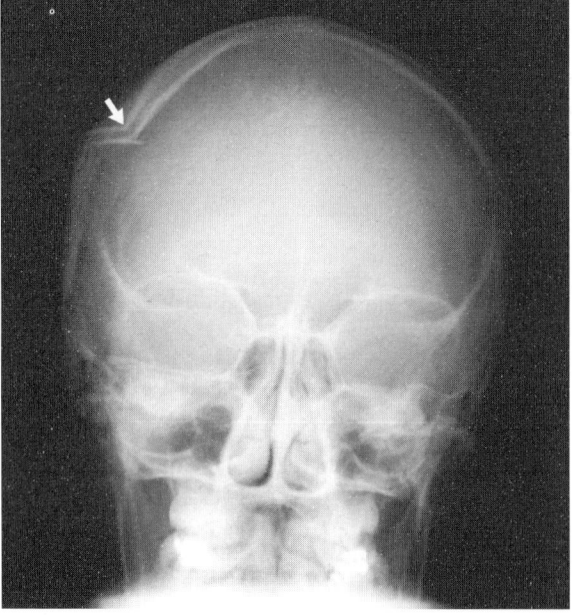

b

Figure 4.21 *Depressed skull fracture.*
(a) Lateral view. The fracture is seen as a white band (arrows) due to overlapping bone fragments. (b) AP view. The configuration of the depressed fracture fragments (arrow) is well shown in this projection.

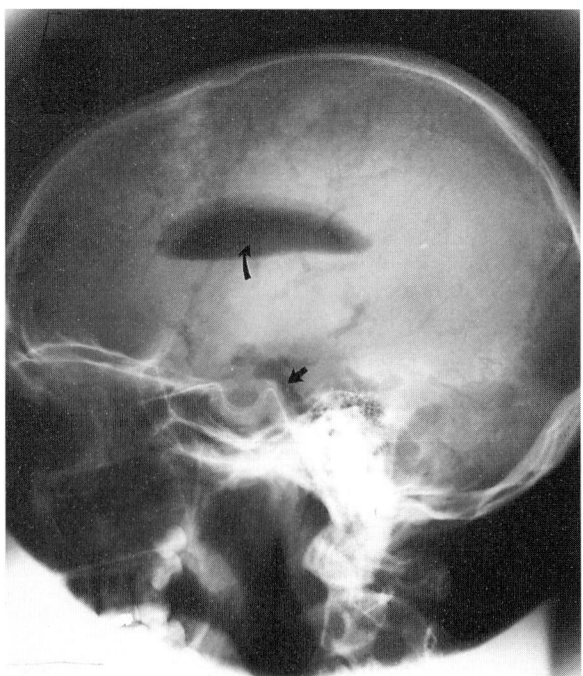

Figure 4.22 *Traumatic pneumocephalus.*
Air is seen in the basal cisterns (straight arrow) and lateral ventricles (curved arrow) following a base of skull fracture involving the sinuses.

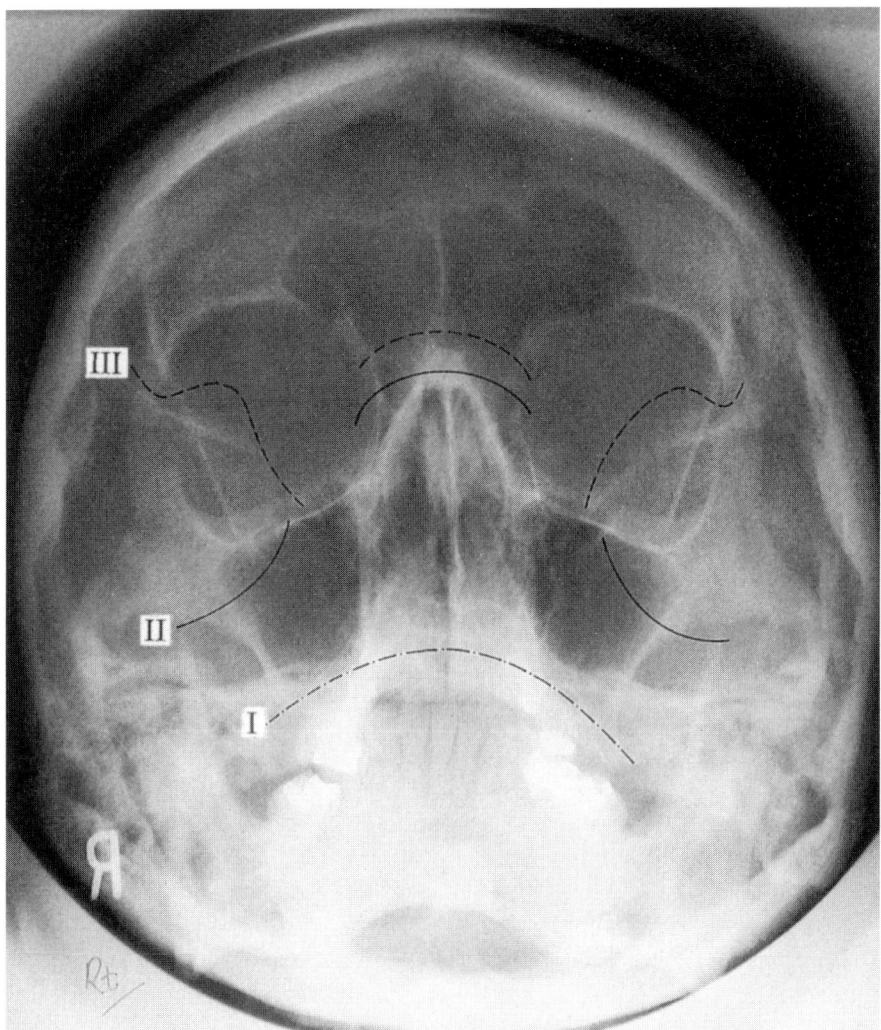

Figure 4.23 *Le Fort fractures.*
A diagrammatic representation of the Le Fort classification of facial features.
Le Fort I _._._._.
Le Fort II ————
Le Fort III ----------

Cervical spine

In all major trauma and head injury cases, the importance of obtaining at least a lateral cervical spine X-ray showing all seven cervical vertebrae cannot be overemphasised.

Facial trauma

Inadequate facial detail is seen on normal skull X-rays and separate facial views must be requested if facial fractures are suspected.

Maxillary fractures

The Le Fort classification provides a useful descriptive guide only; different degrees of fracture may exist on either side of the face (*Fig. 4.23*).

- *Le Fort I:* fracture line through the lower maxillary sinuses and nasal septum with separation of the lower maxilla.

- *Le Fort II:* fracture lines extend from the nasal bones in the midline through the medial and inferior walls of the orbits and the lateral walls of the maxillary sinuses, giving a large triangular separate fragment.

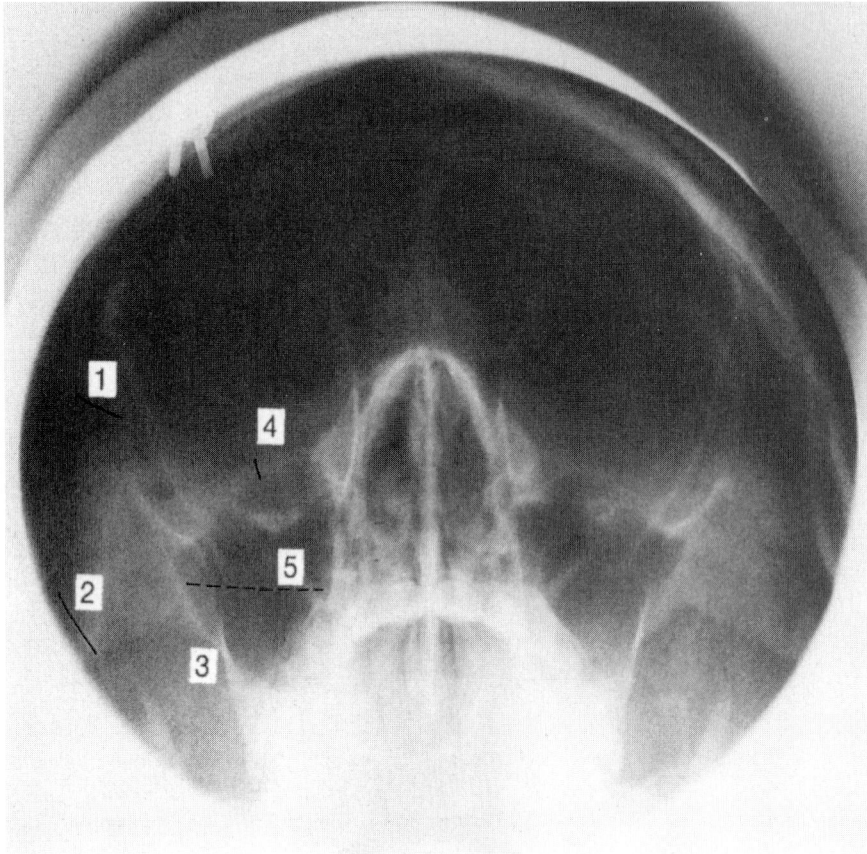

Figure 4.24 *Zygomatic fractures.*
Diagrammatic representation of points to look for in suspected zygomatic fractures:
1. *Diastasis of the zygomatico-frontal articulation in the lateral orbital wall.*
2. *Fracture of the anterior zygomatic arch.*
3. *Fracture of the lateral wall of the maxillary sinus.*
4. *Fracture of the orbital floor.*
5. *Fluid level in the maxillary sinus.*

* *Le Fort III:* fracture lines run horizontally through the orbits and the zygomatic arches, causing complete separation of the facial bones from the cranium.

CT may provide better anatomical definition prior to surgery.

Zygomatic fractures

* Zygomatic fractures occur classically in four places:

    (i)   the inferior orbital margin;

    (ii)   the lateral wall of the maxillary sinus;

    (iii) the anterior end of the zygomatic arch;

    (iv)   the lateral wall of orbit (usually diastasis of the zygomatico-frontal suture) (*Fig. 4.24*).

Blow-out fracture of orbital floor

(a) *Plain films:*

* Soft tissue in the shape of a 'teardrop' in the upper aspect of the maxillary sinus (*Fig. 4.25*).

* May see the actual fracture which will be confirmed by tomograms in the coronal plane.

(b) *CT:*

* Performed in the coronal plane.

* Show the fractures as well as herniation of orbital structures into the maxillary sinus (*Fig. 4.26*).

* Allow delineation of involved structures, especially inferior rectus and inferior oblique muscles.

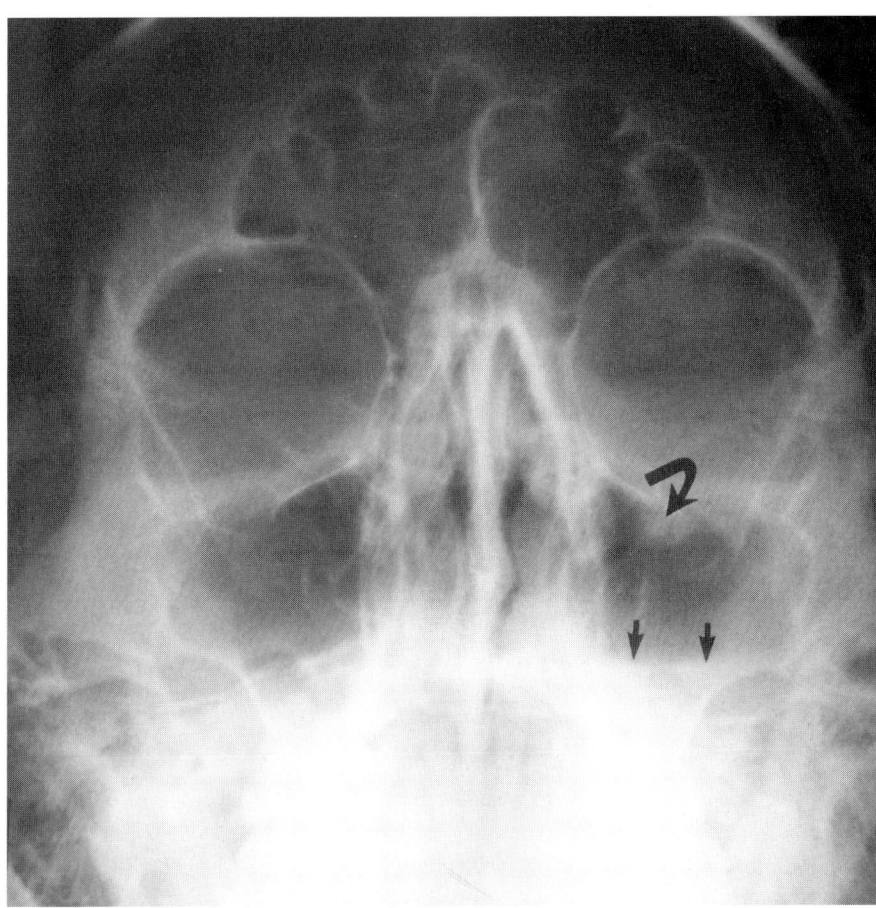

Figure 4.25 *'Blow-out' orbital fracture.*
Note:
- *teardrop shaped mass in the roof of the maxillary sinus (curved arrow)*
- *fluid level in the sinus due to haemorrhage (straight arrows).*

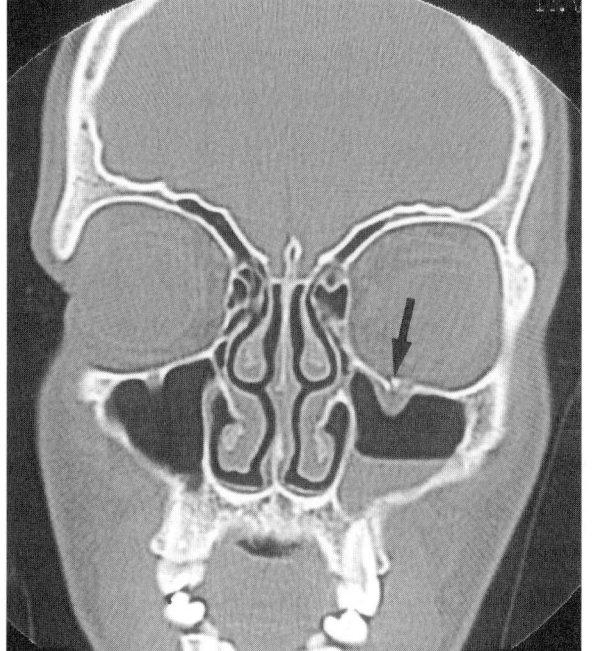

Figure 4.26 *'Blow-out' orbital fracture – CT.*
Note:
- *fracture of the orbital floor (arrow) with downward herniation of orbital fat producing the tear-drop shaped mass in the roof of the maxillary sinus*
- *blood in the sinus.*

(c) *MRI:*

- Herniation of orbital contents well demonstrated by coronal MRI.

Mandibular fractures

- Numerous views may be needed, including OPG (orthopantomogram) which gives a panoramic view of the tooth-bearing part of the mandible with poor definition of the midline and the condyles.

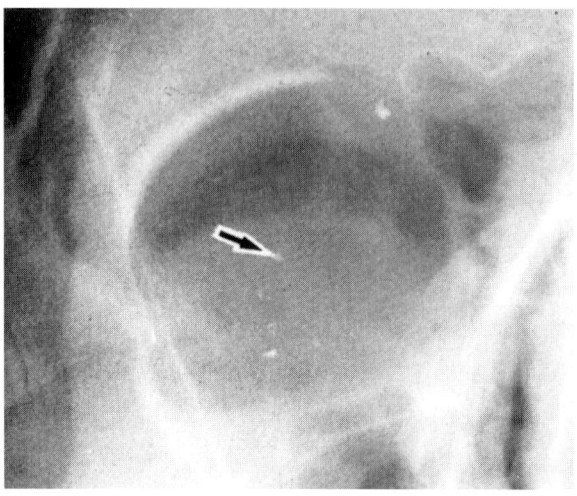 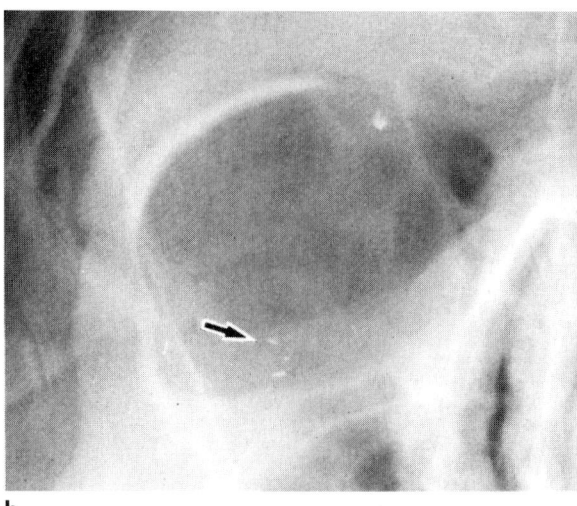

a   b

Figure 4.27 *Orbital foreign body.*
Plain films. There are several metal fragments projected over the right orbit most of which lie in the eyelids. One fragment however shifts significantly with eye movements (arrow). It moves up when the patient looks up and down when the patient looks down indicating that it must lie anteriorly in the eye ball.

- Being U-shaped the mandible often fractures in two places.
- The following areas must be fully imaged in suspected mandibular trauma: midline, body, angle, ramus, condyle, coronoid process.

Associated signs of facial fractures

- Soft tissue swelling.
- Opacification or fluid level of the maxillary or other sinuses.
- Air in the orbit or other soft tissues.

Further assessment of orbital trauma

(a) Plain films:

- Orbital fractures as above.
- Radio-opaque foreign bodies: localise with respect to the bony margins of the orbit; eye movement films give an idea of the position of a foreign body (*Fig. 4.27*).

(b) Ultrasound:

- Foreign bodies: accurate localisation except for very small bodies lying posteriorly; foreign body shows as a dense localised echo, usually with shadowing.
- Ocular trauma: US is particularly good for retinal detachment.

(c) CT:

- Orbital fractures as above.
- Foreign bodies: accurate localisation whether intra- or extraocular.
- Ocular trauma: deformity of the eyeball; intraocular haemorrhage showing as an irregular area of raised attenuation in the vitreous.
- Extraocular trauma: optic nerve separation from the globe or transection; retrobulbar haematoma; extraocular muscle damage.

(d) MRI:

- MRI demonstrates similar lesions to CT, i.e. retrobulbar and intraocular haematoma, deformity of the globe, and as noted above, herniation of orbital structures in blow-out fractures.

- The following disadvantages of MRI make CT preferable for assessing orbital trauma:

(i) Contraindicated by the possibility of a metallic foreign body.

(ii) Less sensitive than CT at detecting fractures.

Spine trauma

The roles of imaging in the assessment of spinal trauma are:

- Diagnosis of fractures/dislocation.

- Assessment of stability/instability.

- Diagnosis of damage to, or impingement on, neurological structures.

- Follow-up:
  (a) Assessment of treatment.
  (b) Diagnosis of long-term complications, e.g. post-traumatic syrinx or cyst formation.

Cervical spine

Plain films

Plain film assessment of the cervical spine should be performed in all trauma patients with neck pain or tenderness, other signs of direct neck injury, or abnormal findings on neurological examination. Cervical spine films should also be performed in all patients with severe head or facial injury or following high velocity blunt trauma or near-drowning.

The following films should be performed:

- Lateral view with patient supine showing all seven cervical vertebrae:
  (i)   traction on the shoulders may be used;
  (ii) traction on the head must *never* be used.

- Other views should also be performed with the patient supine: AP, AP open mouth view to show the odontoid peg, obliques to show the facet joints and intervertebral foramina.

- Functional views, i.e. lateral views in flexion and extension with the patient erect:

(i)   performed where no fractures are seen on the neutral views to diagnose posterior or anterior ligament damage;

(ii) patient must be conscious and co-operative and must themselves perform flexion and extension, i.e. the head must not be moved passively by doctor or radiographer.

Films should be checked in a logical fashion for the following factors:

- Vertebral alignment:

  (i)   Disruption of anterior and posterior vertebral body lines, i.e. lines joining the anterior and posterior margins of the vertebral bodies on the lateral view.

  (ii) Disruption of the posterior cervical line, i.e. a line joining the anterior aspect of the spinous processes of C1, C2 and C3; disruption of this line may indicate upper cervical spine fractures, especially of C2 (*Fig. 4.28*).

  (iii) Facet joint alignment at all levels; abrupt disruption at one level may indicate locked facets.

  (iv) Widening of the space between spinous processes on the lateral film.

  (v)   Rotation of spinous processes on the AP film.

  (vi) Widening of the predental space, i.e. > 5 mm in children; > 3 mm in adults.

- Bone integrity:

  (i)   Vertebral body fractures.

  (ii) Fractures of posterior elements, i.e. pedicles, laminae, spinous processes.

  (iii) Integrity of odontoid peg: anterior/posterior/lateral displacement.

- Disc spaces: narrowing or widening.

- Soft tissue changes:

  (i)   Prevertebral swelling: widening of the retro-tracheal space, i.e. posterior aspect of trachea to C6: > 14 mm in children; > 22 mm in adults.

  (ii) Widening of the retropharyngeal space, i.e. posterior aspect of pharynx to C2: > 7 mm in adults and children.

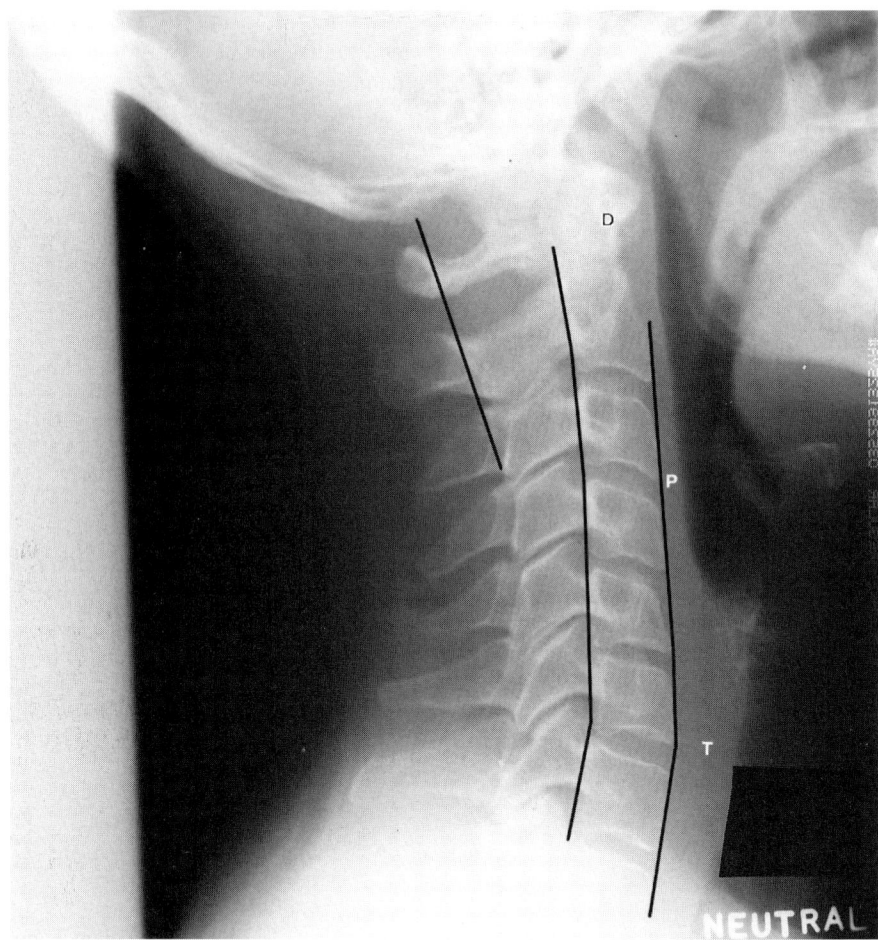

Figure 4.28 *Normal cervical spine.*
Note:
- *anterior vertebral body line*
- *posterior vertebral body line*
- *posterior cervical line*
- *alignment of the facet joints*
- *equal spaces between spinous processes*
- *normal predental space (D)*
- *normal retropharyngeal space (P)*
- *normal retrotracheal space (T).*

Common patterns of injury are as follows:

Flexion (i.e. anterior compression with posterior distraction) (Fig. 4.29):

- Vertebral body compression fracture.

- 'Teardrop' fracture, i.e. small triangular fragment at lower anterior margin of vertebral body.

- Disruption of posterior vertebral line.

- Disc space narrowing.

- Widening of facet joints.

- Widening of space between spinous processes.

Extension (i.e. posterior compression with anterior distraction) (Fig. 4.30):

- 'Teardrop' fracture of upper anterior margin of vertebral body: indicates severe anterior ligament damage.

- Disc space widening.

- Retrolisthesis with disruption of anterior and posterior vertebral lines.

- Fractures of posterior elements, i.e. pedicles, spinous processes, facets, e.g. 'hangman's' fracture – bilateral C2 pedicle fracture (*Fig. 4.31*).

Rotation:

- Anterolisthesis with disruption of posterior vertebral line.

- Lateral displacement of upper vertebral body on AP view.

- Abrupt disruption of alignment of facet joints: locked facets.

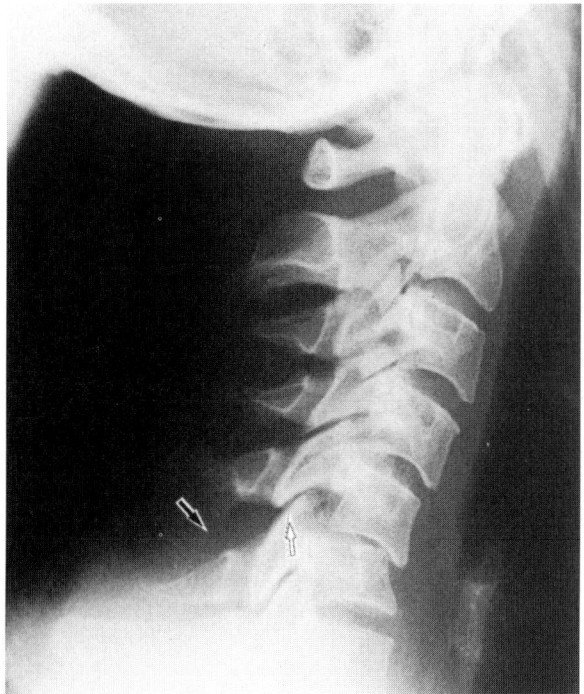

Figure 4.29 *Cervical spine injury.*
This case of unilateral locked facet demonstrates several signs of potentially unstable cervical injury:
- *widening of the space between adjacent spinous processes (solid arrow)*
- *disruption of facet joints (hollow arrow)*
anterior displacement of C5 on C6.

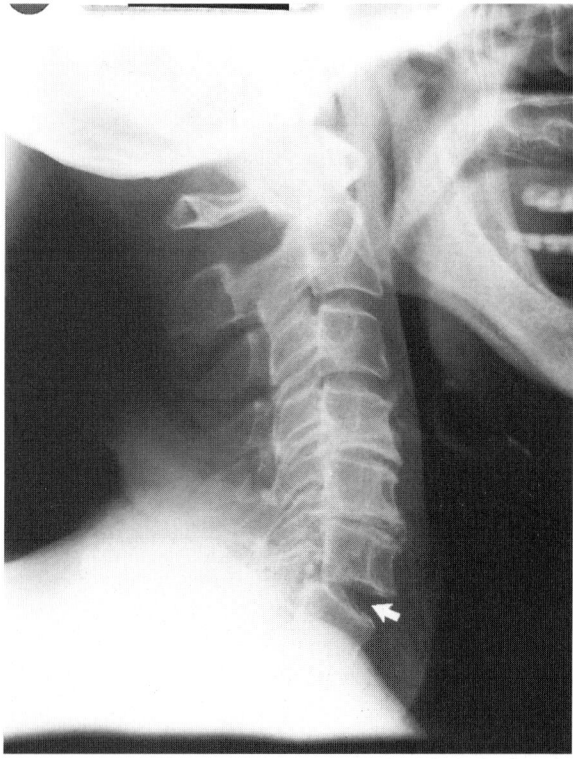

Figure 4.30 *Extension injury at C6/C7.*
Note:
- *disruption of posterior and anterior vertebral body lines*
- *widening of C6/C7 disc space (arrow).*

- Narrow disc space.
- Rotation of spinous processes on AP film.

Instability implies the possibility of increased spinal deformity or neurological damage occurring with continued stress. Signs of instability are:

- Displacement of vertebral body.
- 'Teardrop' fractures of vertebral body.
- Odontoid peg fracture.
- Widening or disruption of alignment of facet joints including locked facets.
- Widening of space between spinous processes.
- Fractures at multiple levels.

CT

- Further delineation of fractures and associated deformity.
- More accurate assessment, especially of neural arches and facet joints (*Fig. 4.32*).
- Accurate estimation of dimensions of spinal canal.

MRI

- Has replaced myelography for the assessment of spinal cord damage:
  (i)   Transection.
  (ii) Swelling/oedema/haemorrhage.
  (iii) Cyst and syrinx formation.
- Soft tissue changes:
  (i) Disc lesions.
  (ii) Spinal canal haematoma.

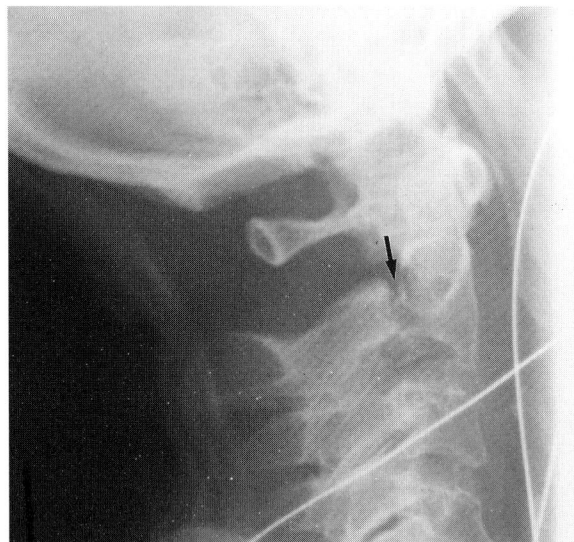

Figure 4.31 *Hangman's fracture.*
Note:
* *disruption of posterior cervical line*
* *fractures of the pedicles of C2 (arrow).*

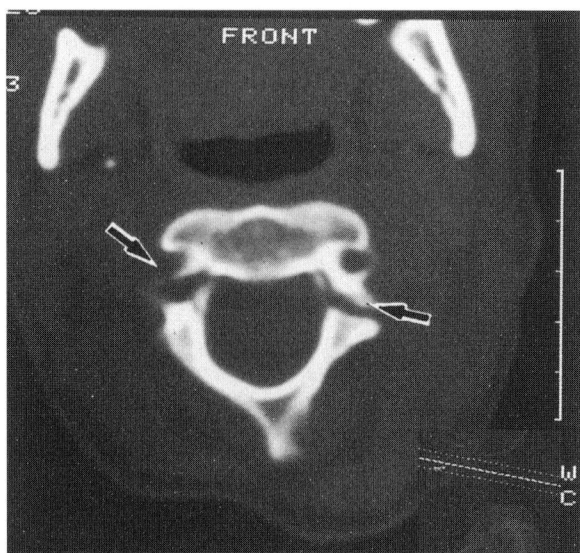

Figure 4.32 *C2 fracture – CT.*
Fractured pedicles of C2 (arrows).

Thoracic and lumbar spine

Plain films

Assessment of plain films of the thoracic and lumbar spine following trauma is similar to that outlined for the cervical spine with particular attention to the following factors:

* Vertebral alignment.

* Vertebral body height.

* Disc space height.

* Facet joint alignment.

* Space between pedicles on AP film: widening at one level may indicate a burst fracture of the vertebral body.

Common patterns of injury are:

Burst fracture:

* Fractures of the vertebral body with a fragment pushed posteriorly into the spinal canal.

Compression fracture:

* Loss of height of vertebral body.

Fracture/dislocation:

* Vertebral body displacement.

* Disc space narrowing or widening.

* Fractures of neural arches, including facet joints.

* Widening of facet joints or space between spinous processes.

Chance fracture (seatbelt fracture):

* Fracture of posterior vertebral body.

* Horizontal fracture line through spinous process, laminae, pedicles, transverse processes (*Fig. 4.33*).

* Most occur at thoracolumbar junction.

* High association with abdominal injury, i.e. solid organ damage, intestinal perforation, duodenal haematoma.

CT

* More accurate delineation of fractures and deformity (*Fig. 4.34*).

* Spinal canal well visualised in cross-section: posterior vertebral fragments impinging on spinal canal.

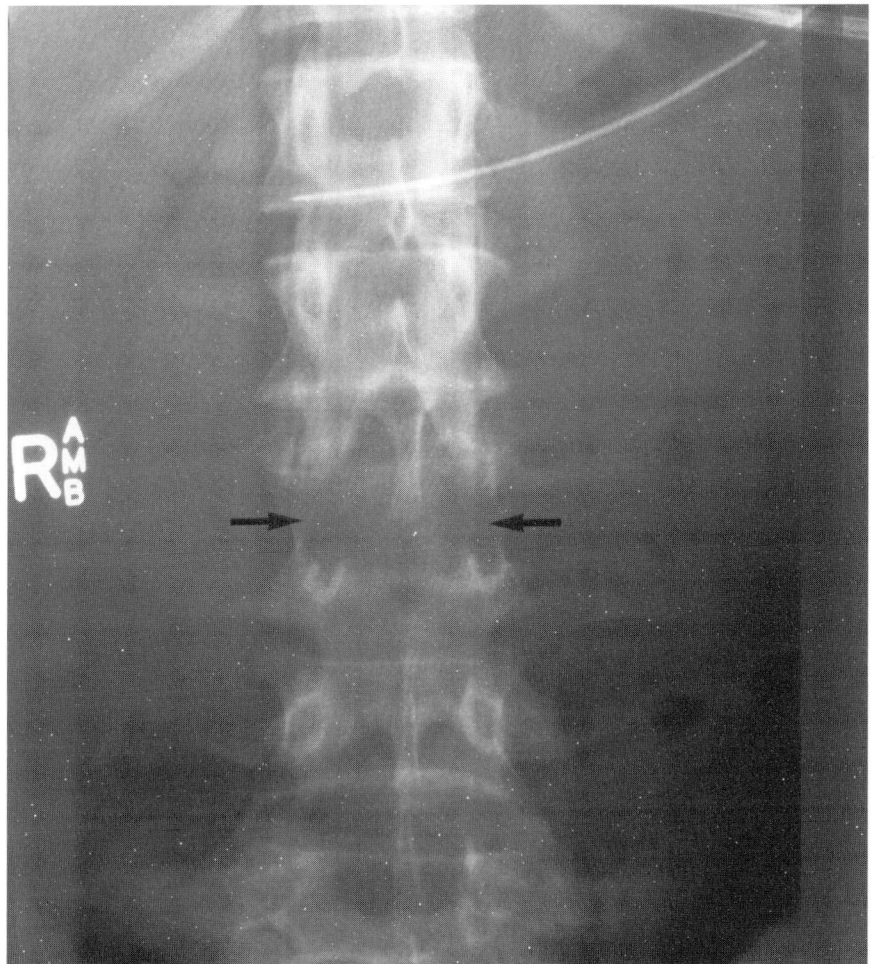

Figure 4.33 *Chance fracture.*
Chance fracture from a high speed motor vehicle accident. Note the horizontal fracture of L3 with splitting of the pedicles and wide separation of the spinous processes (arrows).

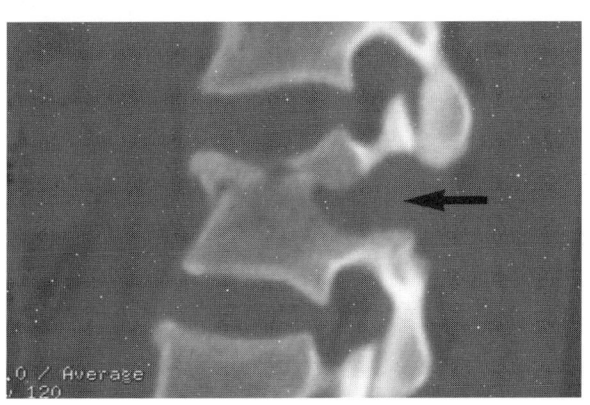

a

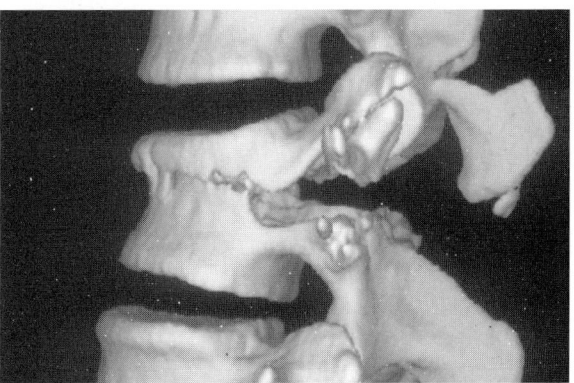

b

Figure 4.34 *Chance fracture – CT.*
(a) Multiplanar reconstruction. Helical CT is performed with sagittal reconstructions. These reconstructions show the horizontal fracture lines through the pedicle and posterior vertebral body (arrow). (b). 3-D reconstruction. A 3-D reconstruction shows the anatomy of the fractures and is of great assistance in planning surgical reduction and repair.

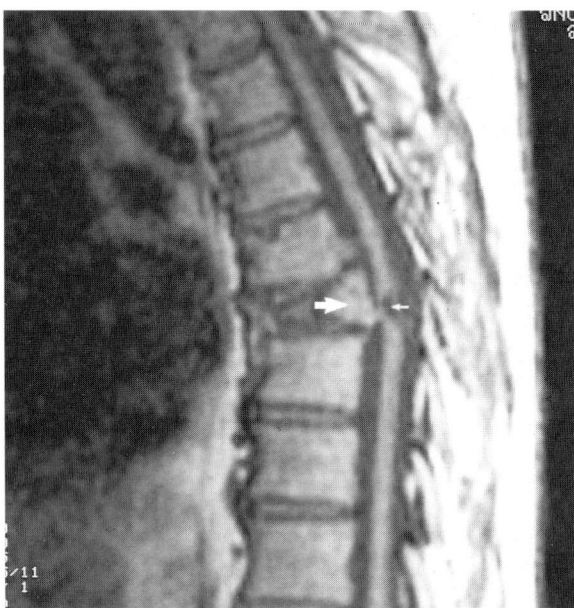

Figure 4.35 *Thoracic spine fracture – MRI.*
Note:
- *localised kyphosis due to a vertebral body crush fracture*
- *bone fragment in the spinal canal impinging on the spinal cord (large arrow)*
- *post-traumatic cyst formation in the spinal cord (small arrow).*

MRI

- Assessment of spinal cord and soft tissues (*Fig. 4.35*).

Limb trauma

General principles

Classification of fractures

Fractures may be classified in a number of ways and are usually described by using a combination of the following terminology.

1. Complete or incomplete:
   - Complete fractures are described as transverse, oblique, or spiral.
   - Incomplete fractures occur in children and are classified as buckle or torus, greenstick, and plastic or bowing (see below).
2. Bone involved and position.
3. Comminution.
   - A comminuted fracture is a fracture associated with more than two fragments.
4. Closed or open (compound).
5. Degree of deformity
   - Angulation.
   - Displacement of fracture fragments.
   - Rotation.
   - Associated joint subluxation or dislocation.

Complications of fractures

1. Delayed union:
   - Occurs due to incomplete immobilisation, infection at the fracture site, pathological fractures, i.e. fractures through an underlying bone lesion, vitamin C deficiency, or in elderly patients.
2. Malunion:
   - Union has occurred, though in a poor position leading to bone or joint deformity, and often to early osteoarthritis.
3. Non-union:
   - This term implies that the bone will never unite without some form of intervention.
   - Two appearances may be seen:
     (i) sclerosis (increased density) of the bone ends with a lucent margin between them;
     (ii) fracture line able to be seen through surrounding callus.
4. Avascular necrosis:
   - Occurs most commonly in three sites: proximal pole of scaphoid (*Fig. 4.36*), femoral head, and body of talus.
   - Due to interruption of blood supply as may occur in fractures of the waist of the scaphoid, femoral neck, and neck of talus.

- The non-vascularised portion of bone becomes sclerotic over 2–3 months; this is due to new bone being laid down on necrosed bone trabeculae.

- Due to weight bearing, the femoral head and talus may show deformity and irregularity as well as sclerosis.

5. Reflex sympathetic dystrophy (Sudeck's atrophy):

- Reflex sympathetic dystrophy may be considered as a severe form of disuse osteoporosis, which may follow trivial bone injury.

- Occurs in bones distal to the site of injury.

- Associated with severe pain and swelling.

- X-ray changes:

    (i) Severe decrease in bone density distal to fracture site.

    (ii) Marked thinning of bone cortex.

- Scintigraphy:

    (i) ^{99m}Tc-MDP.

    (ii) Increased uptake in the limb distal to the trauma site.

6. Myositis ossificans:

- Refers to post-traumatic non-neoplastic formation of bone within skeletal muscle.

- Usually forms within 5–6 weeks of trauma.

- May occur at any site though the muscles of the anterior thigh are most commonly affected.

- Seen on X-ray as bone formation in the soft tissues; this bone has a striated appearance conforming to the structure of the underlying muscle.

Subtle fractures

Obvious fractures are just that – obvious, and can often be diagnosed by the patient holding the X-ray up to the ceiling light! The diagnosis of fractures that display subtle X-ray changes is important and often difficult. There is no substitute for careful history and examination followed by close perusal of the tender region on X-ray. Fractures may be difficult to see for a number of reasons as below.

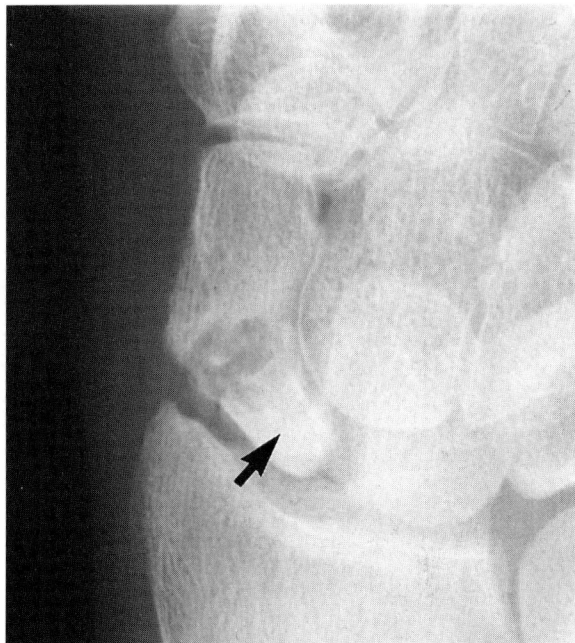

Fig 4.36 *Avascular necrosis complicating scaphoid fracture.*

1. Minimal displacement:

- Often referred to as 'hairline' fractures.

- Oblique fractures of the long bones can be especially difficult, particularly in paediatric patients. A classic example of this is the undisplaced spiral fracture of the tibia in the 1–3 age group, the so-called 'toddler's fracture'.

- Fractures through the waist of the scaphoid can also be difficult in the acute phase. Owing to the risk of avascular necrosis of the proximal pole of the scaphoid it is recommended that regardless of the initial X-ray result, all patients with clinically suspected scaphoid fracture be treated and have a repeat X-ray in 7–10 cases. Bone scintigraphy is useful in doubtful cases.

2. Paediatric fractures:

- Children tend to have softer, more malleable bones, which may not completely fracture.

- Buckle (torus) fracture: bend in the cortex without actual cortical break; common in the distal radius (*Fig. 4.37*).

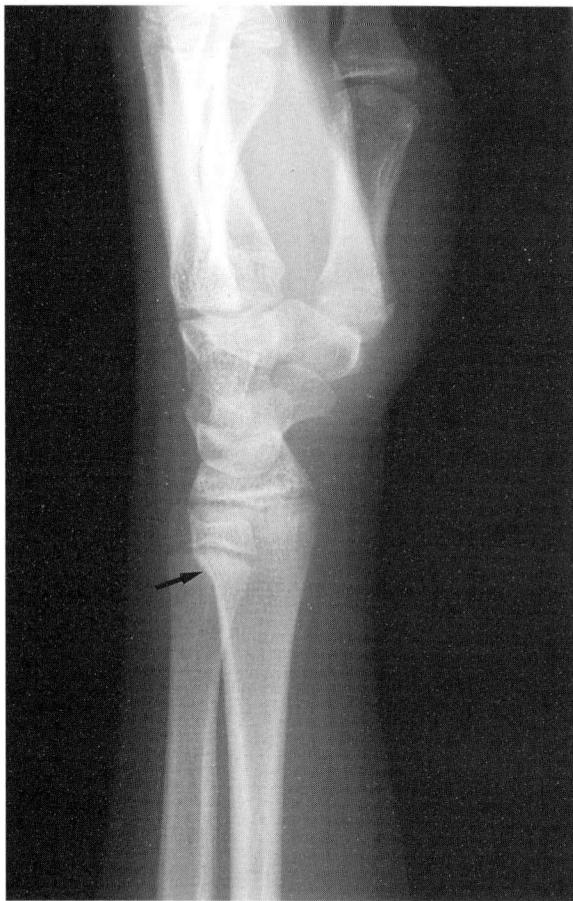

Fig 4.37 *Buckle (torus) fracture.*

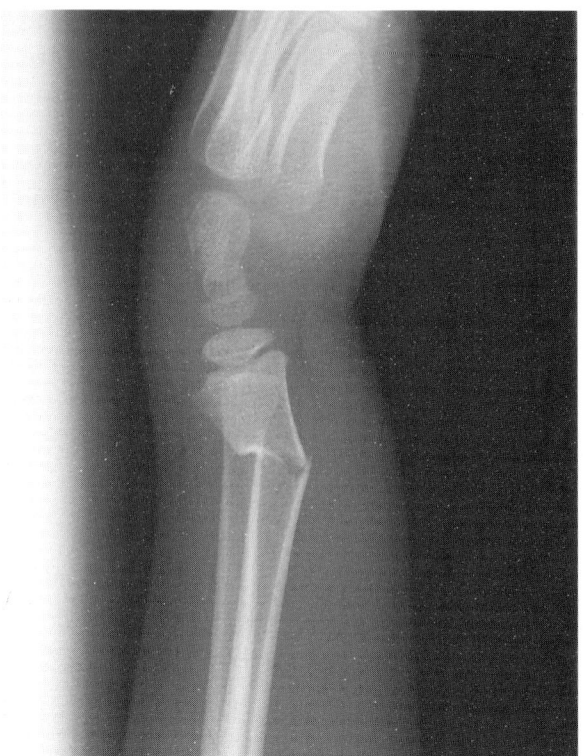

Fig 4.38 *Greenstick fracture.*

- Greenstick fracture: only one cortex is broken with bending of the other cortex (*Fig. 4.38*).

- Plastic or bowing fracture: bending of a long bone without angular deformity.

- Fractures in and around the epiphysis may be difficult to see and are classified by the Salter–Harris system, as follows:
  - (i)   Salter–Harris 1: epiphyseal plate (cartilage) fracture (*Fig. 4.39*).
  - (ii) Salter–Harris 2: fracture of metaphysis with or without displacement of the epiphysis.
  - (iii) Salter–Harris 3: fracture of epiphysis only.
  - (iv) Salter–Harris 4: fracture of metaphysis and epiphysis.
  - (v)   Salter–Harris 5: impaction and compression of the epiphyseal plate.

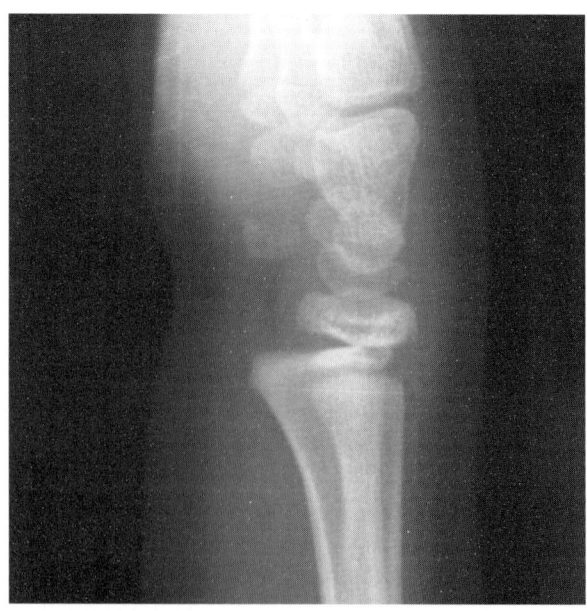

Fig 4.39 *Salter–Harris 1 fracture.*
The distal radial epiphysis is displaced posteriorly from the metaphysis indicating a fracture of the cartilage growth plate.

- Type 2 is the most common form.

- Types 1 and 5 are the most difficult to appreciate as the bones themselves are intact. They are important to diagnose however as untreated disruption of the epiphyseal plate may lead to problems with growth of the bone.

3. Fractures in complex areas:

   - These fractures are difficult to diagnose radiographically due to overlapping structures.

   - Examples include the pelvis, especially the acetabulum; the feet, particularly the tarsal bones; the wrist particularly less common fractures such as fracture of the hook of the hamate.

   - Strategies for diagnosis of suspected fractures in these regions include:
     (i) Further radiographic views: obliques, stress views.
     (ii) Recognition of joint effusions. Effusions are easily recognised in the elbow, knee, and ankle joints. Elbow effusion and lipohaemarthrosis of the knee joint have a very high incidence of associated fractures.
     (iii) Scintigraphy, i.e. bone scan with ^{99m}Tc-MDP. Will be positive within 24 hours of a fracture.
     (iv) CT with fine sections through the area of interest. CT is particularly useful for giving further anatomical detail prior to surgery. This function is especially applicable to the calcaneus and acetabulum where 3D reconstruction may also be useful.

4. Stress fractures:

   - A stress fracture is a fracture occurring in a normal bone due to prolonged, repetitive muscle action on that bone.

   - Stress fractures are particularly common in people engaged in sports, ballet, and gymnastics and a wide range of stress fractures has been described occurring in particular activities.

   - X-rays are often normal at the time of initial presentation.

- After 7–10 days, periosteal thickening is usually visible, as well as a faint fracture line.

- Scintigraphy:
  (i) ^{99m}Tc-MDP.
  (ii) Usually positive at the time of initial presentation.

- CT is useful for stress fractures in complex areas difficult to see with conventional X-rays, e.g. navicular.

Specific areas

In the following section X-ray signs of the more common fracture/dislocations will be discussed. Those lesions that may cause problems with diagnosis will be emphasised. Most fracture/dislocations are diagnosed with conventional X-rays. Other imaging modalities will be described where applicable.

Shoulder

1. Fractured clavicle:

   - Usually involves the middle third.

   - The outer fragment usually lies at a lower level than the inner fragment with the acromio-clavicular joint intact.

2. Acromio-clavicular joint dislocation:

   - Widening of the joint space.

   - Elevation of the outer end of the clavicle.

   - Increased distance between the undersurface of the clavicle and the coracoid process.

   - X-ray signs may be subtle; weight-bearing views may be useful in doubtful cases.

3. Sternoclavicular joint dislocation:

   - Very difficult to see on conventional X-rays.

   - CT is the modality of choice.

4. Anterior dislocation of the shoulder:

   - AP film: Head of humerus overlaps the lower glenoid and the lateral border of the scapula.

   - Lateral film: Head of humerus lies anterior to the glenoid fossa.

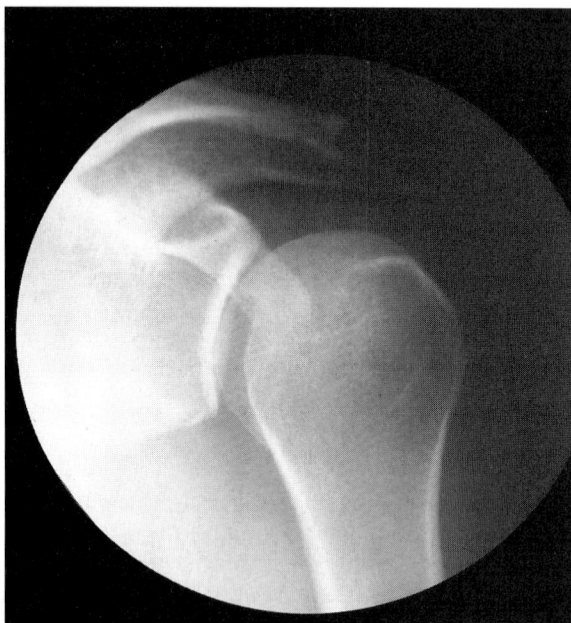

Fig 4.40 *Posterior dislocation of the shoulder.*
The signs of posterior shoulder dislocation on the frontal X-ray may be remarkably subtle. Note that the humeral head has a rounded symmetrical configuration and that there is loss of visualisation of the normal joint space. This is because the humeral head is rotated with the articular surface facing posteriorly.

- Associated fractures:
  (i) Flattening/wedge shaped defect in the posterolateral humeral head (Hill–Sachs deformity).
  (ii) Fracture of the inferior rim of the glenoid (Bankart lesion).
  (iii) Fracture of the greater tuberosity.
  (iv) Fracture of the surgical neck of the humerus.

- Recurrent anterior dislocation may be seen in association with fracture of the glenoid, fracture of the anterior cartilage labrum, and laxity of the joint capsule and glenohumeral ligaments – investigate with CT-arthrogram or MRI.

5. Posterior dislocation of the shoulder:

  - May be easily missed on X-ray.

  - Rare: only 2% of shoulder dislocations.

- Signs on the AP film are often subtle and include:
  (i) loss of parallelism of articular surface of humeral head and glenoid fossa;
  (ii) Medial rotation of the humerus so that the humeral head looks symmetrically rounded like an ice cream cone or an electric light bulb (*Fig. 4.40*).

- Lateral film: Humeral head posterior to the glenoid fossa.

Humerus

1. **Proximal fractures:**

- Surgical neck; displaced or impacted.

- Greater tuberosity.

- Lesser tuberosity.

- Combination of above.

2. **Humeral shaft fracture:**

- Transverse; oblique; simple; comminuted.

Elbow

1. **Elbow joint effusion:**

Fat pads lie on the anterior and posterior surfaces of the distal humerus at the attachments of the synovium of the elbow joint. On a lateral view of the elbow these fat pads are usually not seen. Occasionally the anterior fat pad may be seen applied to the anterior surface of the humerus; this is a normal finding. With an elbow joint effusion the fat pads are lifted off the humeral surfaces and are seen on lateral X-rays of the elbow as dark grey triangular structures. There is a high rate of association of elbow joint effusion with fracture. Recognition of such effusions is therefore very important (*Fig. 4.41*).

Where a joint effusion is present in a setting of trauma and no fracture seen on standard elbow films, consider an undisplaced fracture of the radial head or a supracondylar fracture of the distal humerus.

In this situation, either perform further oblique views or treat and repeat X-rays in 7–10 days.

2. **Supracondylar fracture:**

- May be undisplaced, or displaced anteriorly or posteriorly.

- Posterior displacement is the most common:
  (i)   Variable degree of posterior displacement and angulation.
  (ii) May be associated with injury to brachial artery and median nerve.
- Anterior displacement is very rare.

3.   Fracture and separation of the lateral condylar epiphysis:

- This is a problem for two reasons:
  (i)   The fracture may be missed on X-ray or may look deceptively small as, depending on the age of the child, the growth centre may be predominantly cartilage.
  (ii) Adequate treatment is vital as this fracture may damage the growth plate and the articular surface leading to deformity.

4.   Fracture of the head of the radius:

- Three patterns of fracture are commonly seen:
  (i)   Vertical split.
  (ii)   Small lateral fragment.
  (iii) Multiple fragments.

- May be difficult to see; joint effusion may be the only X-ray sign initially.

5.   Fracture of the olecranon:

- Two patterns of fracture are commonly seen:
  (i)   Single transverse fracture line with separation of fragments due to unopposed action of the triceps muscle.
  (ii) Comminuted fracture.

6.   Other elbow fractures:

- 'T' or 'Y' shaped fracture of the distal humerus with separation of the condyles.
- Fracture and separation of the capitulum – capitulum is sheared off vertically.
- Fracture and separation of the medial epicondylar epiphysis.

Radius and ulna

1.   Mid-shaft fractures:

- Usually involve both radius and ulna.
- Transverse; oblique; angulated; displaced.
- Anteriorly angulated fracture of upper third of the shaft of the ulna is often associated with anterior dislocation of the radial head (Monteggia fracture) (Fig. 4.42).

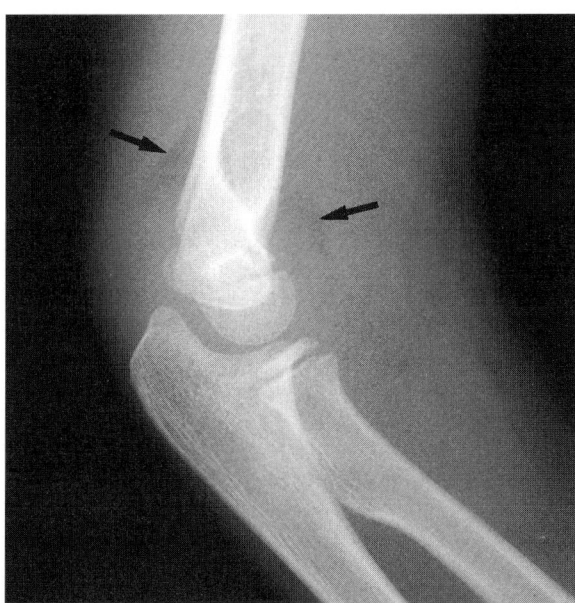

Fig 4.41 Elbow joint effusion.
The anterior and posterior fat pads are elevated from the lower shaft of the humerus (arrows) indicating the presence of a joint effusion. This was associated in this case with an undisplaced supracondylar fracture.

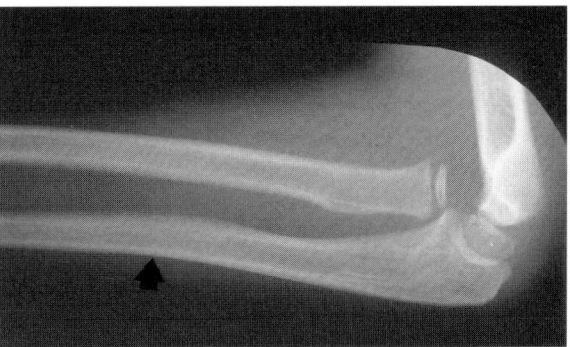

Fig 4.42 Dislocation of the radial head.
There is a plastic (bowing) fracture of the ulna (arrow). This is associated with anterior dislocation of the radial head. This is seen on the lateral view where the radial head should normally align with the round surface of the capitulum. Note that in this case the radial head lies above the capitulum indicating dislocation.

- Fracture of the lower third of the shaft of the radius may be associated with subluxation or dislocation of the distal radio-ulnar joint (Galeazzi fracture).

2. Fracture of the distal radius:

- Most common site of radial injury.

- The classical Colles fracture consists of a transverse fracture of the distal radius with the distal fragment angulated and/or displaced posteriorly, usually associated with avulsion of the tip of the ulnar styloid process.

- The less common Smith's fracture refers to anterior angulation of the distal radial fragment.

- The distal radius is a common fracture site in children with the following patterns seen:
    (i)   Salter–Harris type 2 fracture with posterior displacement and/or angulation of the distal fragment.
    (ii) Buckle fracture of the posterior cortex.
    (iii) Greenstick fracture.

Wrist and hand

1. Scaphoid fracture:

- Two common patterns of fracture are seen:
    (i)   Transverse fracture of the waist of the scaphoid.
    (ii) Fracture and separation of the scaphoid tubercle.

- Fracture of the waist of the scaphoid is a problem for the following reasons:
    (i)   May be difficult to see at initial presentation, even on dedicated oblique views.
    (ii) High incidence of avascular necrosis of the proximal pole due to interruption of its blood supply.

- Further investigations:
    (i)   Repeat X-ray after 10 days to 3 weeks treatment where scaphoid fracture is suspected clinically though not seen on initial X-rays.
    (ii) Scintigraphic bone scan; positive 24 hours following fracture.

2. Lunate dislocation:

- Anterior dislocation of the lunate.

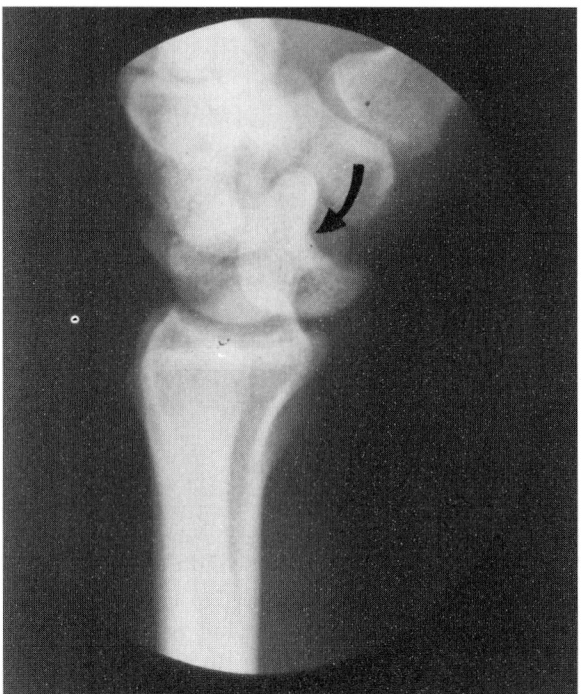

Fig 4.43 *Lunate dislocation.*
Note that the lunate is rotated anteriorly (arrow) while the remainder of the carpal bones align normally with the radius.

- May be difficult to appreciate on the frontal film.

- Easily seen on a properly performed lateral film ('true' lateral) with the lunate rotated and displaced anteriorly (*Fig. 4.43*).

3. Perilunate dislocation:

- Lunate remains attached to radius with the remainder of the carpal bones displaced posteriorly.

- Frontal film:
    (i)   Abnormal overlap of bone shadows.
    (ii) Dissociation of articular surfaces of the lunate and capitate.

- Lateral film:
    (i)   Minimal, if any, rotation of the lunate.
    (ii) Posterior displacement of the remainder of the carpal bones (*Fig. 4.44*).

- May be associated with scaphoid fracture (transscaphoid perilunate dislocation) or fracture of the radial styloid.

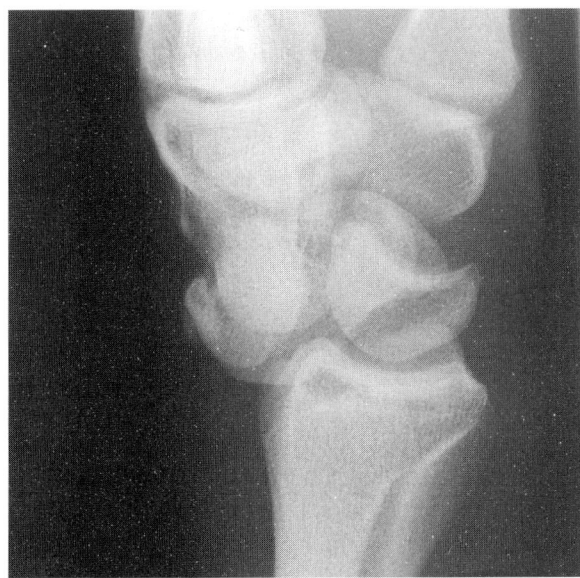

Fig 4.44 *Perilunate dislocation.*
Note on the frontal and oblique X-rays that the carpal bones overlap abnormally and that there is dissociation of the articular surfaces of the lunate and the capitate. The diagnosis is clear on the lateral view where the lunate is seen in normal alignment with the radius, while the other carpal bones are dislocated posteriorly. Compare this appearance with Figure 4.43.

4. Other carpal fractures:

- Avulsion fracture of the posterior surface of the triquetral – only seen on the lateral view.

- Fracture of the hook of hamate.
  (i)   Common injury in golfers and tennis players.
  (ii) May see on a carpal tunnel view.

5. Ligament and cartilage injuries:

- Scapholunate ligament.

- Triquetrolunate ligament.

- Triangular fibrocartilage complex.

- Investigate with MRI or arthrography.

6. Fractures of the base of the first metacarpal:

- Usually unstable.

- Two patterns of fracture are seen:
  (i)   Transverse fracture of the proximal shaft with lateral bowing.

(ii) Oblique fracture extending to the articular surface at the base of the first metacarpal.

Pelvis

1. Pelvic ring fracture:

- In general fractures of the pelvic ring occur in two separate places though there are exceptions.

- Three common patterns of injury are seen:
  (i)   Separation of the pubic symphysis with widening of a sacro-iliac joint or fracture of the posteromedial aspect of the iliac bone (*Fig. 4.9*).
  (ii) Fractures of the superior and inferior pubic rami, which may be uni- or bilateral.
  (iii) Unilateral fracture of the pubic rami anteriorly, and the iliac bone posteriorly.

- Pelvic ring fractures have a high rate of association with urinary tract injury (see above) and with severe blood loss; angiography and embolisation may be required in such cases.

2. Hip dislocation:

- Anterior dislocation: rare injury easily recognised on X-ray and usually not associated with fracture.

- Posterior dislocation:
  (i)   Most common form of hip dislocation.
  (ii) Femoral head dislocates posteriorly and superiorly.
  (iii) Usually associated with small or large fractures of the posterior acetabulum, and occasionally fracture of the femoral head.

3. Fractures of the acetabulum:

- Three common fracture patterns are seen:
  (i)   Fracture through the anterior acetabulum associated with fracture of the inferior pubic ramus.
  (ii) Fracture through the posterior acetabulum extending into the sciatic notch associated with fracture of the inferior pubic ramus.
  (iii) Horizontal fracture through the acetabulum.

- Acetabular fractures are difficult to define on X-rays owing to the complexity of the anatomy and overlapping bony structures.

- CT with multiplanar and 3D reconstruction is useful for definition of fractures and for planning of operative reduction.

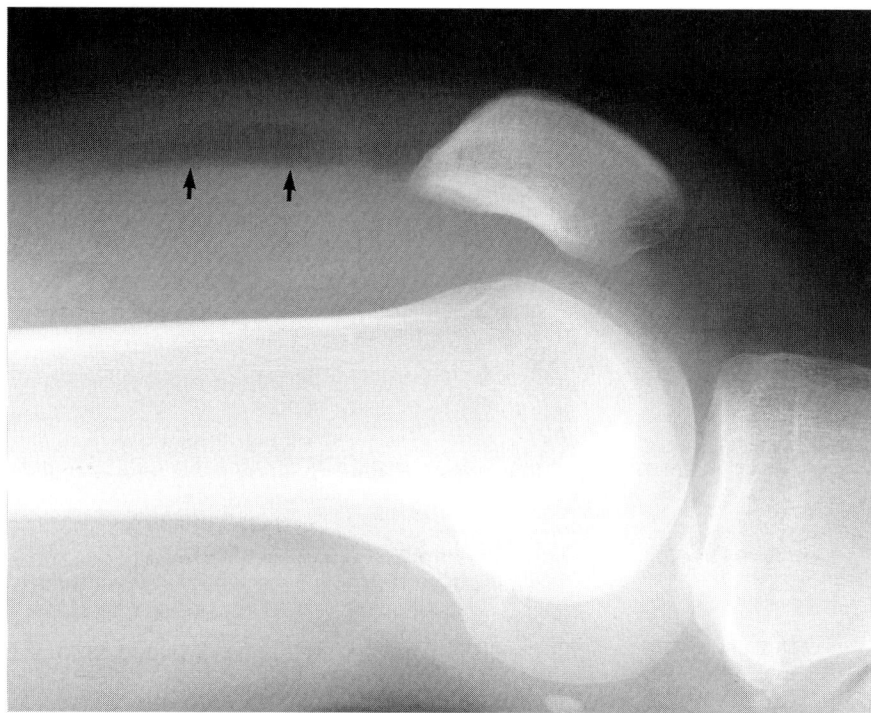

Fig 4.45 *Knee joint lipohaemarthrosis. Note low-density fat floating on higher-density blood in the suprapatellar pouch of the knee joint. This produces a fluid–fluid level (arrows) and indicates release of fat into the knee joint from a fracture. In this case, there was a fracture of the upper tibia.*

- Combinations of the above fracture patterns may be seen as well as extensive comminution, and central dislocation of the femoral head.

Femur

1. Upper femur:

- Fractures of the upper femur are particularly common in the elderly and have a strong association with osteoporosis.

- Femoral neck fracture:
  - (i) Usually consists of a fracture across the femoral neck with varying degrees of angulation and displacement.
  - (ii) The occasional undisplaced or mildly impacted fracture may be difficult to recognise on X-ray; these fractures may be seen as a faint sclerotic band passing across the femoral neck.
  - (iii) Complicated by avascular necrosis in 10% of cases with a higher rate for severely displaced fractures.

- Intertrochanteric fracture: varies in appearance from an undisplaced oblique fracture to comminuted fractures with marked displacement of the lesser and greater trochanters.

- Subtrochanteric fracture: refers to fracture below the lesser trochanter.

2. Femoral shaft:

- These fractures are easily recognised on X-ray.

- Common patterns include transverse, oblique, spiral, and comminuted fractures with varying degrees of displacement and angulation.

- Often associated with severe blood loss, and occasionally with fat embolism.

Knee

1. Lower femur:

(i) *Supracondylar fracture:*

- Usually consists of a transverse fracture above the femoral condyles with posterior angulation of the distal fragment best appreciated on the lateral X-ray.

(ii) *Fractures of the femoral condyles:*

- Fracture and separation of a femoral condyle with varying degrees of vertical displacement.

- 'T' or 'Y' shaped fracture with a vertical fracture line extending upwards from the articular surface causing separation of the femoral condyles.

2. Patella:

- Three common patterns are seen:
  (i)   Undisplaced fracture.
  (ii) Displaced transverse fracture.
  (iii) Complex comminuted fracture.
- All patterns may be associated with haemarthrosis.
- Should not be confused with bipartite patella:
  (i)   Anatomical variant with a fragment of bone separated from the superolateral aspect of the patella.
  (ii) Unlike an acute fracture, the bone fragments in bipartite patella are corticated, i.e. have a well-defined white margin.

3. Tibial plateau:

- Common patterns of injury include:
  (i)   Crush fracture of the lateral tibial plateau.
  (ii) Fracture and separation of one or both tibial condyles.
  (iii) Complex comminuted fracture of the upper tibia.
- Minimally crushed or displaced fractures of the upper tibia may be difficult to recognise on X-ray.
- Often the only clue is the presence of a joint effusion or lipohaemarthrosis (*Fig. 4.45*); oblique views may be required to diagnose subtle fractures.

Tibia and fibula

- Fracture of the tibial shaft is usually associated with fracture of the fibula.
- Fractures may be transverse, oblique, spiral, and comminuted with varying degrees of displacement and angulation.
- Fractures of the tibia are often open (compound) with an increased incidence of osteomyelitis, compartment syndrome, and vascular injury.
- In particular, injury to the popliteal artery and its major branches requires emergency angiography and treatment.

- Isolated fracture of the tibia is a relatively common injury in children aged 1 to 3 ('toddler's fracture').
  (i)   Often undisplaced and therefore very difficult to see.
  (ii) Usually best seen as a thin oblique lucent line on the lateral X-ray; this film in particular must be closely perused in a limping child.
  (iii) Scintigraphic bone scan may be useful in difficult cases.
- Tibial stress fracture is a common injury in athletes.

Ankle and foot

1. Common ankle fractures:

- Injuries may include fractures of the distal fibula (lateral malleolus), fractures of distal tibia medially (medial malleolus) and posteriorly, talar shift and displacement, fracture of the talus, separation of the distal tibio-fibular joint, and ligament rupture with joint instability.
- Salter–Harris fractures of the distal tibia and fibula are common in children.
- Pattern of fracture seen on X-ray depends on mechanism of injury.

(i) *Adduction:*
- Vertical fracture of the medial malleolus, avulsion of the tip of the lateral malleolus, medial tilt of the talus.

(ii) *Abduction:*
- Fracture of the lateral malleolus, avulsion of the tip of the medial malleolus, separation of the distal tibio-fibular joint.

(iii) *External rotation:*
- Spiral or oblique fracture of the lateral malleolus, lateral shift of the talus.

(iv) *Vertical compression:*
- Fracture of the distal tibia posteriorly or anteriorly, separation of the distal tibio-fibular joint.

2. Fractures of the talus:

- Small avulsion fractures of the talus are commonly seen in association with ankle fractures and ligament damage.

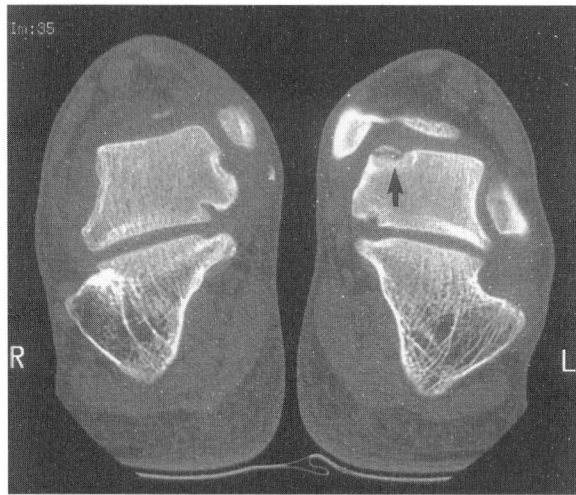

Fig 4.46 *Talar dome fracture – CT.*
An osteochondral fracture of the articular surface of the talus is well shown on this CT in the coronal plane. Note the defect in the articular surface with a small irregular bone fragment (arrow).

- Osteochondral fractures of the upper articular surface of the talus are common sports related injuries. These fractures may be difficult to see on X-ray and often require assessment with scintigraphy and CT (*Fig. 4.46*).

- Fracture of the neck of the talus:
  (i) may be widely displaced and associated with disruption of the subtalar joint;
  (ii) complicated by avascular necrosis of the body of the talus, particularly when the fracture is displaced.

3.   *Fractures of the calcaneus:*

- Fractures of the calcaneus may show considerable displacement and comminution, and may involve the subtalar joint.

- Boehler's angle is the angle formed by a line tangential to the superior extra-articular portion of the calcaneus and a line tangential to the superior intra-articular portion.
  (i) Boehler's angle normally measures 25–40 degrees.
  (ii) Reduction of this angle is a useful sign of a displaced intra-articular fracture of the calcaneus as these fractures may be difficult to see on X-ray (*Fig. 4.47*).

- CT is useful to define fractures and to assist in planning of surgical reduction.

- Calcaneal fractures, particularly when bilateral, have a high association with spine and pelvis fractures.

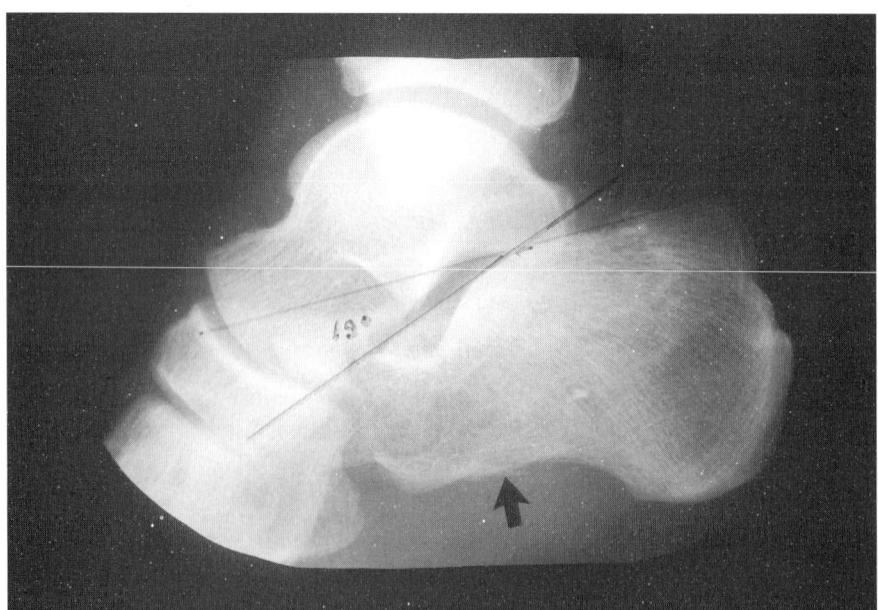

Fig 4.47 *Fracture of the calcaneus.*
Lines drawn as shown form Boehler's angle. It should measure 25 to 40 degrees. In this case it is abnormal at 19°. This indicates a fracture of the intra-articular portion of the calcaneus. A fracture line can be seen inferiorly (arrow).

4. *Other fractures of the foot:*

- Fractures of the other tarsal bones are less common than fractures of the talus and calcaneus.

- Tarsal fractures are often quite complex and associated with ligament disruption and dislocations.

- Metatarsal fractures are usually transverse.

- The growth centre at the base of the fifth metatarsal lies parallel to the shaft and should not be mistaken for a fracture; fractures in this region usually lie in the transverse plane.

- Stress fractures of the foot are common particularly involving the metatarsal shafts, and less commonly the navicular and talus.

Further Reading

1. Cohen AM, Crass JR. Traumatic aortic injuries: current concepts. *Seminars in US, CT, and MRI* 1993; 14:71–84.

2. Editorial. Diagnosing splenic trauma. *Clinical Radiology* 1991; 43:297–300.

3. Fagan J, Rogers F. Spinal trauma. *Current Imaging* 1990; 2:31–41.

4. Felson B. (ed.) The normal skull and its variations. *Seminars in Roentgenology* 1974; 9(2).

5. Kerns SR, Gay SB. CT of blunt chest trauma. *AJR* 1990; 154:55–60.

6. Marnocha KE, Maglinte DDT. Plain-film criteria for excluding aortic rupture in blunt chest trauma. *AJR* 1985; 144:19–21.

5 Liver, biliary system and pancreas

Investigation of liver masses

Helical CT of the liver

The ability to visualise a mass in the liver on CT, i.e. lesion conspicuity, is due to the difference in density between the lesion and the surrounding liver. Lesions that are of low attenuation such as liver cysts are well seen on non-contrast enhanced CT; lesions containing calcification such as mucin-producing metastases (*Fig. 5.1*) and hydatid cysts are also well seen. Unfortunately a large percentage of liver malignancies are of equal or similar attenuation to liver tissue and are therefore difficult if not impossible to see on an unenhanced CT. Intravenous contrast material is used to improve lesion conspicuity.

The liver receives a dual blood supply. The hepatic artery supplies 20% whilst the portal vein supplies 80% of hepatic blood flow. Following intravenous injection of a bolus of contrast there are three phases of contrast enhancement. An early arterial phase begins at around 25 seconds following commencement of injection. After blood has circulated through the mesentery, intestine, and spleen there is a later portal venous phase of enhancement beginning at around 70 seconds following commencement of injection. Given that 80% of the liver's blood supply is from the portal vein it follows that maximum enhancement of liver tissue will occur in the later portal venous phase. After several minutes there is redistribution of contrast to the extracellular space giving the third or equilibrium phase of contrast enhancement.

Most liver tumours are supplied by the hepatic artery. Furthermore, most tumours are hypovascular, i.e. receive less blood supply than surrounding liver. It follows then that maximum lesion conspicuity for most liver tumours including metastases will occur in the portal venous phase of contrast enhancement. Please note that this is due to liver enhancement, not enhancement of the lesion. These hypovascular lesions are seen as low attenuation masses well visualised against high attenuation enhancing liver (*Fig. 5.2*).

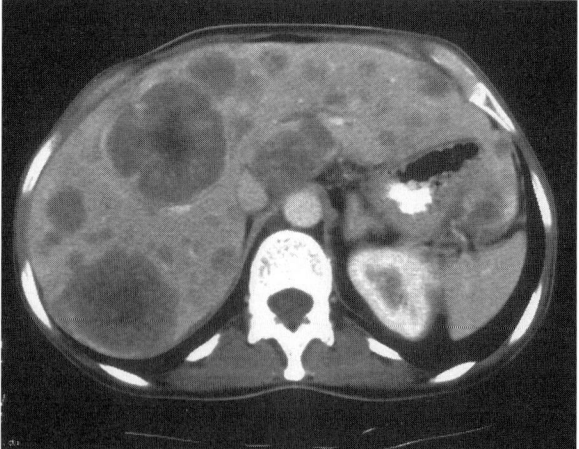

Figure 5.2 *Liver metastases – CT. Contrast-enhanced helical CT, portal-venous phase. Liver tissue shows dense enhancement. The hypovascular metastases which are supplied by the hepatic artery are well seen as low attenuation masses in the portal-venous phase of contrast enhancement.*

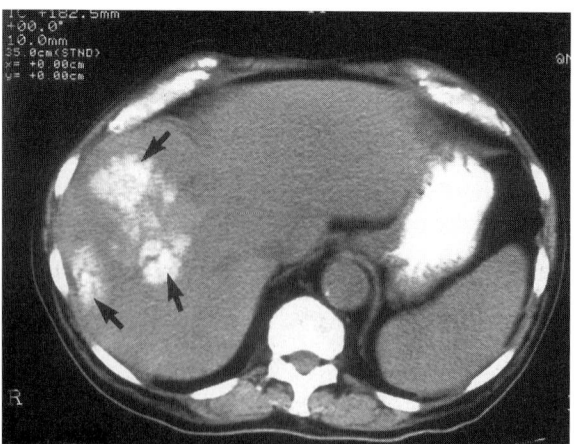

Figure 5.1 *Calcified liver metastases – CT. Non-contrast CT. Calcified metastases are well seen as high attenuation masses in the liver (arrows).*

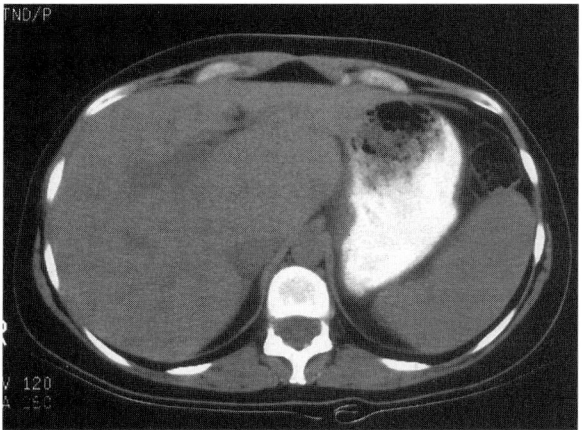

a

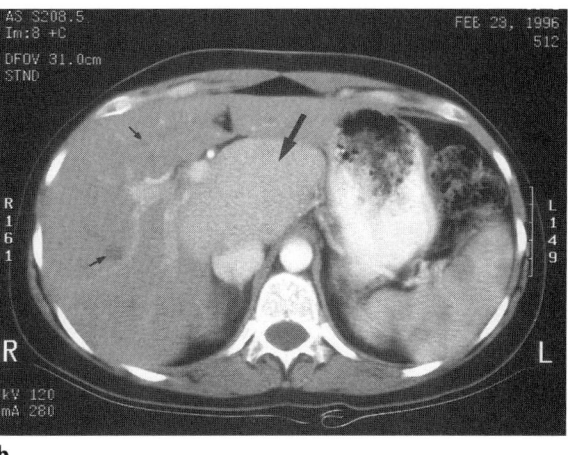

b

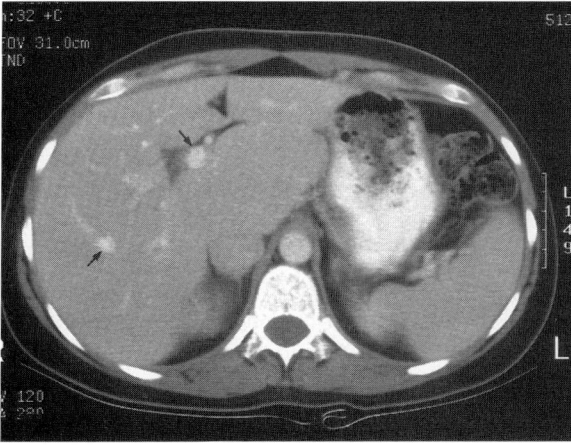

c

Figure 5.3 *Focal nodular hyperplasia – CT.*
Focal nodular hyperplasia is a good example of a hypervascular mass supplied by the hepatic artery and therefore best seen in the arterial phase of contrast enhancement. (a) Non-contrast CT. The mass is of equal density to surrounding liver and could easily be missed. (b) Contrast CT – arterial phase. The mass is well seen (large arrow) due to dense enhancement compared with relatively unenhanced surrounding liver tissue. Note other normal features of the arterial phase:
* *patchy enhancement of the spleen.*
* *unenhanced hepatic veins (small arrows) not to be confused with metastases.*
(c) Portal-venous phase. The mass is once again of equal density to surrounding liver tissue. Note that the spleen now shows homogeneous enhancement and that the hepatic and portal veins are now filled with contrast (arrows).

A minority of liver tumours are hypervascular, i.e. receive more blood supply than surrounding liver. For these tumours maximum lesion conspicuity will occur in the arterial phase of contrast enhancement. This is due to enhancement of the lesion, not the liver. These lesions are seen as high attenuation masses compared with the relatively low attenuation liver tissue (*Fig. 5.3*).

Examples of hypervascular lesions best seen in the arterial phase are:

* Small hepatocellular carcinomas.

* Focal nodular hyperplasia.

* Hypervascular metastases.

Helical CT has two principal advantages for liver scanning:

* Speed.

* Overlapping reconstructions.

The speed of helical CT allows imaging of the entire liver in around 20 seconds, i.e. during a single breath-hold. This means that the entire liver may be scanned during the separate phases of contrast enhancement. This technique is termed 'dual phase' liver CT. Overlapping reconstruction implies that all of the liver is accurately imaged so that even small lesions of the order of 1 cm should be seen.

Helical CT is now the imaging investigation of choice

for assessment of liver masses. It is the most sensitive technique for the presence of a mass. It is also useful for the following:

- Good anatomical localisation.
- Definition of tumour margins.
- Characterisation of contents, e.g. fluid, necrosis, fat, calcification, gas etc.
- Diagnosis of complications, e.g. venous invasion, arteriovenous shunting.
- Biopsy guidance.

Ultrasound

US is often the first investigation performed for a suspected liver mass as it is non-invasive and relatively cheap. As with CT it gives good anatomical localisation. It is highly sensitive for fluid filled lesions such as cysts and abscesses though less accurate than CT for characterisation of solid lesions. Being non-invasive US is particularly useful for masses requiring follow-up:

- Haemangioma, to confirm lack of growth.
- Metastases and other tumours receiving chemotherapy.
- Abscess, following drainage/antibiotic therapy.

Intraoperative US is now widely used in the diagnosis and management of metastases.

Scintigraphy

- ^{99m}Tc-labelled sulphur colloid compounds which are taken up by Kupffer cells in the liver (not hepatocytes), as well as by the spleen and, to a lesser extent, the bone marrow.
- Lesions larger than 1 cm can be seen.
- Especially useful for the diaphragmatic surface which may be difficult to image with other techniques.
- Generally complements US and CT.
- May occasionally find metastases missed by other modalities.

- Most masses appear as filling defects except for focal nodular hyperplasia which usually contains Kupffer cells and therefore shows tracer uptake.

Plain films

- Not useful as a primary investigation for suspected liver mass.
- Presence of a liver mass on an AXR may be inferred by various secondary signs, e.g. elevation of the right diaphragm, displaced hepatic flexure.
- Occasionally more specific signs may be seen, e.g. gas in an abscess, calcification in hepatocellular carcinoma, some metastases, hydatid cyst.

Angiography

- More often used for liver masses than in other organs, not so much for diagnostic purposes but as a surgical 'road map'.
- This includes outlining the arterial supply, portal vein (hepatocellular carcinoma and some metastases may invade the portal vein), and occasionally the IVC.
- Angiography may also be used for selective infusion of chemotherapy or embolisation.

Imaging findings of the more common liver masses

Metastases

(a) US:

- Multiple, occasionally solitary.
- Variable echotexture.
- Hyperechoic suggests gastrointestinal primary, though may be seen with others, e.g. TCC, choriocarcinoma (*Fig. 5.4*).
- Other primaries such as lung and breast tend to have hypoechoic metastases.

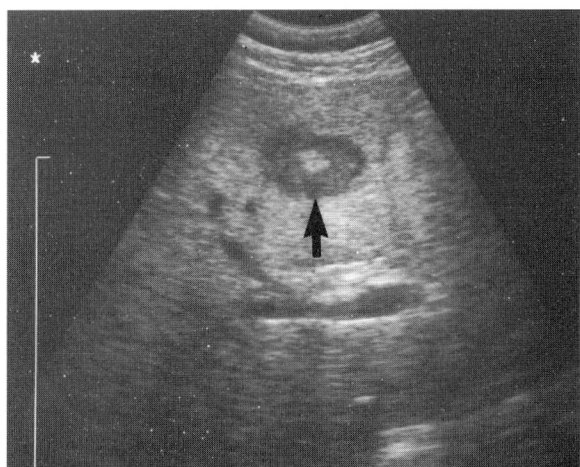

Figure 5.4 *Liver metastasis – US.*
A solitary metastasis from colonic carcinoma is seen as a target-like lesion in the liver (arrow) with a hyperechoic centre and a hypoechoic rim.

(b) Intraoperative US:

- Highly accurate technique for detection and localisation of hepatic metastases.

- Used at time of initial surgery for carcinoma of the colon.

- Also used with partial hepatic resection to localise metastases and to identify vascular structures in the liver.

(c) CT:

- Iso-intense or of slightly less attenuation than liver on non-enhanced CT.

- Most are best seen on the portal venous phase as low attenuation lesions (*Fig. 5.2*).

- May see peripheral rim enhancement and central low attenuation due to necrosis.

- Hypervascular metastases from melanoma, pancreatic islet cell tumour, renal cell carcinoma are best seen as enhancing lesions on the arterial phase.

(d) CT arterial portography:

- Highly accurate technique for detection of hepatic metastases.

- Arterial catheter positioned in the superior mesenteric artery (SMA); must be placed distal to any aberrant hepatic artery branches.

- Contrast is infused into the SMA and thus into the portal vein producing excellent enhancement of hepatic parenchyma.

- Rarely used in current practice due to the high level of accuracy of other less invasive and less expensive techniques, particularly dual-phase helical CT and intra-operative US.

Hepatocellular carcinoma

(a) US:

- Single mass; multiple masses; diffuse infiltration.

- Heterogeneous echotexture: areas of necrosis, haemorrhage, calcification.

(b) CT:

- Appearance depends on tumour pattern and size.

- Single mass; multiple masses; diffuse infiltration.

- Small tumours of 3 cm or less tend to be hypervascular and best seen as small enhancing masses on the arterial phase of contrast enhancement.

- Larger tumours of 5 cm or more tend to be best seen as low attenuation masses on the portal venous phase.

- Portal vein invasion: enlarged non-enhancing portal vein.

- Arteriovenous shunting: early filling of portal vein on arterial phase (*Fig. 5.5*).

Simple cyst

- Must differentiate from cystic metastases, especially where simple cysts are multiple.

- Cystic metastases usually have a thin irregular wall with some contrast enhancement.

(a) US:

- Well-defined margin.

- Anechoic contents.

- Acoustic enhancement.

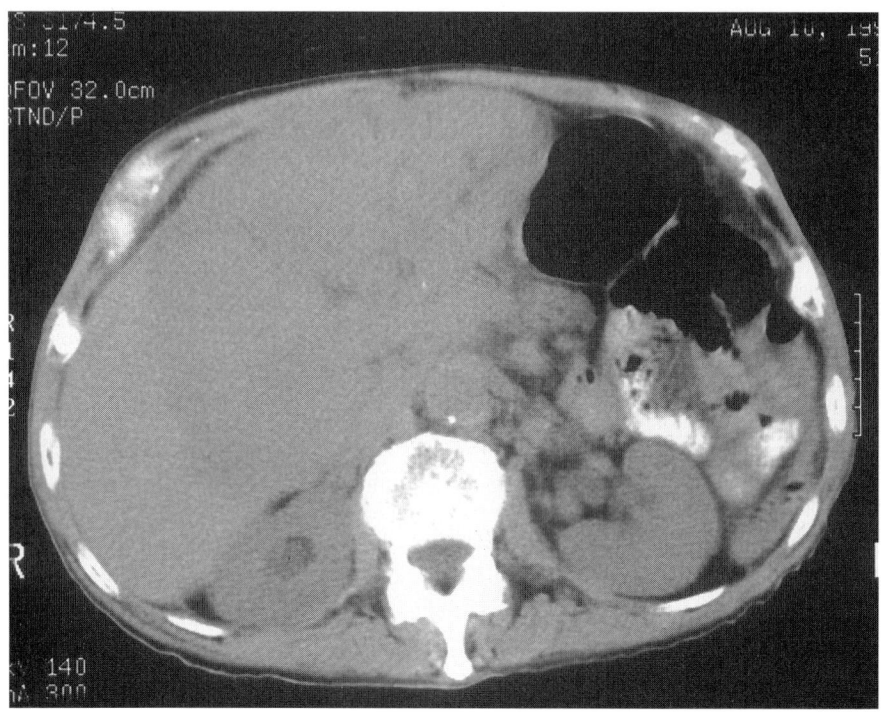

a

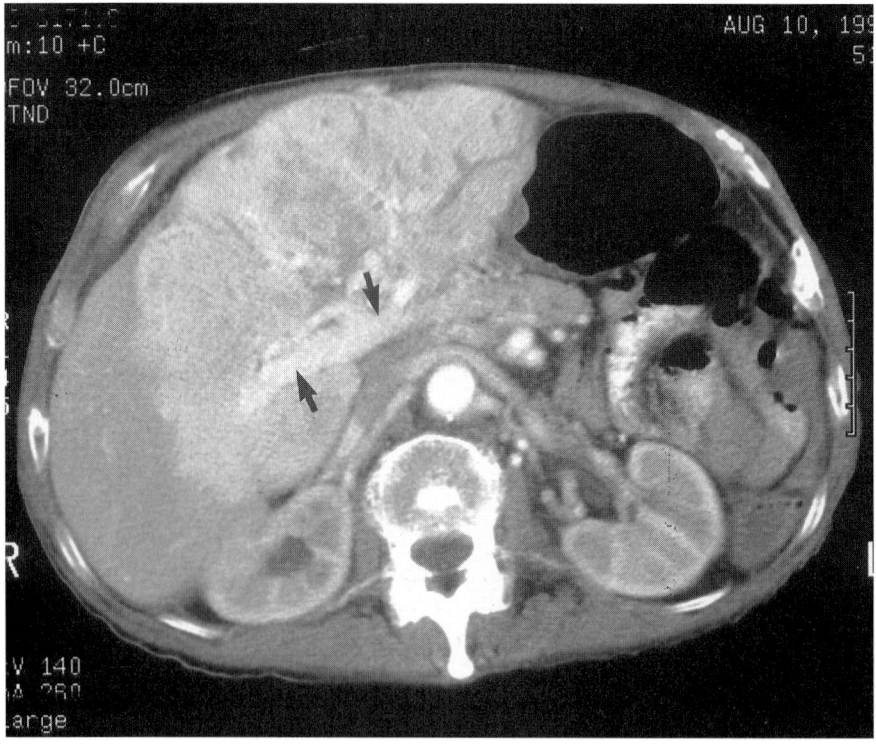

b

Figure 5.5 *Hepatocellular carcinoma – CT.*
(a) Non-contrast CT. A large mass of slightly lower attenuation than normal hepatic parenchyma is seen replacing most of the liver. (b) Contrast CT – arterial phase. The mass is hypervascular and shows dense enhancement during the arterial phase of contrast enhancement. Early filling of the portal vein indicates arteriovenous shunting (arrows).

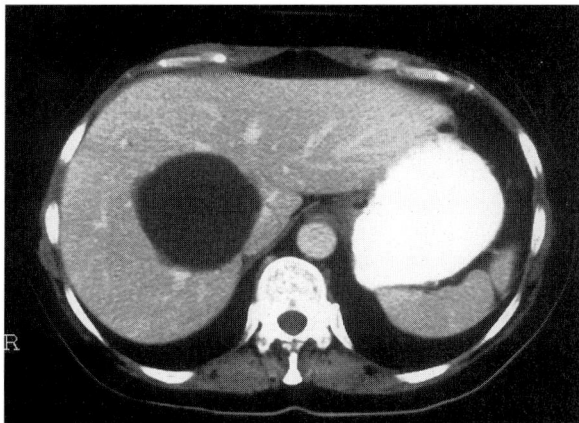

Figure 5.6 *Liver cyst – CT.*
Note the features of a simple cyst:
- *well defined margin*
- *homogeneous low attenuation fluid contents.*

(b) CT:

- Well-defined margin.

- Cyst wall too thin to be seen.

- Homogeneous low attenuation contents.

- No contrast enhancement (*Fig. 5.6*).

Pyogenic abscess

(a) US:

- Ill-defined irregular margin.

- Hypoechoic centre, though may contain echogenic debris or gas.

- Variable acoustic enhancement (*Fig. 5.7*).

(b) CT:

- Low-attenuation contents.

- Irregular enhancing wall.

Hydatid cyst

(a) US:

- Simple cyst or a large cyst with multiple septations and echogenic debris.

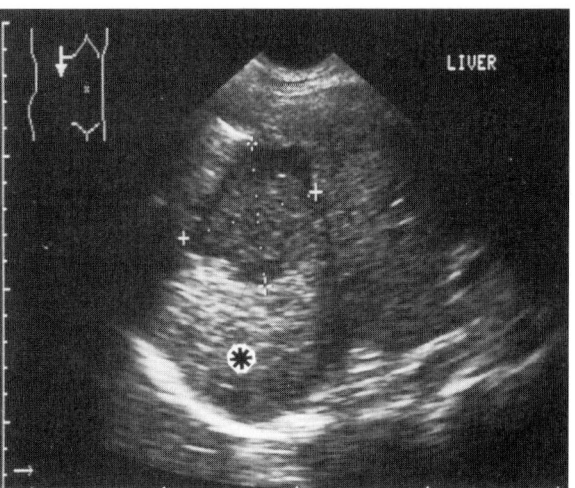

Figure 5.7 *Liver abscess – US.*
Abscess seen as an area of reduced echogenicity in the liver. Note the following features:
- *irregular wall*
- *echogenic contents due to inflammatory debris*
- *acoustic enhancement (*).*

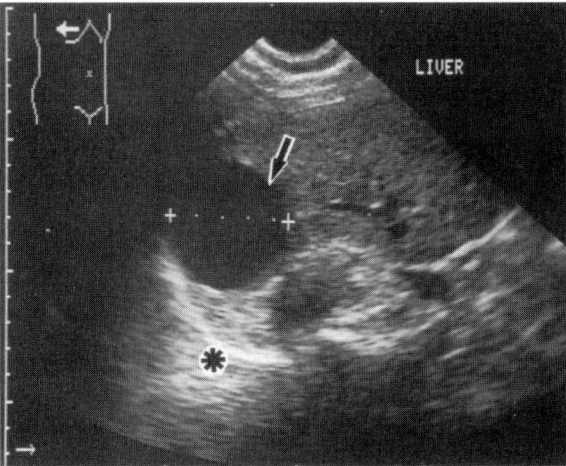

Figure 5.8 *Amoebic abscess.*
Hypoechoic lesion in the posterior aspect of the right lobe of the liver. Note the well defined wall (arrow) and acoustic enhancement (*).

(b) CT:

- Simple or multiloculated cyst.

- Low-attenuation contents; calcification well shown on CT.

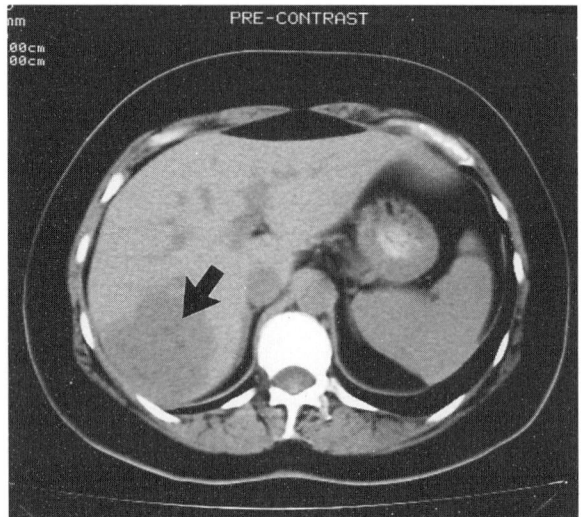

a

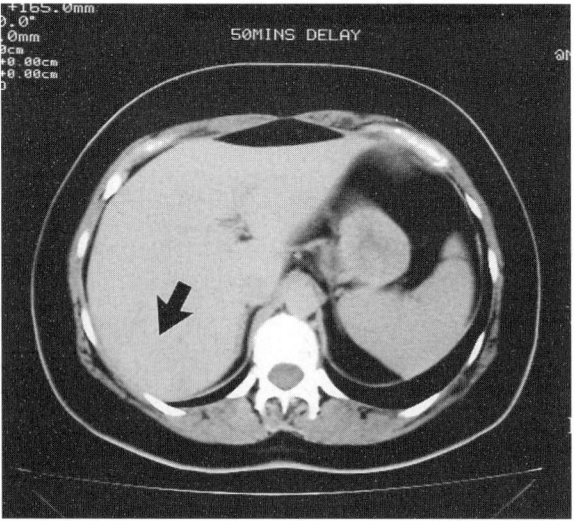

c

Figure 5.9 *Liver haemangioma – CT.*
(a) Pre-contrast scan. Note:
- *large mass in the right lobe of the liver (arrow)*
- *low attenuation compared with surrounding normal liver.*

(b) Immediate post-contrast scan. Note:
- *contrast in aorta, IVC and portal vein branches*
- *dense contrast enhancement of the periphery of the mass (arrow).*

(c) 50-minute post-contrast scan. The mass is now uniformly enhanced (arrow), so its density is equal to that of normal liver tissue. This is a typical enhancement pattern for haemangioma of the liver.

Amoebic abscess

(a) US:

- Well-defined, usually with homogeneous hypo-echoic contents.

- Most common peripherally in the posterior segment of the right lobe (*Fig. 5.8*).

(b) CT:

- Well-defined, low attenuation mass.

Haemangioma

- Most common benign hepatic mass.

- Usually asymptomatic though large lesions may bleed.

- Multiple in up to 20%.

- Greatest significance in clinical practice is to differentiate haemangioma from a more sinister liver mass, especially in a patient with a primary tumour elsewhere. In these patients haemangioma is often seen as an incidental finding. If seen initially on US it is suggested that CT be performed to define the enhancement pattern. If this is typical of haemangioma then this is usually adequate. Doubtful lesions may be followed up with a further US or CT to confirm lack of growth; MRI and/or scintigraphy may occasionally be used in these cases.

(a) US:

- Commonly subcapsular in the right lobe.
- Homogeneous hyperechoic mass with a well-defined margin.

(b) CT:

- Low-attenuation mass on non-enhanced CT.
- Early peripheral nodular enhancement on the arterial phase continuing into the portal venous phase.
- Later scans show central enhancement so that the mass achieves a similar density to liver (*Fig. 5.9*).

(c) MRI:

- Low signal mass on T1-weighted images.
- Hyperintense high signal mass on T2-weighted images.

(d) Scintigraphy:

- ^{99m}Tc-labelled red blood cells.
- Focal area of increased activity.

Hepatic adenoma

- Occur most commonly in young women in association with oral contraceptives.
- May be asymptomatic or present with pain due to mass effect or haemorrhage.

(a) US:

- Well-defined mass of similar echogenicity to liver.
- Altered echogenicity with bleeding.

(b) CT:

- Well-defined mass of less attenuation than liver.

Focal nodular hyperplasia

- Rare benign tumour with no malignant potential and no tendency to haemorrhage.
- Often asymptomatic, i.e. incidental finding; occasionally presents with mild abdominal pain due to mass effect.
- Usually not treated, therefore important to differentiate from other types of liver mass such as adenoma and hepatocellular carcinoma.

(a) US:

- Well-defined mass of similar or equal echogenicity to liver.
- Hyperechoic central scar seen in around 50%.

(b) CT:

- Equal attenuation to liver on non-enhanced CT.
- Central scar seen as a central focus of low attenuation.
- Dense enhancement on arterial phase.
- Often iso-intense on portal venous phase (*Fig. 5.3*).

(c) Scintigraphy:

- ^{99m}Tc sulphur colloid.
- Often contain sufficient functioning Kupffer cells to give uptake of tracer; this is compared with most other liver masses which usually show no uptake of sulphur colloid.

Jaundice

Ultrasound

- Initial investigation of choice to differentiate obstructive from non-obstructive jaundice, i.e. distinguish dilated from non-dilated bile ducts.
- Common bile duct:
  (i) Normal < 6 mm
  (ii) Equivocal 6–8 mm
  (iii) Dilated > 8 mm.

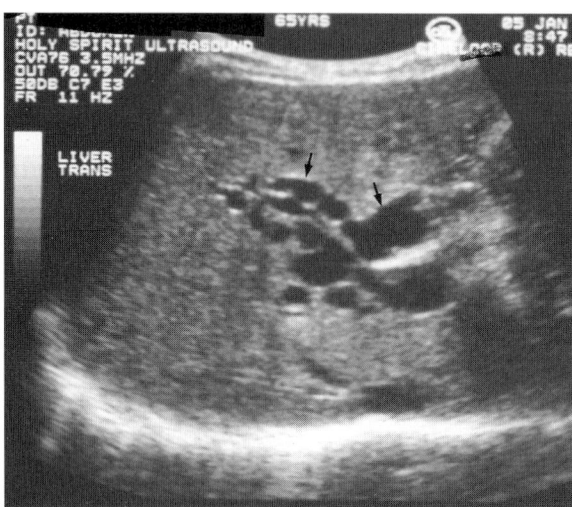

Figure 5.10 *Dilated bile ducts – ultrasound. Dilated intrahepatic bile ducts seen as branching fluid-filled structures in the liver (arrows).*

- Dilated intrahepatic bile ducts show a stellate branching pattern radiating from the porta, often best seen in the left hepatic lobe (*Fig. 5.10*).

- Site and cause of obstruction defined in only 25% as the lower duct is often obscured by overlying intestinal gas.

- Associated dilatation of the main pancreatic duct suggests obstruction at the level of the pancreatic head/ampulla.

- In the absence of ductal dilatation, diffuse or focal liver diseases may be seen (e.g. metastases, fatty infiltration, cirrhosis).

- Guidance for biopsy.

Endoscopic retrograde cholangiopancreatography (ERCP)

- Defines site and nature of obstruction.

- May be combined with sphincterotomy, basket stone extraction, stent insertion.

- Dilated common bile duct > 10 mm.

Percutaneous transhepatic cholangiogram (PTC)

- For obstructive jaundice where:
  (i)   ERCP has failed to outline the ductal system or to adequately define the obstructing lesion.

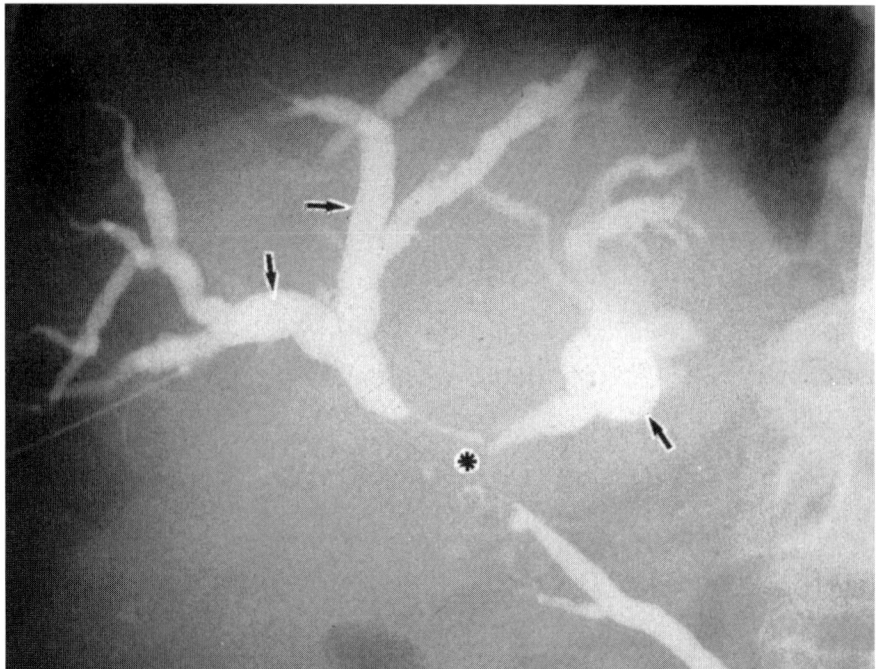

Figure 5.11 *Hepatocellular carcinoma – PTC. The tumour is causing compression of the bile ducts at the porta (*). The proximal ducts are dilated (arrows).*

(ii) ERCP is technically impossible due to tumour or surgery deforming the second part of the duodenum.

(iii) A high obstructing lesion as suggested on US or CT examination suggests PTC to be the preferred procedure (*Fig. 5.11*).

- Preceding an interventional procedure: stent insertion, biliary drainage, stone extraction.

CT

- Parameters of dilatation as for ultrasound, i.e. common bile duct > 8 mm is dilated.

- Dilated intrahepatic ducts show a low attenuation branching pattern radiating from the porta.

- As with ultrasound, main pancreatic duct dilatation localises the obstruction to the lower common bile duct.

- Site and cause of obstruction suggested on CT in 90% of cases.

- In the absence of bile duct dilatation, the liver can be assessed by CT for diffuse diseases causing jaundice (e.g. fatty infiltration, cirrhosis, metastases) or focal lesions (e.g. hepatocellular carcinoma).

- Guidance for biopsy.

Cholescintigraphy: HIDA scan

- ^{99m}Tc-labelled iminodiacetic acid (IDA) compounds.

- Taken up by liver cells and rapidly excreted in bile, therefore used to delineate the biliary system and gallbladder.

- Limited role in jaundice owing to impaired excretion and poor visualisation of the bile ducts in the presence of elevated bilirubin.

- Findings may be as follows:
  (i)   Failure of liver uptake indicates severe liver dysfunction.
  (ii) Liver uptake with non-visualisation of bile ducts indicates cholestasis or a high obstruction.
  (iii) Visualisation of bile ducts but not duodenum indicates low obstruction (*Fig. 5.12*).

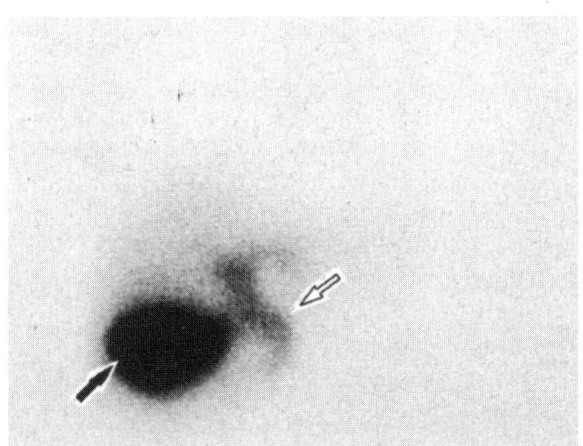

Figure 5.12 *Low biliary obstruction – HIDA scan. Note the following features:*
- *distended gallbladder (black arrow)*
- *bile ducts well outlined (white arrow)*
- *no tracer was seen in the bowel even on delayed images indicating obstruction at the lower end of the common bile duct.*

Findings in common surgical causes of jaundice

Bile duct calculus

(a) US:

- Hyperechoic focus in the duct (*Fig. 5.13*).

- May or may not show acoustic shadowing.

(b) ERCP:

- Filling defect in the bile duct: single/multiple; mobile/impacted; round/faceted.

(c) CT:

- Appearance varies with density and therefore depends on composition: may be heavily calcified (high attenuation), mainly cholesterol (low attenuation), or mixed (attenuation similar to soft tissue) (*Fig. 5.14*).

- Gallstones are often surprisingly difficult to see on CT.

Table 5.1 *Suggested protocol for investigation of jaundice*

Ultrasound

Dilated ducts	Non-dilated ducts
– Level and/or cause in 25%	↓
Cholangiography:	US of liver
¬ ── ERCP	CT
PTC	↓
+ Stents/biliary drainage	Biopsy
Sphincterotomy	
Basket stone removal	
↓	
CT	
Level and/or cause in 90%	
↓	
└─→HIDA scan	
(Limited role).	

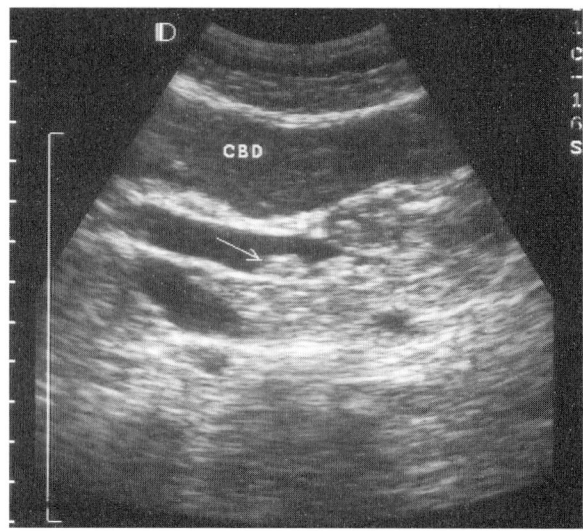

Figure 5.13 *Common bile duct stones – US. The common bile duct is dilated. Stones are seen as hyperechoic foci in the lower common bile duct (arrow).*

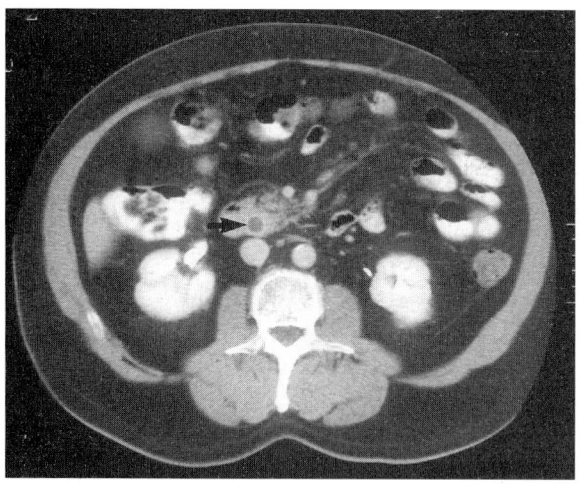

a

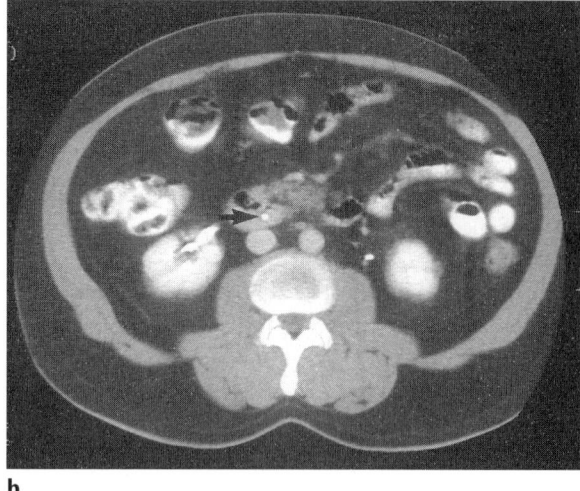

b

Figure 5.14 *Common bile duct stone – CT.*
(a) The dilated common bile duct is seen as a well defined low attenuation area in the pancreatic head (arrow). (b) An obstructing gallstone is seen as a high attenuation focus at the lower end of the common bile duct (arrow).

Carcinoma of the head of the pancreas

(a) US:

• Dilated bile ducts.

• Dilated pancreatic duct.

• Distended gallbladder.

• May see a mass in the pancreatic head though US is generally unreliable for direct visualisation of pancreatic tumours.

• May also see liver metastases and lymphadenopathy.

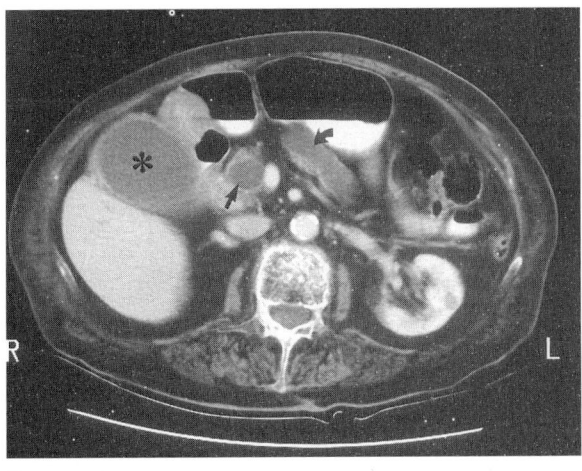

a

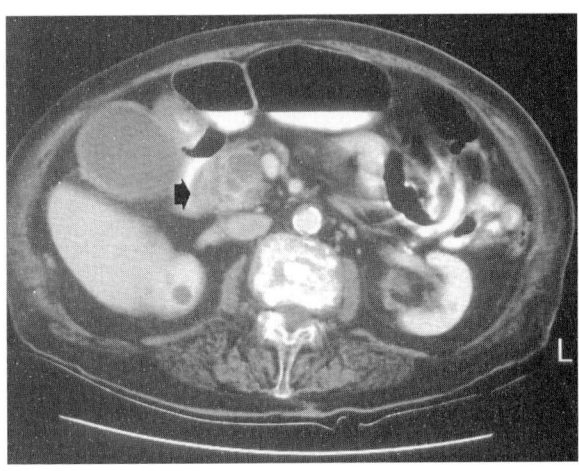

b

Figure 5.15 *Carcinoma head of pancreas – CT.*
(a) Note the following features:
- *dilated common bile duct (straight arrow)*
- *dilated pancreatic duct (curved arrow)*
- *distended gallbladder (*).*
(b) Enlarged irregular head of pancreas (arrow).

(b) CT:

- Dilated bile ducts and pancreatic duct.

- Enlarged, irregular head of pancreas (*Fig. 5.15*).

- Advanced tumours may show invasion of adjacent structures and encasement of mesenteric vessels.

- With small tumours the pancreatic head is not enlarged; a focal area of altered density may be seen.

(c) ERCP:

- Stricture of lower end of common bile duct; usually a smooth tapering stricture ('rat's tail') (*Fig. 5.16*).

Carcinoma of the ampulla of Vater

(a) US:

- Dilated bile ducts.

- Dilated pancreatic duct.

- Distended gallbladder.

- Soft tissue mass usually not visualised.

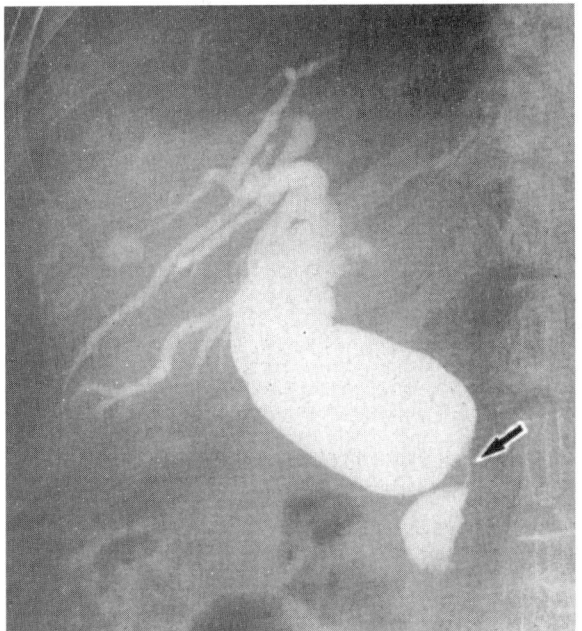

Figure 5.16 *Carcinoma head of pancreas.*
Mass encircling and compressing the lower common bile duct (arrow). The duct above is grossly dilated.

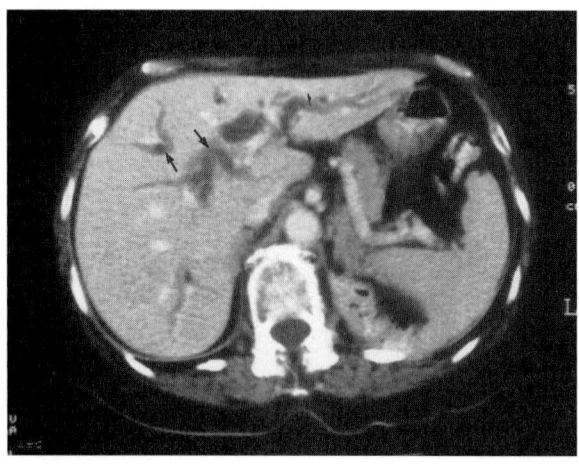
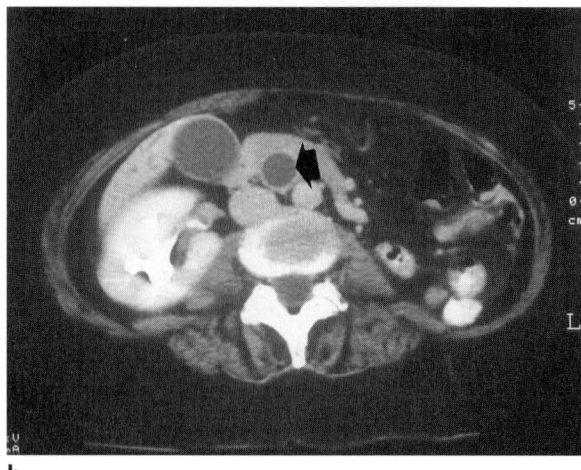

a   b

Figure 5.17 *Carcinoma ampulla of Vater – CT.*
(a). Dilated intrahepatic bile ducts seen as low attenuation branching structures in the liver (arrows). (b) The lower end of the common bile duct is markedly dilated with no apparent mass or stone (arrow). This finding may be due to a small carcinoma of the head of pancreas or carcinoma of the ampulla of Vater. In this case the latter tumour was found at ERCP.

(b) CT:

- Dilated bile ducts and pancreatic duct.

- Abrupt termination of the lower end of the dilated bile duct (*Fig. 5.17*).

- Soft tissue mass usually not seen.

- Abrupt termination of dilated common bile duct without an apparent mass or calculus on CT is highly suggestive of carcinoma of the ampulla or a small carcinoma of the pancreatic head.

(c) ERCP:

- Rapid termination of CBD at its lower end.

- May see a small filling defect at the ampulla.

Cholangiocarcinoma

(a) US:

- Dilated bile ducts which terminate at a soft tissue mass in or around the duct.

(b) CT:

- Abrupt transition from dilated to absent duct.

(c) ERCP:

- Stricture or filling defect in the bile duct.

- May not be able to fill dilated system from below.

(d) PTC:

- Abrupt termination of dilated bile ducts (*Fig. 5.18*).

Carcinoma of the gallbladder

(a) US:

- Irregular thickening of the gallbladder wall.

- Soft tissue mass replacing gallbladder and invading adjacent liver.

(b) CT:

- Irregular soft tissue mass replacing gallbladder.

- Liver metastases.

(c) ERCP:

- Extrinsic duct compression.

- Direct invasion of the duct with irregular narrowing and proximal dilatation.

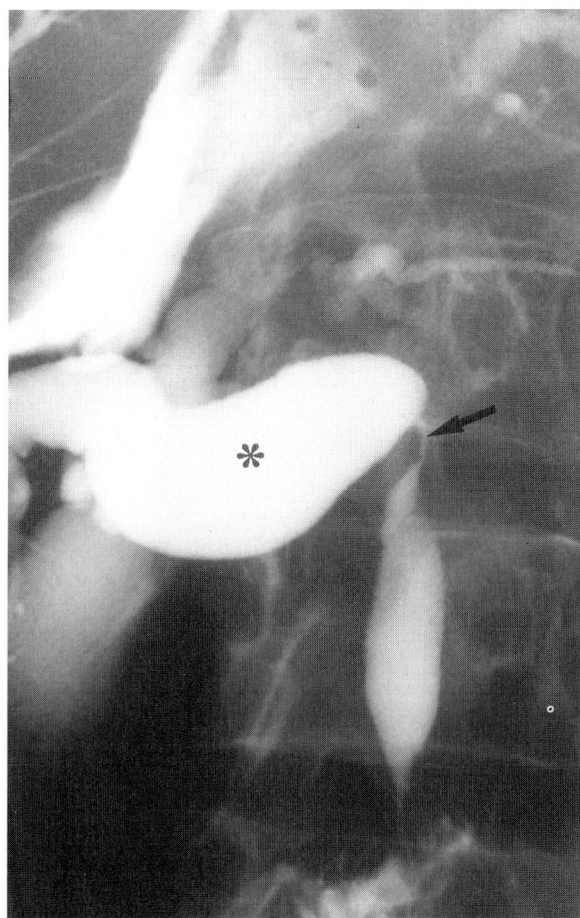

Figure 5.18 *Cholangiocarcinoma – PTC. There is severe dilatation of the intrahepatic bile ducts and of the common hepatic duct (*). A cholangiocarcinoma is causing a tight stricture of the upper common bile duct (arrow).*

Extrinsic bile duct compression by a liver mass (*Fig. 5.11*)

- See above for notes on hepatic masses.

Laparoscopic cholecystectomy

Laparoscopic surgery is now a well-established technique in general surgery. Its most widely practised and accepted applications are cholecystectomy, fundoplication, and removal of small adrenal tumours. Other applications such as hernia repair, appendicectomy, colectomy, etc. continue to be explored and developed. Imaging impacts on laparoscopic cholecystectomy in five ways:

1. Imaging of acute cholecystitis (*see* Chapter 1).

2. Visualisation of bile ducts prior to surgery.

3. Operative cholangiogram.

4. Visualisation of bile ducts post-surgery.

5. Complications of surgery.

Visualisation of bile ducts prior to and following laparoscopic cholecystectomy

Visualisation of the biliary system prior to surgery is required for two reasons:

1. Presence of bile duct stones.

2. Diagnosis of bile duct variants which may complicate surgery.

Bile duct visualisation following surgery is required to exclude or detect bile duct stones in patients with persistent or recurrent symptoms.

Conventional US and CT techniques have a relatively low sensitivity for detection of bile duct calculi, especially where the bile ducts are not dilated. Furthermore, anatomical variants of the biliary system may be difficult to appreciate. ERCP has been the 'gold standard' for opacification of the biliary system. It has the advantage of therapeutic applications such as sphincterotomy. It is however invasive, highly operator dependent, and not always possible technically. Two relatively non-invasive techniques are now available for reliable delineation of the biliary system:

1. 3D Helical CT cholangiography.

2. Magnetic resonance cholangiopancreatography (MRCP).

These techniques are gaining wide acceptance for assessment of the bile ducts, pre- and post-laparoscopic cholecystectomy.

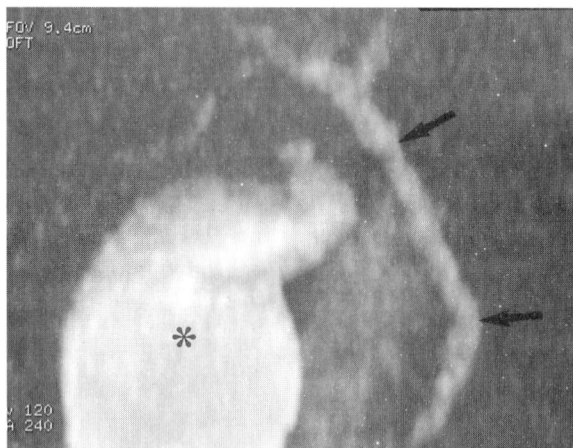

Figure 5.19 *3-D CT cholangiography – normal study. The bile ducts (arrows) and gallbladder (*) are well demonstrated.*

3D Helical CT cholangiography (*Fig. 5.19*)

Indications:

(a) Pre-laparoscopic cholecystectomy.

- Outline variants of the biliary system which may increase the risk of bile duct injury.

- Diagnose bile duct stones.

(b) Post-laparoscopic cholecystectomy. Diagnose missed stones in patients with recurrent symptoms.

(c) Pancreatitis where ERCP is not suitable.

Method:

- Slow infusion of cholangiographic agent to opacify bile ducts.

- Helical CT acquisition and 3D reconstructions performed.

Limitations:

- Poor bile duct opacification in jaundiced patients.

- Poor opacification of the cystic duct when obstructed by a calculus.

- Depending on their composition, some calculi may be very difficult to see against the contrast in the bile ducts.

- Allergy to contrast material.

Magnetic resonance cholangiopancreatography (MRCP) (*Fig. 5.20*)

Technique:

- Heavily T2-weighted images.
  - (i) Stationary fluids such as bile are high signal.
  - (ii) Moving fluids and solids are low signal.

- 3D or multiplanar reconstructions.

Indications:

- Pre-laparoscopic cholecystectomy.
  - (i) Bile duct calculi.
  - (ii) Bile duct variants.
  - (iii) Avoid intra-operative exploration of common bile duct.

- Failed ERCP.

- Depending on availability of technique and cost considerations may in the future replace diagnostic ERCP in the assessment of jaundiced patients with dilated bile ducts on US.

Advantages:

- Non-invasive.

- No radiation.

- No i.v. contrast.

- Simultaneous imaging of ducts proximal and distal to obstruction.

- Unaffected by bilirubin levels.

Disadvantages:

- Cost and relative unavailability of MRI.

- Patients unsuitable for MRI, e.g. cardiac pacemakers, claustrophobia.

- Limited spatial resolution, therefore difficulty visualising:
  - (i) Stones < 3 mm.
  - (ii) Tight biliary stenosis.
  - (iii) Small peripheral bile ducts.
  - (iv) Small side branches of pancreatic duct.

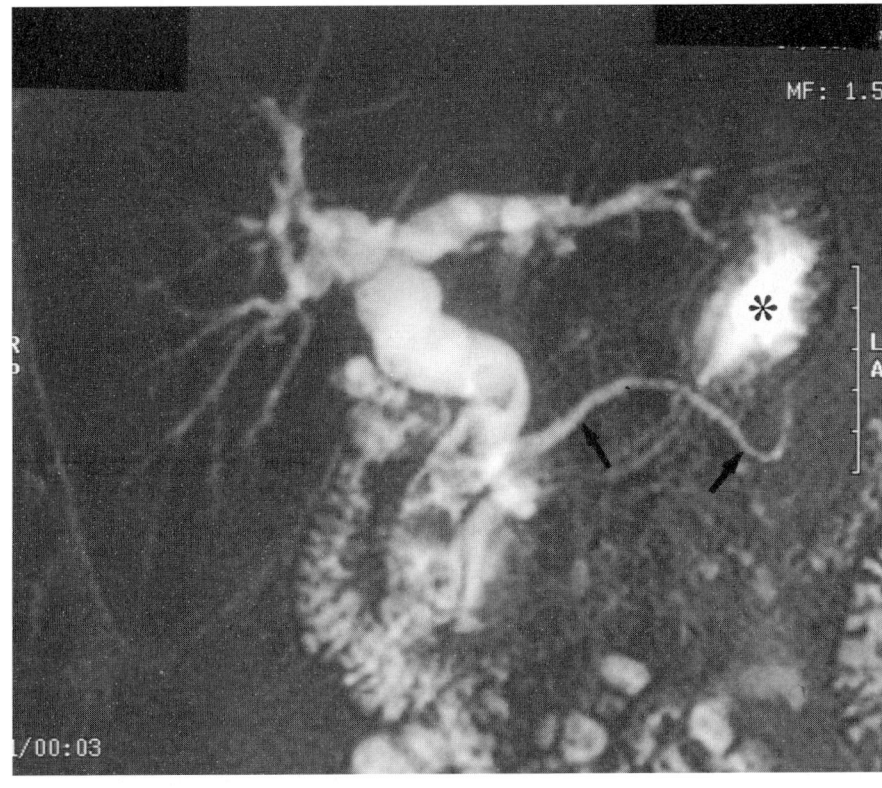

Figure 5.20 *MRCP – biliary calculi.*
Post-cholecystectomy patient. Note the following findings:
- *dilated bile ducts with several large calculi in the common bile duct*
- *pancreatic duct (arrows)*
- *stomach (*), duodenum, and small bowel loops are also seen.*

- No therapeutic applications, i.e. unable to perform sphincterotomy, insert stents, etc.

Imaging of complications of laparoscopic cholecystectomy

Biliary obstruction

- Causes:
  - (i) Incorrect clip placement, i.e. clip placed on CHD/CBD.
  - (ii) Retained calculus.
  - (iii) Partial resection of accessory right hepatic duct.
  - (iv) Miscellaneous: thermal injury, post-operative biliary fibrosis.

- Imaging:
  - (i) Biliary dilatation: US/CT.
  - (ii) Retained calculus: ERCP, sphincterotomy, basket removal.
  - (iii) Bile duct stricture: ERCP/PTC, biliary drainage, stent insertion.

Bile leak

- Imaging:
  - (i) Fluid collection: US/CT, percutaneous drainage (*Fig. 5.21*).
  - (ii) Confirm bile leak: HIDA scan, PTC, biliary drainage.

Imaging of pancreatic masses

CT is the investigation of choice for imaging of pancreatic masses. Helical CT using a dual phase technique is preferable, i.e. fine sections through the pancreas during the arterial phase of contrast enhancement followed by scans of the liver and pancreas during the portal venous phase. Most large pancreatic tumours will be seen on US examination. Smaller masses (< 2 cm) however are frequently missed on US due to overlying intestinal gas or obesity. This particularly applies to small carcinomas of the pancreatic head

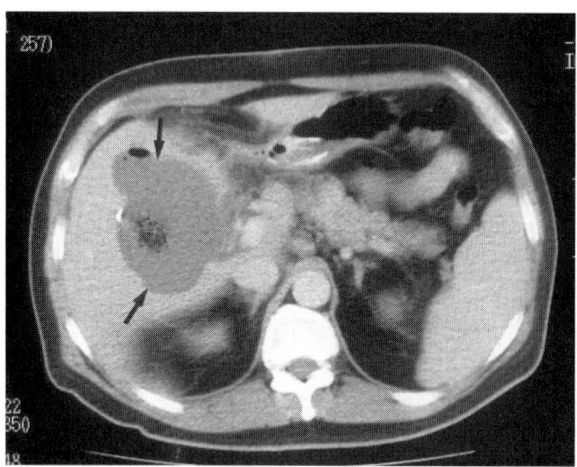

Figure 5.21 *Abscess post-laparoscopic cholecystectomy. Irregular fluid collection containing a small amount of gas lying beneath the liver in the gallbladder fossa (arrows). This was successfully drained percutaneously.*

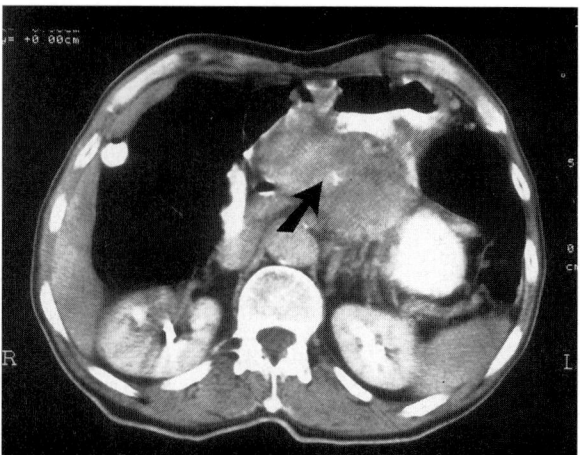

Figure 5.22 *Carcinoma body of pancreas – CT. A large soft tissue mass is seen arising from the body of the pancreas (arrow). Tumours at this site do not cause biliary obstruction and so are usually quite large at the time of presentation.*

and islet cell tumours. MRI has been widely described in the assessment of pancreatic tumours and it may occasionally be useful in difficult cases.

Adenocarcinoma of the pancreas

* The commonest pancreatic neoplasm.

* Location: 60% pancreatic head; 25% body; 15% tail.

(a) CT:

* Dilatation of bile ducts and pancreatic duct.

* Soft tissue mass (*Figs 5.22 and 5.15*).

* Invasion of adjacent organs.

* Encasement of mesenteric vessels.

* Lymphadenopathy, liver metastases, ascites.

(b) US:

* Biliary and pancreatic duct dilatation.

* Hypoechoic mass (*Fig. 5.23*).

(c) ERCP:

* 'Rat tail' stricture of lower CBD.

For further notes on staging of adenocarcinoma of the pancreas, *see* Chapter 12.

Pseudocyst

* Occur secondary to acute pancreatitis, chronic pancreatitis, and pancreatic trauma.

* Location:
  (i) Majority within the pancreas.
  (ii) Also in lesser sac, mesentery, rarely in mediastinum or within other organs, e.g. liver or spleen.

(a) US:

* Well-defined unilocular cyst.

* Anechoic contents or low level echoes due to cellular debris or haemorrhage.

* Guidance of percutaneous drainage.

(b) CT:

* Well-defined cyst with low attenuation contents (*Fig. 5.24*).

* Guidance of percutaneous drainage.

Serous microcystic neoplasm

* Benign neoplasm composed of multiple small cysts measuring up to 2 cm diameter and separated by soft tissue septa.

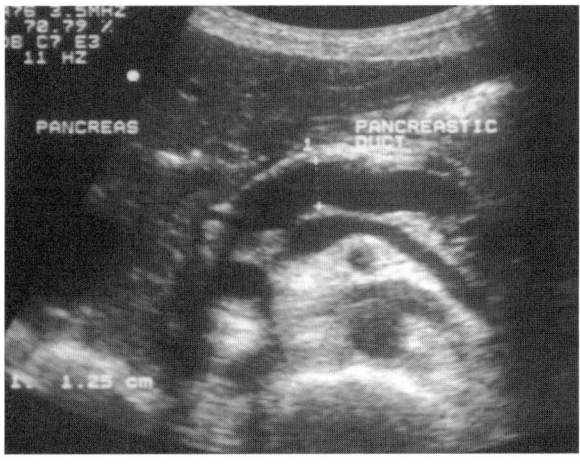

a

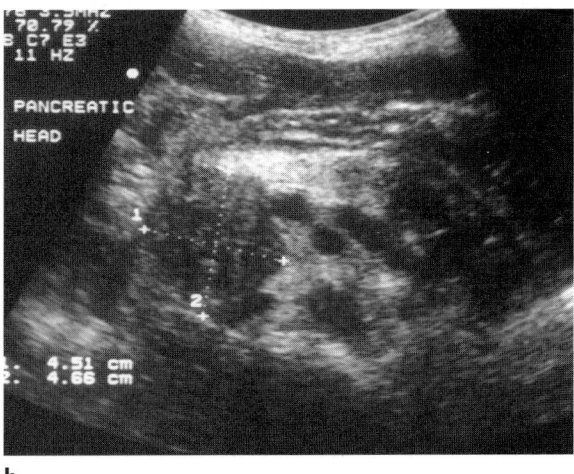

b

Figure 5.23 *Carcinoma head of pancreas – US.*
(a) Marked dilatation of the pancreatic duct is well shown. (b). The tumour is seen as a hypoechoic mass in the head of the pancreas.

- Occur anywhere in the pancreas though slightly more common in the pancreatic head.

(a) US:

- Usually a hyperechoic mass.

- Cysts over 1 cm may be seen as hypoechoic areas.

(b) CT:

- Complex mass with multiple low attenuation cysts (*Fig. 5.25*).

Mucinous macrocystic neoplasm

- May be benign tumour with malignant potential (cystadenoma) or frankly malignant tumour which metastasises to the liver (cyst-adenocarcinoma).

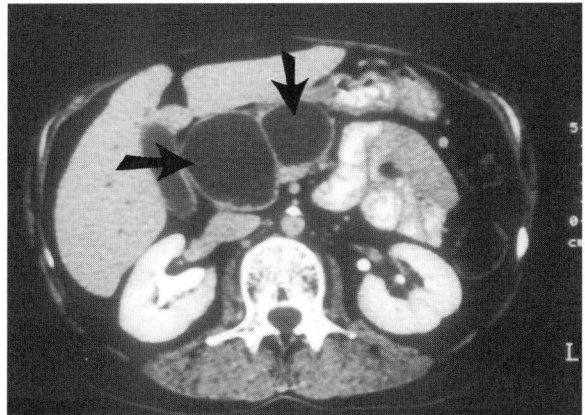

Figure 5.24 *Pancreatic pseudocysts – CT.*
Two well defined low attenuation cysts in the pancreatic head and neck (arrows). Note the following features:
- *thin wall*
- *homogeneous low attenuation fluid contents.*

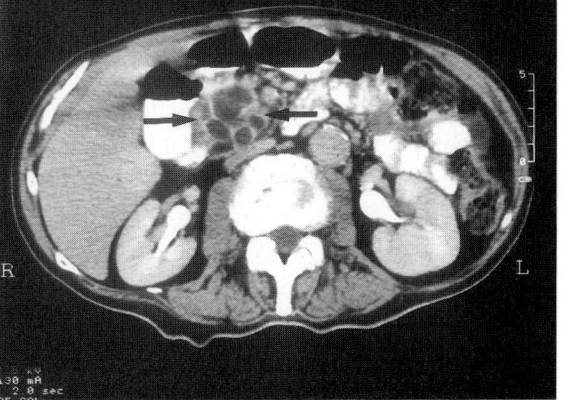

Figure 5.25 *Serous microcystic neoplasm – CT.*
Complex mass of the pancreatic head containing multiple small cysts (arrows).

- Occur most often in the tail of the pancreas.

(a) US:

- Large single cyst or multiple cysts over 2 cm diameter separated by thick soft tissue septa.

(b) CT:

- Uni-/multilocular cystic mass with individual cysts over 2 cm diameter.

- Soft tissue masses may be seen with malignant tumours.

- Invasion of adjacent structures, e.g. spleen.

Islet cell tumours of the pancreas

Rare subset of pancreatic tumours which usually produce ectopic hormones.

(a) Clinical presentation:

- Endocrine syndrome depending on the hormone produced.

- Non-functioning islet cell tumours (the third most common type after insulinoma and gastrinoma) may present with a soft tissue mass, jaundice, or liver metastases.

(b) Insulinoma:

- Most common islet cell tumour.

- Usually solitary, small (1–2 cm), benign adenoma.

- Whipple's triad: symptoms of hypoglycaemia with fasting, documented hypoglycaemia, relief of symptoms with i.v. glucose infusion.

(c) Gastrinoma:

- Second most common islet cell tumour.

- Zollinger–Ellison syndrome: gastric hypersecretion; severe, recurrent peptic ulceration; diarrhoea.

- Tend to be larger than insulinoma; may be up to 15 cm.

- Malignant in 60%; frequently multiple and extrapancreatic.

- Most extrapancreatic tumours occur in the

'gastrinoma triangle' formed by the porta superiorly, the second and third parts of the duodenum inferiorly, and the junction of the neck and body of the pancreas medially.

(d) Glucagonoma:

- Rare.

- High incidence of malignancy and liver metastases.

- Diabetes mellitus, dermatitis, painful glossitis.

(e) Somatostatinoma:

- Rare.

- High incidence of malignancy.

- Diabetes mellitus, gallbladder disease, steatorrhoea.

(f) VIPoma:

- Rare.

- Release of vasoactive intestinal polypeptide.

- Verner–Morrison syndrome: severe watery diarrhoea, hypokalaemia, hypochlorhydria.

(g) The presence of a functioning islet cell tumour is usually strongly suspected on clinical presentation and biochemistry.

(h) The main roles of imaging are:

- Localisation of the tumour to facilitate surgical removal.

- Diagnosis of multiple tumours.

- Diagnosis of evidence of malignancy.

(i) Numerous imaging modalities are available for the assessment of islet cell tumours.

(j) US:

- Reasonable sensitivity for larger tumours; small tumours less than 2 cm are frequently missed.

- Well defined hypoechoic mass.

(k) Intra-operative US:

- Excellent detection of even tiny tumours down to about 3 mm.

- Delineate relationship of tumour to pancreatic duct and major blood vessels.

(l) Endoscopic US:

- Accurate though not widely available technique.

(m)   CT:

- Most widely used and accepted method.

- Helical CT using dual phase technique and fine sections is preferable.

- As well as tumour detection, helical CT is also highly accurate for signs of malignant behaviour, i.e. liver metastases, invasion of surrounding structures, and vascular invasion.

(n) MRI:

- May be useful in difficult or equivocal cases, or in patients allergic to iodinated contrast material.

(o) Angiography:

- Selective injection of coeliac, superior mesenteric, splenic, hepatic, and gastroduodenal arteries.

- Tumour seen as a dense blush of contrast.

- Rarely used.

(p) Transhepatic portal venous sampling (TPVS):

- Transhepatic catheterisation of portal and splenic veins.

- Samples for hormone analysis from pancreatic veins as well as from portal, splenic, superior mesenteric, and inferior mesenteric veins.

- Highly invasive; problems with multiple tumours and variations of venous drainage.

- Rarely used.

(q) Selective arterial stimulation testing (SAST):

- Sampling catheter placed in right hepatic vein via femoral vein approach.

- Second catheter via femoral artery to selectively catheterise pancreatic arteries.

- Drugs to stimulate hormone production (secretagogues) injected into small arterial branches and 1–2 minutes later blood obtained from hepatic vein.

- Increased hormone concentration in the hepatic vein identifies the arterial supply of the tumour thereby localising it.

- Less invasive than TPVS.

- May be used prior to surgery where other imaging modalities are negative.

(r) Choice of imaging modality will depend on clinical presentation as well as local expertise and availability. In general spiral CT and intra-operative US would be the imaging investigations of choice for localisation of small tumours especially insulinoma. Spiral CT is also useful for detection of larger masses as well as signs of malignancy such as liver metastases, local invasion, and vascular invasion. MRI and SAST may be used in difficult cases with angiography and TPVS rarely used in clinical practice.

Imaging in portal hypertension

Ultrasound

- Signs of liver cirrhosis are increased echogenicity of liver parenchyma (due to associated fatty infiltration), irregular liver surface, and/or loss of normal liver architecture (i.e. loss of visibility of hepatic vessels).

- Enlarged spleen.

- Enlarged portal vein > 13 mm.

- Decreased or reversed portal vein flow on Doppler studies.

- Varices may be seen in the splenic hilum and around the head of the pancreas, and the recanalised umbilical vein may be seen in the falciform ligament.

- Ascites.

CT

Signs of liver cirrhosis: irregular contour; decreased density with fatty change or increased density with haemochromatosis; enlarged caudate lobe.

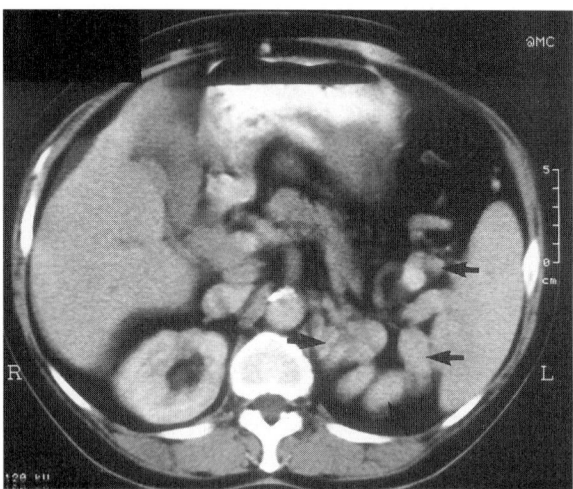

Figure 5.26 *Portal hypertension – CT.*
Varices are seen as multiple, tortuous, enhancing blood
vessels (arrows) above the left kidney and near the
splenic hilum.

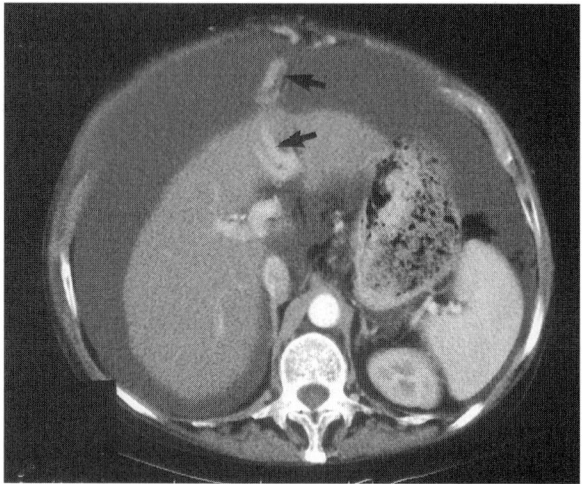

Figure 5.27 *Portal hypertension – CT.*
There is a large amount of ascites seen as low
attenuation fluid surrounding the liver, stomach and
spleen. Note the recanalised umbilical vein (arrows)
secondary to portal hypertension.

- Enlarged spleen.

- Varices: discrete round or tubular structures which
  enhance with contrast (*Fig. 5.26*).

- Ascites (*Fig. 5.27*).

Scintigraphy

- ^{99m}Tc sulphur colloid.

- Decreased, patchy liver uptake.

- Increased bone marrow uptake.

- Enlarged spleen (*Fig. 5.28*).

Angiography

- To demonstrate anatomy and flow pattern of the
  portal vein and its feeding branches.

- Aim to outline portal system and measure
  pressures and flow rates.

- Complemented, and often superseded, by Doppler
  studies.

- Techniques:

  (i)   Indirect: venous phase of arterial injection into
        coeliac trunk, splenic artery, and superior
        mesenteric artery.
  (ii) Direct: trans-hepatic or trans-splenic.
  (iii) Operative cannulation of superior mesenteric
        vein.

- Angiography also used post-operatively to demonstrate shunt patency.

Summary of interventional procedures of the liver and biliary tree

Liver biopsy

- CT or US guidance.

- Core biopsy often required as fine-needle aspiration
  may not provide sufficient material for diagnosis.

- Two basic indications:
  (i)   Localised mass/masses: imaging guidance to
        confirm position of needle in mass.

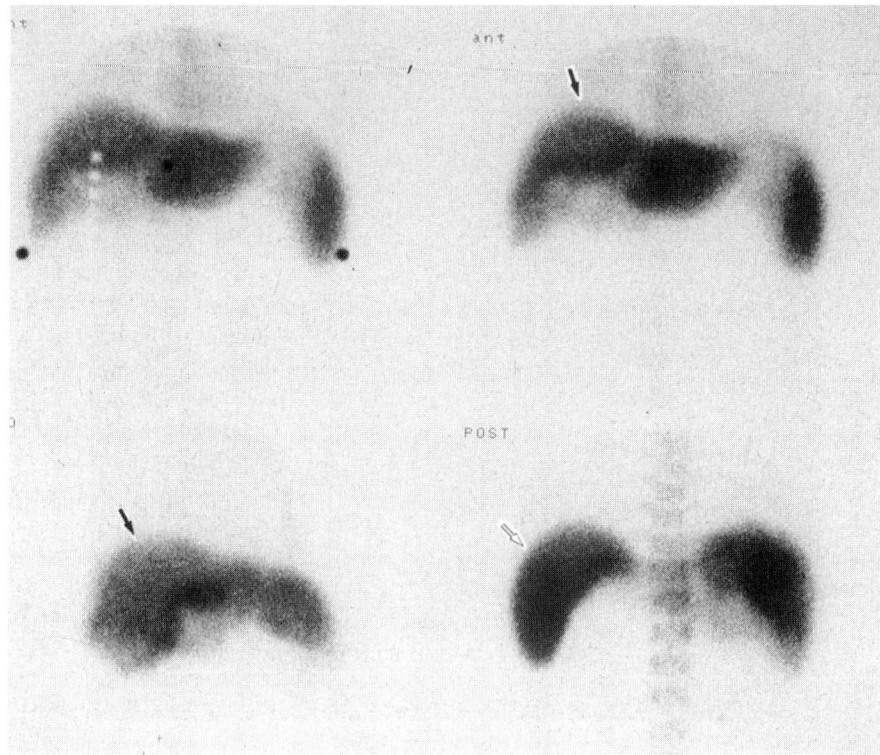

Figure 5.28 *Portal hypertension – scintigraphy. ^{99m}Tc sulphur-colloid. Note:*
- *patchy hepatic uptake (solid arrows)*
- *splenomegaly (hollow arrow)*
- *increased activity in the vertebral column. (Courtesy of Dr F. Smith, Aberdeen.)*

(ii) Diffuse liver disease: imaging guidance not strictly required though may increase safety and diagnostic yield.

- Imaging is also required prior to biopsy to exclude a vascular mass such as haemangioma or AVM.

Non-surgical management of bile duct stones

(a) ERCP:

- Sphincterotomy.

- Basket removal.

(b) Basket removal through T-tube tract:

- T-tube should be *in situ* for at least 4 weeks post-surgery to ensure a 'mature' tract able to accept wires and catheters.

- T-tube cholangiogram to assess position and number of stones.

- Wire through T-tube; T-tube removed.

- Steerable catheter and wire manipulated to stone; basket sheath over guide wire.

- Stone engaged in basket and removed.

- Rare complications include pancreatitis, cholangitis, and bile leak.

(c) Flexible choledochoscope through T-tube tract:

- May be accompanied by intracorporeal lithotripsy.

(d) Chemical dissolution:

- Not widely practised or accepted.

Non-surgical management of malignant biliary obstruction

Indications:

- Performed for symptomatic relief, i.e. relief of pruritus, pain, cholangitis.

- Non-resectable tumour of bile ducts, head of pancreas, or liver.

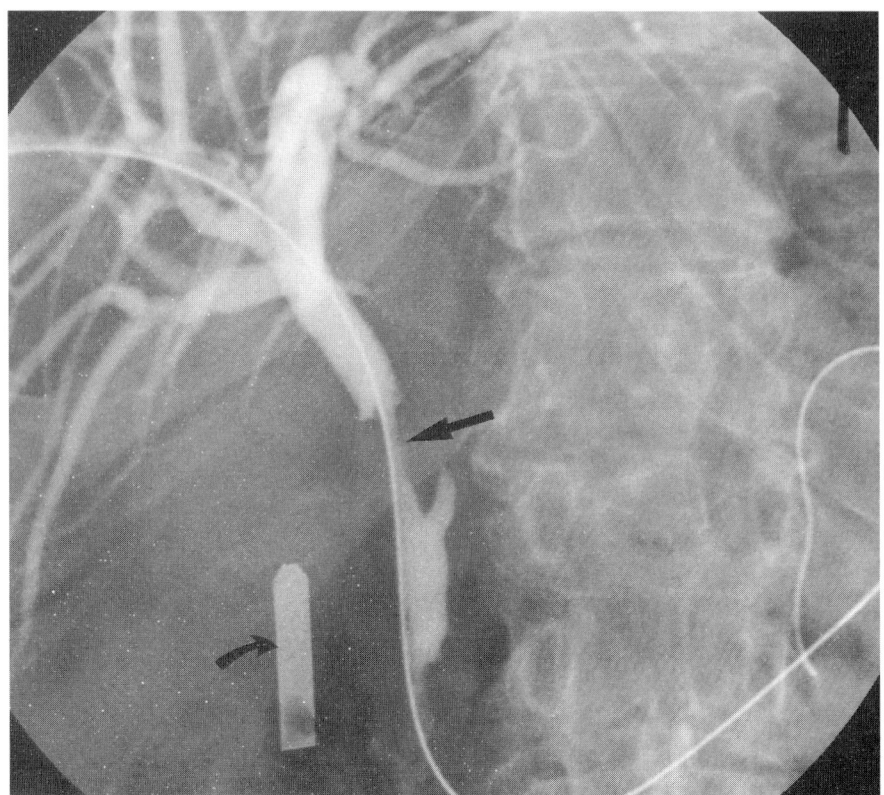

Figure 5.29 *Biliary stent insertion.*
(a) Pre-stent insertion. The biliary system has been opacified by PTC. There is a stricture of the upper common bile duct due to a cholangiocarcinoma (straight arrow). A wire has been passed through the obstruction and into the duodenum. A marker placed on the skin will help with subsequent stent positioning (curved arrow). (b) Biliary stent. This image shows the biliary stent in position. This is a plastic stent with mushroom-shaped tips which help to maintain its position (Miller stent).

a

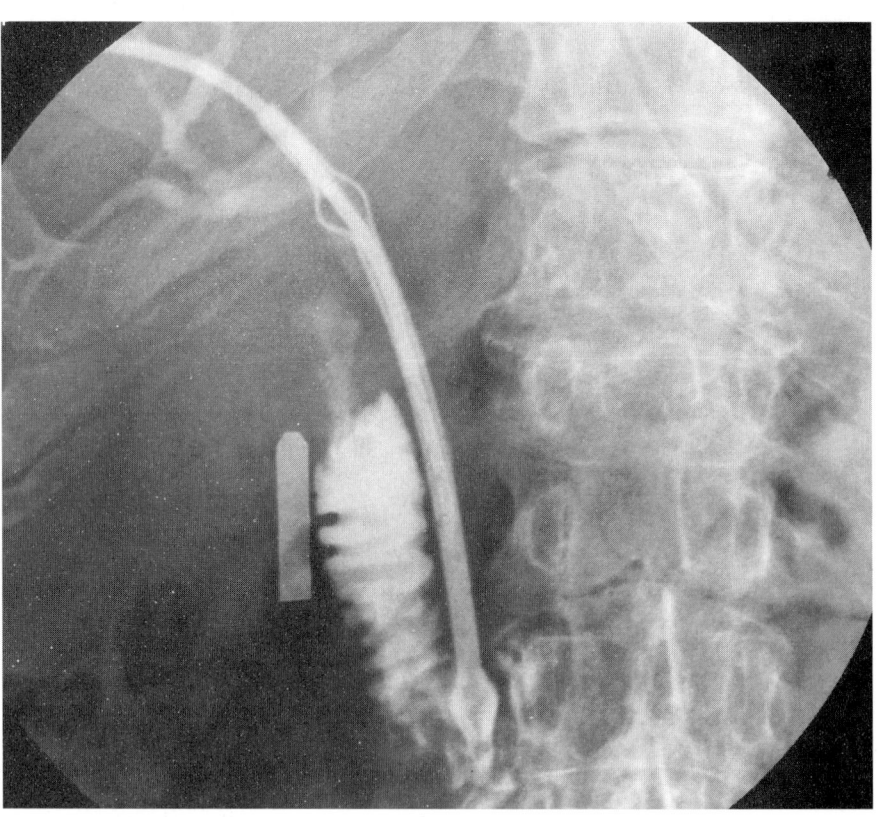

b

- Medical risk factors which make surgery impossible.

Method:

- Endoscopic, i.e. 'from below' for mid to low biliary obstruction.

- Percutaneous, i.e. 'from above' or combined percutaneous–endoscopic for high obstruction or where the second part of duodenum is inaccessible due to tumour or prior surgery.

- Regardless of approach the basic technique is the same:

  opacify ducts by ERCP or PTC; pass wire across obstruction; insert stent or internal–external drain (*Fig. 5.29*).

- Occasionally in severe obstruction a 2-stage procedure is required, i.e. drainage tube above obstruction for a few days; after decompression of the biliary system a wire is passed across the obstruction and a stent inserted.

- Internal biliary stents are plastic or self-expanding metal and are better accepted by patients as they avoid the problems of external biliary drains such as skin irritation, pain, bile leaks, and risk of dislodgement.

Percutaneous cholecystostomy (gallbladder drainage)

Indications:

- Acute cholecystitis where the surgical risks are unacceptable.

Technique:

- US guidance.

- Transhepatic approach preferable due to reduced risk of bile leak.

- Puncture gallbladder, wire through needle, drainage catheter over wire.

Post-procedure:

- Non-resolution of pyrexia within 48 hours may indicate gangrene of the gallbladder requiring surgery.

- Cholecystogram once acute illness has settled: stones causing cystic duct obstruction may require surgery; otherwise the catheter is removed.

Liver embolisation

- Via catheter selectively placed in the hepatic artery or its branches.

Indications:

- Metastases.
  (i) Selective delivery of chemotherapy.
  (ii) Occasionally to reduce bulk and therefore relieve mass effect of large lesions.

- Non-resectable hepatocellular carcinoma for palliation of symptoms.

- AVM or false aneurysm.

- Haemostasis in bleeding adenoma or haemangioma.

TIPSS – *See* Chapter 3 (page 56)

Further Reading

1. Baron RL. Understanding and optimizing use of contrast material for CT of the liver. *AJR* 1994; **163**:323–331.

2. Bluemke DA, Soyer P, Fishman EK. Helical (Spiral) CT of the liver. *Radiological Clinics of North America* 1995; **33**: 863–886.

3. Buetow PC, Miller DL, Parrino TV, Buck LJ. Islet cell tumours of the pancreas: clinical, radiologic, and pathologic correlation in diagnosis and localisation. *RadioGraphics* 1997; **17**:453–472.

4. Buetow PC, Pantongrag–Brown L, Buck JL *et al*. Focal nodular hyperplasia of the liver: radiologic–pathologic correlation. *RadioGraphics* 1996; **16**:369–388.

5. Guiband L, Bret PM, Reinhold C *et al*. Bile duct obstruction and choledocholithiasis: diagnosis with MR cholangiography. *Radiology* 1995; **197**:109–115.

6. McGahan JP, Stein M. Complications of laparoscopic cholecystectomy: imaging and intervention. *AJR* 1995; **165**:1089–1097.

7. Pieters PC, Miller WJ, DeMeo JH. Evaluation of the portal venous system: complementary roles of invasive and noninvasive imaging strategies. *RadioGraphics* 1997; **17**:879–895.

8. Raymond HW, Zwiebel WJ (eds.) Laparoscopic cholecystectomy: impact on radiology. *Seminars in US, CT, and MRI* 1993; **14**(5).

9. Reinhold C, Bret PM, Guibaud L *et al*. MR Cholangio-pancreatography: potential clinical applications. *RadioGraphics* 1996; **16**:309–320.

6 Urology

Investigation of a renal mass

The goals of imaging a suspected renal mass include:

- Confirmation of presence and site of mass.
- Differentiation of benign from malignant.
- Accurate characterisation of features.
- Assess metastatic disease.
- Assess contralateral kidney.

Ultrasound provides a cheap, safe and reliable screening test for a renal mass suspected clinically or found on IVP during investigation of haematuria/renal colic. It is the initial investigation of choice for assessment of a renal mass, followed by CT.

Ultrasound

- Will differentiate a simple cyst from either a complicated cyst or a solid mass.
  (i) Features of a simple cyst: (a) well-defined thin wall; (b) anechoic; (c) acoustic enhancement (*Fig. 6.1*).
  (ii) Any lesion not fitting the above parameters requires further assessment.
  (iii) A complicated cyst refers to a cyst with: (a) internal echoes which may be due to haemorrhage or infection; (b) soft tissue septa; (c) associated soft tissue mass (*Fig. 6.2*).
  (iv) A solid lesion may show areas of increased echogenicity due to calcification or fat, or areas of decreased echogenicity due to necrosis.

- Where renal cell carcinoma is suspected, ultrasound is also used to look for:
  (i) Invasion of renal vein and IVC.
  (ii) Lymphadenopathy.
  (iii) Metastases in the liver and contralateral kidney.

- Ultrasound may be used as a guide for:
  (i) Biopsy of solid lesions or complicated cysts.

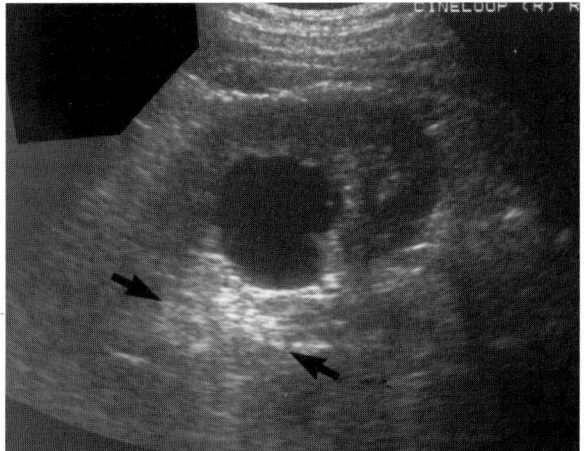

Figure 6.1 *Simple renal cyst – ultrasound.*
Note the following features of a simple cyst on US:
- *anechoic (black) contents*
- *well defined posterior wall*
- *acoustic enhancement (arrows).*

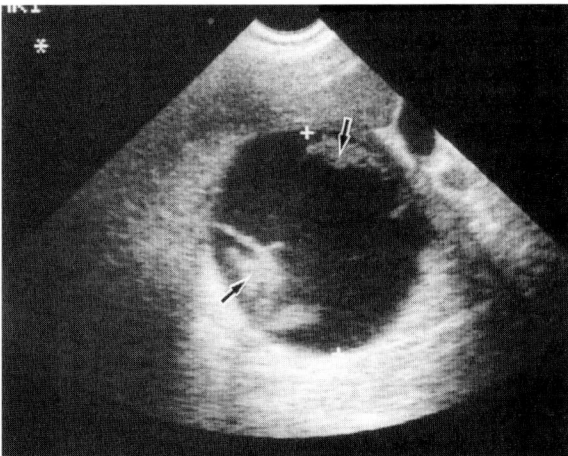

Figure 6.2 *Complicated renal cyst.*
The cyst contains echogenic areas (arrows) in this case due to haemorrhage.

(ii) Cyst aspiration for diagnostic and therapeutic purposes.

(iii) Cyst ablation by injection of ethanol.

CT

- Contrast-enhanced CT is used for further characterisation of a solid lesion or complicated cyst.

- CT is more accurate than US for characterisation of internal contents of a mass as well as for staging of renal cell carcinoma.

- May show areas of calcification, fat, necrosis, or marked enhancement with a vascular lesion.

- For renal cell carcinoma, CT is also used to assess:
    (i) Invasion of local structures seen as tumour tissue extending into perirenal and pararenal fat and into surrounding muscles and organs.
    (ii) Vascular invasion seen as increased calibre and decreased density of renal vein or IVC with failure to enhance with contrast.
    (iii) Lymphadenopathy.
    (iv) Metastases in liver and contralateral kidney.

- CT can be used to guide biopsy, or cyst aspiration and ablation.

- The majority of renal masses will be adequately characterised and staged with US and/or CT. Other imaging investigations are only occasionally performed.

MRI

MRI gives similar information to CT. Its potential advantages are:

- Accurate for assessing vascular invasion.

- Iodinated contrast is not required.

- Multiplanar imaging gives more accuracy in assessing the renal pole and for showing invasion of surrounding structures.

Angiography

This is performed rarely for renal cell carcinoma in the following situations:

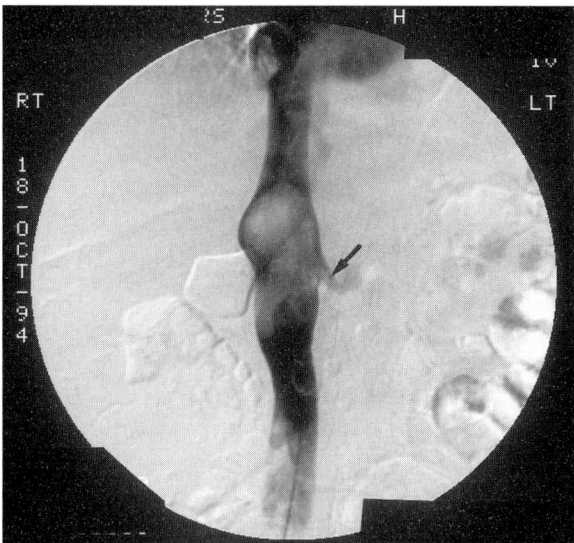

Figure 6.3 *Renal cell carcinoma – cavogram. Cavogram is still occasionally performed to confirm tumour invasion of the IVC where CT and US are equivocal, or to assist with surgical planning. This case shows a large tumour mass in the IVC. Note that there is normal reflux of contrast into the left renal vein (arrow). The right renal vein is occluded with tumour and therefore is not seen.*

- Prior to tumour embolisation.

- As a surgical 'road map'.

- Where results of the above imaging modalities are equivocal with respect to vascular invasion (*Fig. 6.3*).

US and CT features of the more common renal masses

Renal cell carcinoma

(a) *US:*

- Heterogeneous mass; heterogeneity due to haemorrhage, necrosis, calcification (*Fig. 6.4*).

- May be generally hyperechoic or less commonly hypoechoic.

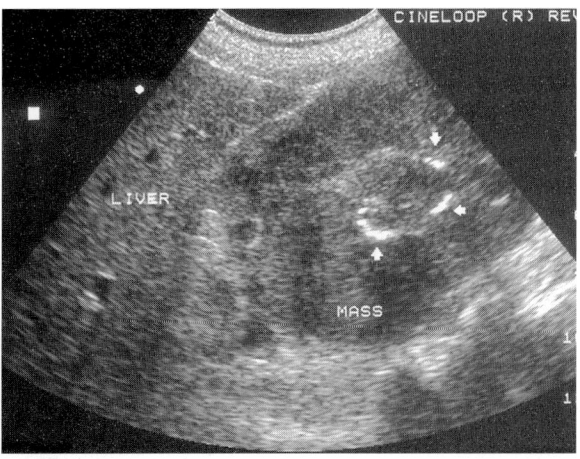
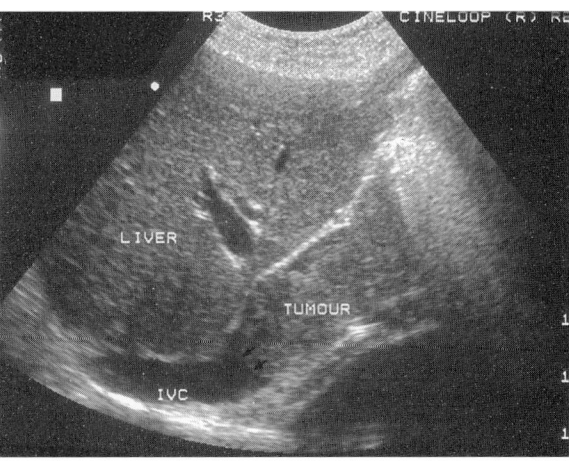

a   b

Figure 6.4 *Renal cell carcinoma – US.*
(a) Carcinoma of the right kidney. US shows a large heterogeneous tumour beneath the liver. Note hyperechoic areas due to calcification (arrows). (b) US shows tumour invading the IVC. The distal extent of tumour invasion is well seen (arrows). Note that the upper IVC is clear.

(b) *CT:*

- Heterogeneous mass, often iso-intense to kidney on non-contrast CT.

- Low-attenuation areas due to necrosis.

- Calcification well seen on CT.

- Less enhancement than kidney therefore better seen on post-contrast scans (*Fig. 6.5*).

- Signs of spread: invasion of local structures, e.g. psoas muscle, invasion of renal vein and IVC, lymphadenopathy, metastases in liver, lungs, and contralateral kidney.

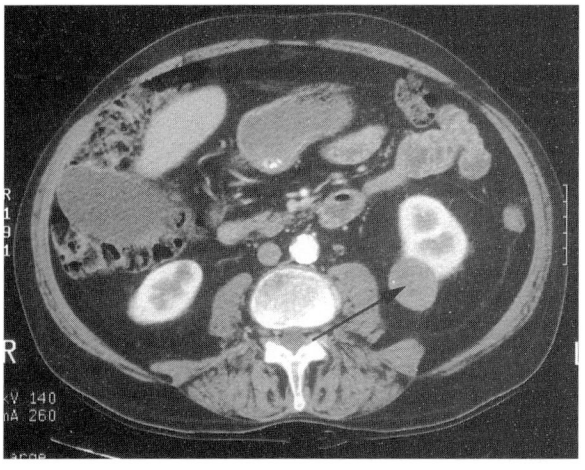
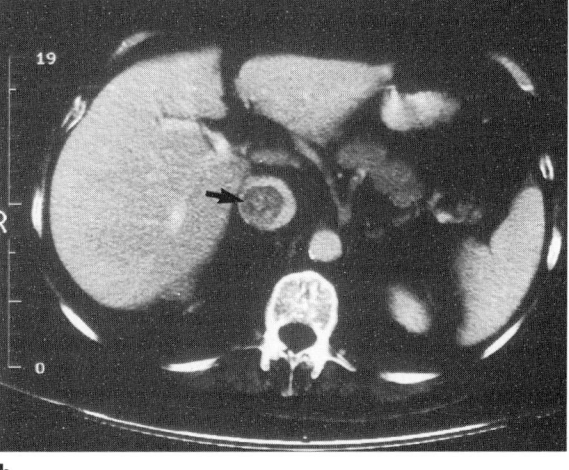

a   b

Figure 6.5 *Renal cell carcinoma – CT.*
(a) Carcinoma of the left kidney. The low attenuation mass (arrow) is best seen on a contrast-enhanced scan due to enhancement of the kidney. (b) IVC invasion. A separate case shows IVC invasion. There is a mass in the IVC (arrow) well outlined by surrounding contrast-enhanced blood.

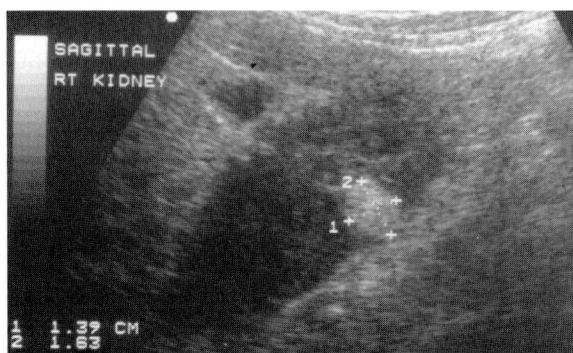

Figure 6.6 *Angiomyolipoma (AML) – US. A small AML is seen as a hyperechoic mass in the renal cortex.*

Angiomyolipoma (AML)

- Two types:
  - (i) Sporadic – most common in females, 40–60 years; usually solitary and unilateral.
  - (ii) Associated with tuberous sclerosis – multiple and bilateral.

- Small AMLs are asymptomatic and often seen as incidental findings on imaging; larger lesions may present with acute pain or haematuria.

(a) *US:*

- Heterogeneous mass with markedly hyperechoic areas due to fat content (*Fig. 6.6*).

(b) *CT:*

- Heterogeneous mass.

- Low-attenuation areas due to fat are virtually diagnostic of AML (*Fig. 6.7*) though fat may rarely be seen in renal cell carcinoma.

Oncocytoma

(a) *US:*

- Well-defined hypoechoic mass.

- Central hyperechoic scar occasionally seen.

(b) *CT:*

- Low attenuation mass with well-defined pseudocapsule.

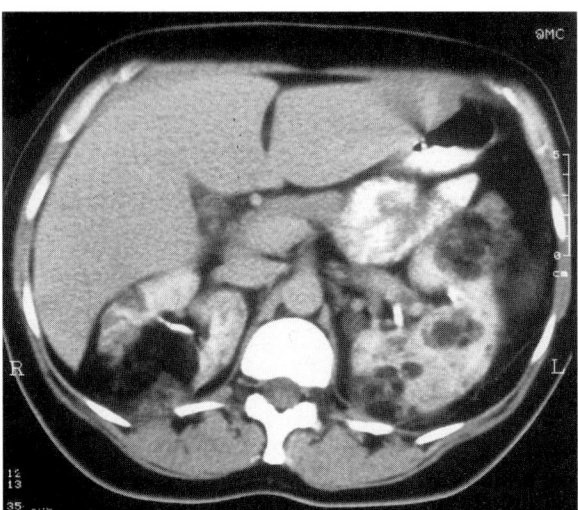

Figure 6.7 *Tuberous sclerosis – CT. Multiple angiomyolipomas are seen in both kidneys. The low attenuation fat content of these tumours is well seen on CT.*

- Central scar seen in about 30% of cases.

Lymphoma

- Three patterns of renal involvement are seen: diffuse infiltration, single/multiple masses, direct invasion from perirenal disease.

(a) *US:*

- Single/multiple anechoic/hypoechoic masses.

- Enlarged, diffusely hypoechoic kidney.

(b) *CT:*

- Single/multiple low attenuation masses.

- No enhancement with contrast.

- Enlarged low attenuation kidney with diffuse involvement.

Multilocular cystic nephroma

- Rare, benign neoplasm occurring in young males (3 months–4 years) and older females (50–60 years).

- Occasional development of nephroblastoma in children or sarcoma in adults.

(a) *US:*

- Anechoic lesion containing multiple echogenic septae.

(b) *CT:*

- Low attenuation lesion containing multiple higher attenuation septae.

- Septae may show contrast enhancement.

Inflammatory masses

Nephronia (acute focal bacterial nephritis)

(a) *US:*

- Ill-defined hypoechoic mass.

(b) *CT:*

- Low-attenuation mass with ill-defined margins.

Abscess

(a) *US:*

- Hypoechoic/anechoic fluid collection with ill-defined walls.

(b) *CT:*

- Low-attenuation centre.

- Ill-defined wall which may show contrast enhancement (*Fig. 6.8*).

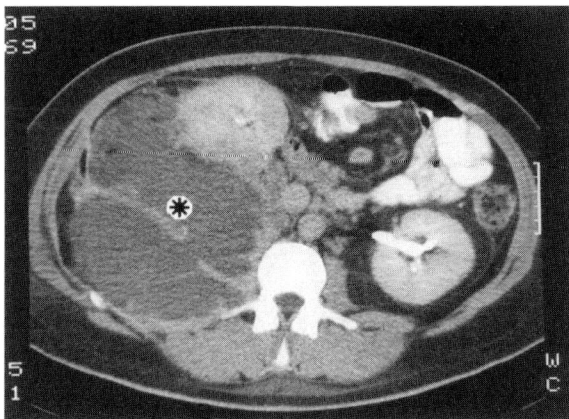

Figure 6.8 *Perinephrenic abscess – CT. Huge perinephric collection (*) with anterior displacement of the right kidney.*

Metastases

- The most common primary sites for renal metastases are lung, breast and stomach.

- Multiple heterogeneous masses are seen on US/CT.

Biopsy and the indeterminate renal mass

Occasionally a renal mass will be encountered which cannot be definitively classified with imaging. A common example is a cyst complicated by haemorrhage or infection. This will appear as a well-defined hypoechoic lesion on US and as a high to intermediate attenuation lesion on CT, and as such may be difficult to differentiate from a solid mass.

Biopsy of renal masses is usually not indicated:

- Interpretation of a 'non-malignant' result is difficult.

- Biopsy may alter radiological parameters for further follow-up, e.g. haemorrhage into a cyst.

Biopsy of a solitary renal mass may be indicated in the following uncommon situations:

- High suspicion for lymphoma.

- Known or previous primary carcinoma elsewhere, especially lung, breast, or stomach.

- Where a positive biopsy result would indicate a non-operative approach.

Generally, a decision will be made to either remove or observe an indeterminate renal mass. A suggested imaging protocol for observation would be:

- Repeat imaging in 6 months.

- If increased in size then remove.

- If unchanged go to annual follow-up.

Painless haematuria

Intravenous pyelogram (IVP)

In combination with cystoscopy, IVP remains the best initial screening test for painless haematuria. It

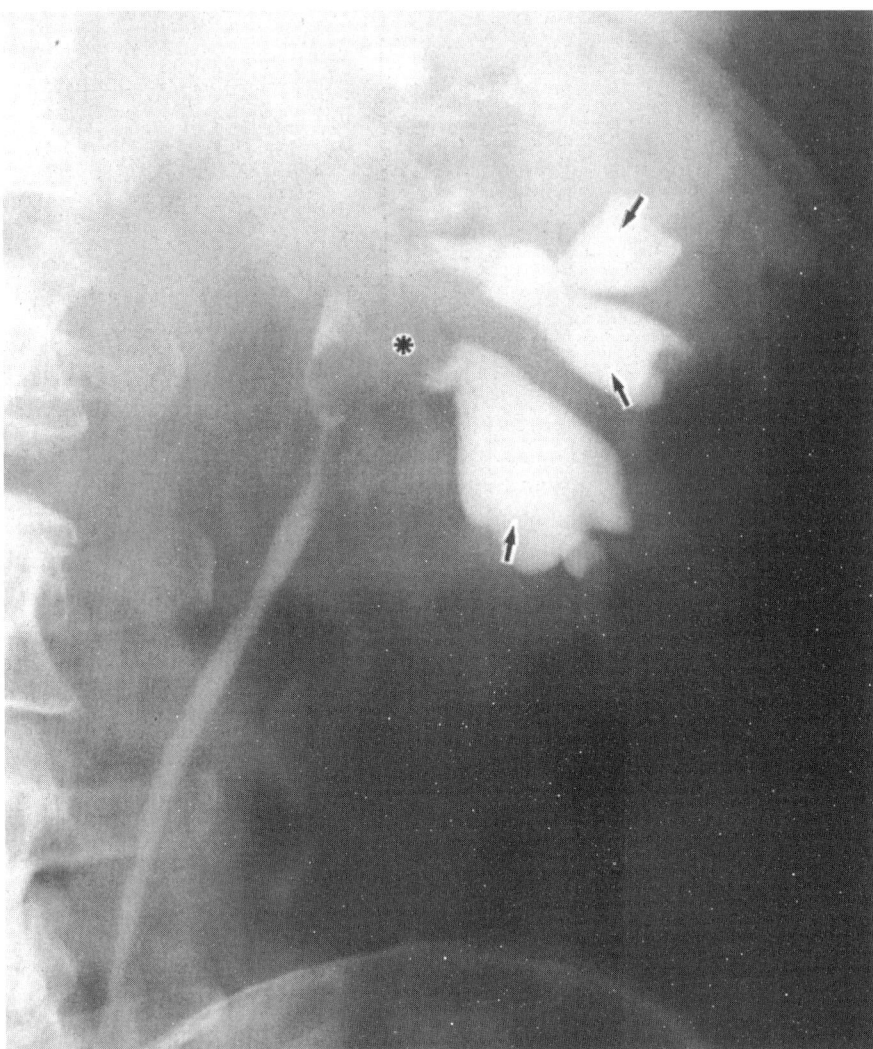

Figure 6.9 *Transitional cell carcinoma (TCC) of the renal pelvis – IVP.*
Irregular filling defect in renal pelvis (*). Dilated and blunted calyces (arrows) due to obstruction.

provides visualisation of the calyces, renal pelvis and ureter with an anatomical resolution not possible with other imaging modalities; a small transitional cell carcinoma (TCC) will not be seen on ultrasound or CT unless the pelvicalyceal system is dilated.

- Signs of a TCC on IVP:
  (i) Lucent filling defect (D.D. blood clot, sloughed papilla, uric acid or xanthine calculus) (*Fig. 6.9*).
  (ii) Dilatation of the urinary tract above the tumour.
  (iii) Obstructed kidney may show delayed opacification.
  (iv) Often multiple so the whole urinary tract must be closely examined.

- Fine section non-contrast CT is sometimes useful to further delineate a lucent filling defect; all stones will be of high attenuation on CT, even stones that are lucent on IVP and plain films (*Fig. 6.10*).

- A suspected TCC can be further investigated by retrograde or antegrade pyelogram (*Fig. 6.11*).

- Imaging by ultrasound and CT can be performed to further delineate tumour extent, assess complications like hydronephrosis, and assess local invasion, lymphadenopathy, and other metastases.

- A renal mass found on IVP will be investigated as above, i.e. ultrasound followed by further imaging as indicated.

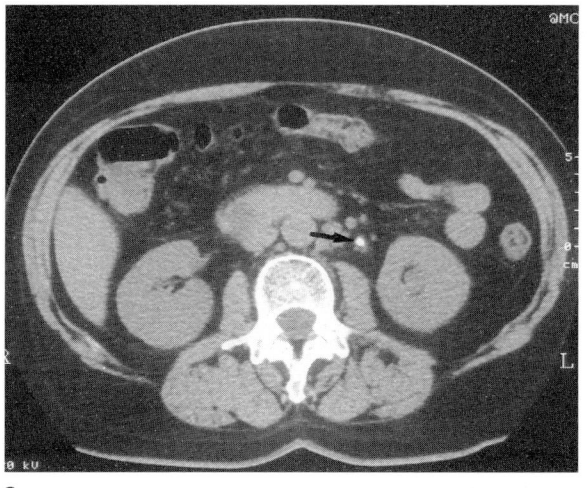 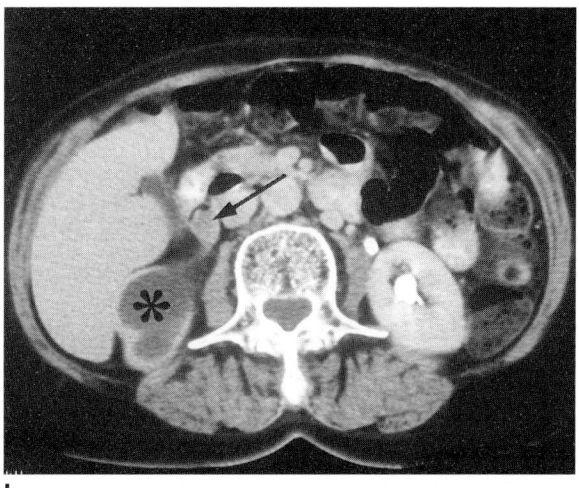

a   b

Figure 6.10 *CT of ureteric filling defects.*
(a) Ureteric stone. A small stone is well seen as a high attenuation focus in the upper left ureter (arrow). (b) Ureteric TCC. There is dilatation of the right renal collecting system (*). A low attenuation mass is seen in the upper right ureter (arrow). Compare this appearance with the stone in (a).

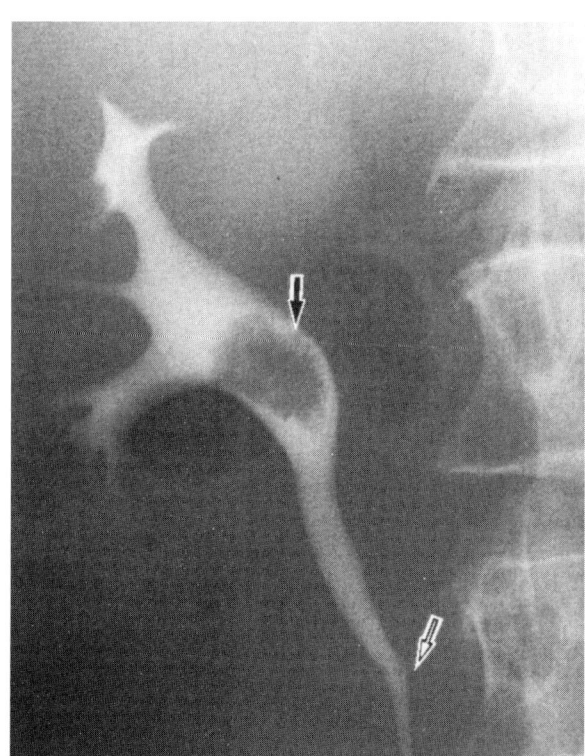

Figure 6.11 *TCC – retrogram pyelogram.*
The tumour is seen as an irregular filling defect in the renal pelvis (black arrow). Note the tip of the retrograde catheter (white arrow) in the upper ureter.

- If IVP and/or cystoscopy show a bladder tumour, CT is warranted for staging, i.e. to assess perivesical spread, lymphadenopathy and metastases to other sites.

US

- For a renal mass to be visible on IVP it must distort the renal outline or deform/invade the collecting system. A small mass may therefore be missed on IVP.

- If IVP and cystoscopy are negative, US is warranted as it is more sensitive than IVP for showing small renal masses lying outside the collecting system.

- If all imaging is negative then medical causes of haematuria such as glomerulonephritis should be considered.

- After exclusion of bleeding disorder renal biopsy may be performed, most safely under US control.

Imaging in prostatism

- The symptoms of prostatism include frequency, nocturia, poor stream, hesitancy etc.

Table 6.1 *Investigation of haematuria: suggested protocol*

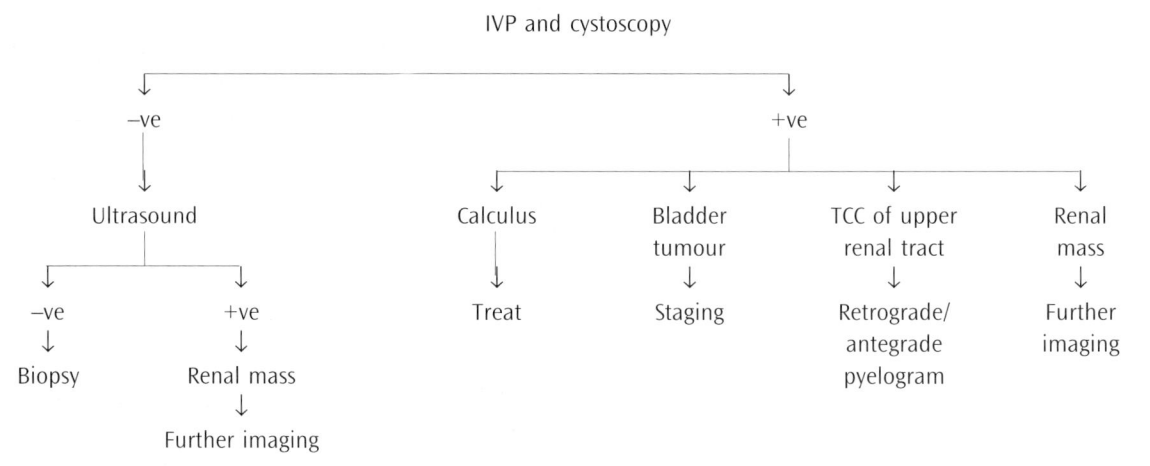

The primary imaging investigations in the assessment of prostatism are plain abdomen X-ray and urinary tract ultrasound.

• IVP is no longer recommended for routine use in prostatism.

Urinary tract ultrasound

(a) Bladder ultrasound:

• Measure volume pre- and post-micturition.

• Calculate residual volume by the simple formula:

volume = height × width × length × 0.50.

• Morphological changes:
 (i) Bladder wall thickening.
 (ii) Trabeculation and diverticula.
 (iii) Calculi (*Fig. 6.12*).

(b) Renal ultrasound:

• Hydronephrosis.

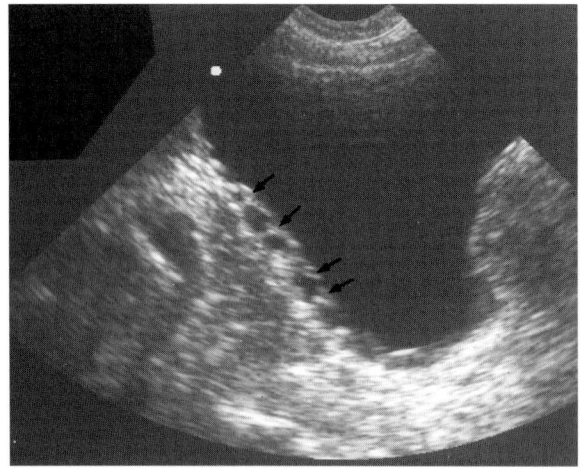

a

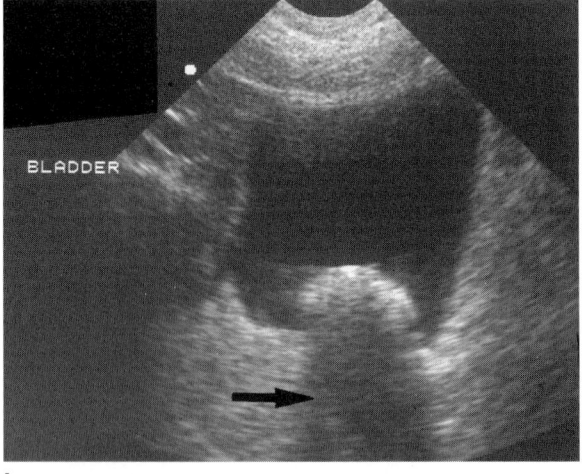

b

Figure 6.12 *Bladder changes in prostatism – US.*
(a) Bladder trabeculation. Note the hypertrophied muscle bands producing irregularity of the bladder wall (arrows).
(b) Bladder calculus. A bladder calculus is well seen as a large hyperechoic focus in the bladder lumen casting a prominent acoustic shadow (arrow).

- Asymptomatic congenital anomalies and tumours.
- Calculi.

(c) Prostate ultrasound:

- Measure prostate volume = height $\times$ width $\times$ length $\times$ 0.50.

AXR

For calculi in kidneys and ureters which may not be seen on ultrasound.

Investigation of a scrotal mass

Ultrasound

- US is the first investigation of choice for a scrotal mass.
- The primary role of US is to differentiate intratesticular from extratesticular masses; in most cases this is sufficient to distinguish malignant and benign lesions.
- Most (90%) intratesticular masses are malignant.
- Exceptions include:
  (i)   testicular abscess;
  (ii) TB;
  (iii) testicular infarct;
  (iv) benign tumour, e.g. Sertoli–Leydig;
  (v)   sarcoid.
- Most intratesticular tumours are hypoechoic compared with surrounding testicle, although some may be hyperechoic, particularly in the presence of haemorrhage or calcification.
- Seminomas are usually hypoechoic and may be seen as a localised hypoechoic mass well outlined by surrounding hyperechoic testicular tissue (*Fig. 6.13*); occasionally with a large tumour the entire testicle is replaced by abnormal hypoechoic tissue.
- Other tumour types such as choriocarcinoma, embryonal cell carcinoma, teratoma, and mixed tumours usually show a heterogeneous echotexture.

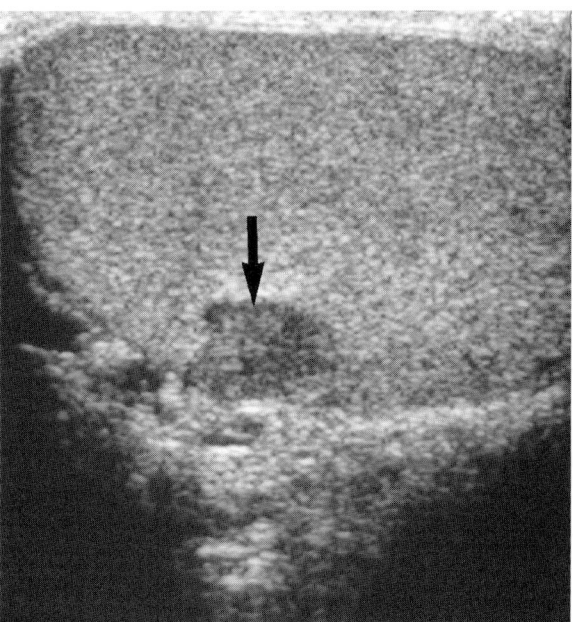

Figure 6.13 *Testicular tumour – US.*
A small seminoma is seen as a hypoechoic mass well outlined against normal surrounding hyperechoic testicular tissue (arrow).

- Lymphoma of the testis is hypoechoic and homogeneous and may be focal or diffuse.
- For notes on staging of testicular tumours, *see* Chapter 12.
- Most (90%) extratesticular lesions are benign; the more common of these are outlined below.

(a) Hydrocele:

- Anechoic fluid surrounding the testicle.
- May be congenital, idiopathic, or secondary to inflammation, torsion, trauma, or tumour.

(b) Varicocele:

- Dilated veins of the pampiniform plexus producing a tortuous nest of veins well seen on US (*Fig. 6.14*).
- Vascular nature of the mass is confirmed with colour Doppler.
- Occur mostly on the left.
- Present with a clinically obvious mass or with infertility.

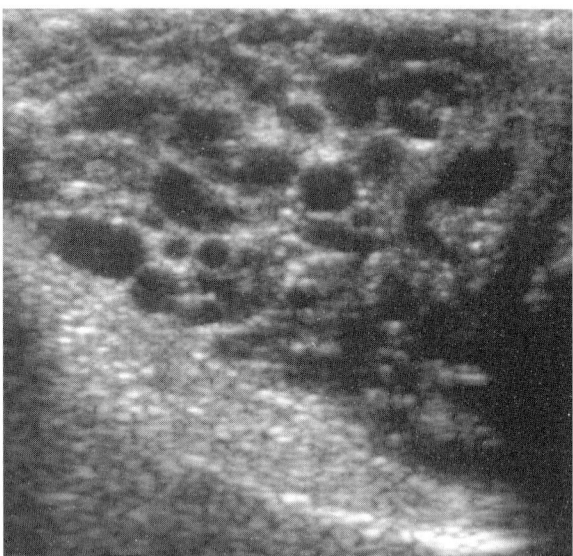

Figure 6.14 *Varicocele – US.*
A nest of dilated tortuous veins is well demonstrated on US examination.

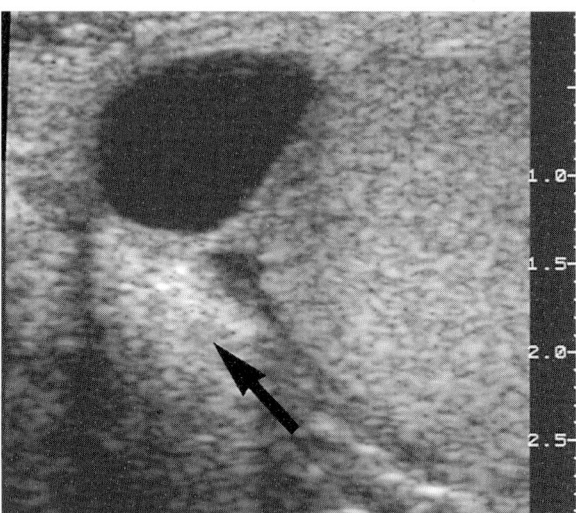

Figure 6.15 *Epididymal cyst – US.*
Note the following features:
- *well defined anechoic cyst above the testis*
- *acoustic enhancement (arrow).*

- Small varicoceles are often incidental findings on scrotal US.

- Caused by venous incompetence in most cases; rarely may be caused by obstruction of the left renal vein by tumour or thrombosis.

- May be amenable to therapeutic embolisation (see below).

(c) Spermatocele/epididymal cyst:

- Well-defined anechoic simple cyst in the head of the epididymis, i.e. posterolaterally at the superior pole of the testis (*Fig. 6.15*).

Acute scrotum

The main differential in this situation is torsion versus acute epididymo-orchitis. The need for early exploration in suspected torsion gives imaging a role only in doubtful cases where it is quickly available. Acute epididymo-orchitis is usually caused by bacterial infection or mumps.

Scrotal haematoma, usually related to trauma, is the next most common cause of acute scrotum. Rarely, haemorrhage into a testicular tumour may present with acute pain.

Ultrasound

(a) Epididymo-orchitis:

- Enlarged, hypoechoic epididymis.

- Enlarged, hypoechoic testis.

- Fluid around the testis.

- Increased blood flow in the testis/epididymis on colour Doppler.

- Abscess formation: intra- or extratesticular.

(b) Torsion:

- Testis may be normal in appearance or enlarged and hypoechoic.

- Epididymis usually enlarged and hypoechoic.

- Decreased spermatic cord Doppler signal.

- Lack of blood flow in the testis on colour Doppler.

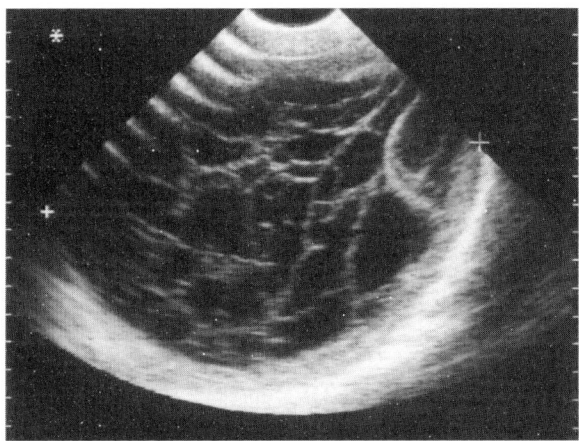

Figure 6.16 *Scrotal haematoma.*
Large haematoma following trauma. Note the multiple echogenic septations.

(c) Haematoma:

- Hypoechoic collection with loculations and septations (*Fig. 6.16*).

- Reduction in size over time.

- Chronic haematomas may calcify producing hyperechoic areas with shadowing.

Scintigraphy

- Very quick method (takes about 10 minutes).

- Inject ^{99m}Tc-pertechnetate and take images during perfusion and serial static images for 10 minutes.

- Epididymo-orchitis: increased uptake.

- Torsion: Well-defined area of decreased uptake, sometimes with a surrounding 'halo' of increased uptake on the static images (*Fig. 6.17*).

Adrenal imaging

CT

CT is the investigation of choice for imaging the adrenal glands. This includes fine sections pre- and post-contrast injection. Scintigraphy may occasionally

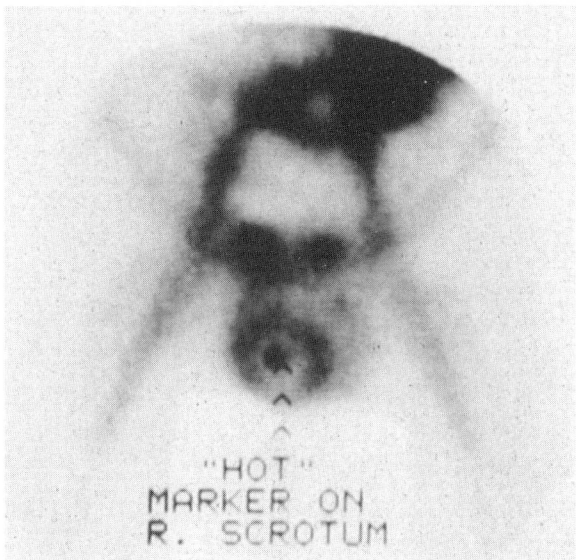

Figure 6.17 *Testicular torsion – scintigraphy.*
^{99m}Tc-pertechnetate. A 'hot' marker has been placed on the right scrotum as indicated. Surrounding the marker is a halo of increased activity indicating peripheral hyperaemia. The central 'cold' area within the halo represents the non-perfused testicle.

be useful. Whilst adrenal masses may be seen on US, CT is more accurate for diagnosis and characterisation (*Fig. 6.18*). More specialised techniques, such as adrenal vein sampling and percutaneous biopsy, may rarely be required.

Indications for adrenal imaging:

(a) Endocrine syndromes.

- Cushing syndrome.

- Conn syndrome.

- Phaeochromocytoma.

- Primary adrenal insufficiency.

(b) Neoplasms with a high incidence of spread to the adrenals, especially lung and breast.

(c) Miscellaneous indications.

- Investigation of calcification seen on AXR.

- Neonatal haemorrhage.

- Palpable mass.

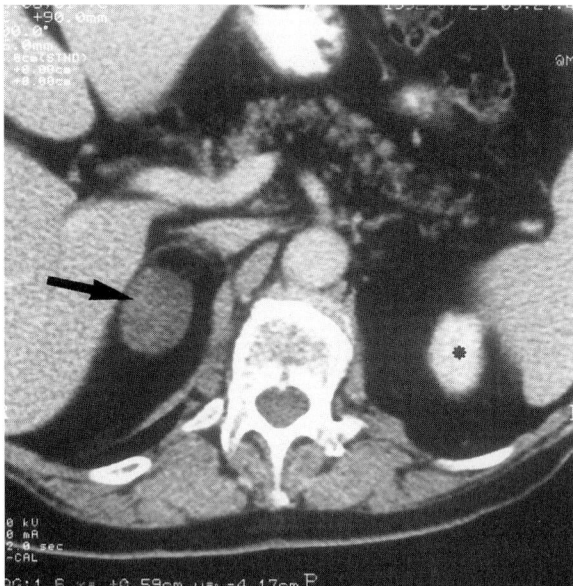

Figure 6.18 *Adrenal adenoma – CT.*
There is an adenoma of the right adrenal gland (arrow).
The upper pole of the left kidney is also seen on this
section (*). Note the CT features of adrenal adenoma:
* *small size*
* *smooth contour*
* *low attenuation.*

In the above situations, and in incidental adrenal masses seen on CT, it is important to differentiate benign from malignant, specifically adrenal adenoma from adrenal metastasis or carcinoma. It should be noted that about 50% of adrenal masses seen in patients with primary carcinoma elsewhere are in fact benign adenomas, not metastases.

CT features of benign non-hyperfunctioning adrenal adenomas:

* Size < 3 cm.

* Well-defined, smooth contour.

* Low density on unenhanced scans.

CT features of carcinoma:

* Size > 5 cm.

* Higher density on unenhanced scans.

* Low density centrally due to necrosis.

* Direct evidence of malignancy: liver metastases, lymphadenopathy, venous invasion.

CT features of a metastasis:

* Tend to be larger though size not a reliable indicator.

* Higher density on unenhanced scans.

* When an adrenal mass is the only evidence of metastasis in a patient with a lung, breast, or other primary tumour, percutaneous biopsy under CT guidance is often required for definitive diagnosis.

Cushing syndrome

(a) Bilateral adrenal hyperplasia (70%).

* Normal appearance or diffuse thickening of limbs of both adrenals.

(b) Unilateral adrenocortical adenoma (20%).

* Small well-defined mass usually < 5 cm.

(c) Adrenal carcinoma (10%).

* Mass usually > 5 cm.

* Central necrosis.

* Metastatic spread: liver metastases, lymphadenopathy.

Primary hyperaldosteronism (Conn syndrome)

* Solitary unilateral adenoma (70%) – usually a small mass of 1–2 cm.

* Multiple adenomas (20%).

* Bilateral adrenal hyperplasia (10%).

* Adrenal carcinoma (rare).

* When bilateral disease is seen or suspected on CT, or when CT is normal, bilateral selective adrenal vein sampling for aldosterone levels may be helpful to localise a small abnormality and therefore guide surgery.

Phaeochromocytoma

* Presents in two situations:

(i) Symptomatology related to excess catecholamine production: paroxysmal or sustained hypertension, headaches, sweating, flushing, nausea and vomiting, abdominal pain.

(ii) Part of a syndrome, e.g. multiple endocrine neoplasia, familial phaeochromocytomas, tuberous sclerosis, von Hippel–Lindau disease, neurofibromatosis.

- 10% multiple.
- 10% malignant.
- 10% extra-adrenal.
- 90% occur in adrenal medulla.
  (i) Usually large tumours up to 12 cm, average around 5 cm.
  (ii) Intravenous contrast use is not recommended in patients when phaeochromocytoma is suspected as it may precipitate a hypertensive crisis unless alpha-adrenergic blocking drugs have been administered.
- When the adrenals are normal and phaeochromocytoma is suspected on clinical grounds, whole body scintigraphy with iodine labelled metaiodobenzylguanidine (^{131}I-/^{123}I-MIBG) is useful.

Primary adrenal insufficiency (Addison disease)

(a) Idiopathic adrenal atrophy most common cause (probably autoimmune).
- Adrenal glands reduced in size.

(b) Bilateral adrenal haemorrhage.
- *Newborn:* birth trauma, hypoxia, sepsis.
- *Adults:* anticoagulation therapy, sepsis, surgery, trauma.
- *CT:* high attenuation mass in acute haemorrhage.

(c) TB/sarcoid.
- Soft tissue masses.
- Cysts.
- Calcification.

Myelolipoma

- Benign cortical neoplasm containing myeloid tissue and fat.
- Asymptomatic: usually incidental finding on US or CT.

(a) *US:*
- Well-defined hyperechoic mass.

(b) *CT:*
- Low-attenuation fat content well seen on CT.

Interventional radiology of the urinary tract

Percutaneous nephrostomy

Indications:
- Relief of urinary tract obstruction.
  (i) Stones (*Fig. 6.19*).
  (ii) Carcinoma: bladder, ureteric TCC, prostate.

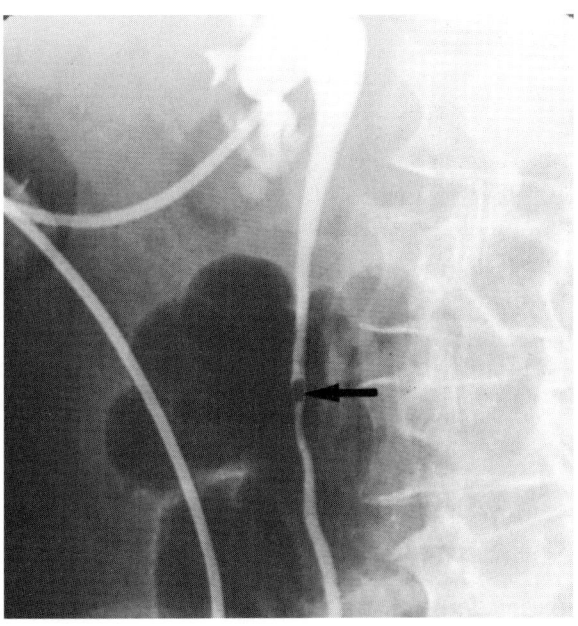

Figure 6.19 *Ureteric calculus – nephrostogram. Nephrostomy inserted for relief of right renal obstruction due to a ureteric calculus. Nephrostogram performed several days later shows the nephrostomy tube well positioned and the calculus in the ureter (arrow).*

- Pyonephrosis.
- Leakage of urine from upper urinary tract post-surgery or trauma.

Contraindications:

- Bleeding diathesis.

Technique:

- Local anaesthetic and sedation usually adequate; may require general anaesthetic in children or complicated cases.
- Antibiotic cover.
- Perform with US and fluoroscopic guidance or under CT control.
- Puncture collecting system; pass wire; dilate tract; insert nephrostomy over wire.

Complications:

- *Haematuria:* usually mild and transitory and occurs in most patients.
- *Vascular trauma:* very rare with imaging guidance.

Ureteric stents

Indications:

- Malignant obstruction of urinary tract: bladder/prostate/cervix.
- Pelviureteric junction obstruction.
- Other benign obstructions of the urinary tract, e.g. retroperitoneal fibrosis, radiotherapy.
- Post-ureteric surgery.
- Extracorporeal shockwave lithotripsy (ESWL) of large renal calculi.
  (i) Promote passage of fragments.
  (ii) Relieve ureteric obstruction by fragments.

Technique:

- Retrograde insertion via cystoscopy.
- Antegrade insertion: puncture kidney; guide wire passed down ureter into bladder; stent over guide wire pushed into position.

- Upper pigtail should lie in the renal pelvis or upper pole calyx; lower pigtail should lie in the bladder.

Extracorporeal shockwave lithotripsy (ESWL).

- Technique of choice for most renal stones.
- Stone localised by fluoroscopy and/or US.

Percutaneous nephrolithotomy (PCNL)

Indications:

- Failed ESWL.
- Staghorn calculus.
- Cysteine, matrix calculus.

Technique:

- General anaesthetic.
- Insert retrograde catheter.
  (i) Opacify collecting system.
  (ii) Prevent calculus fragments passing down ureter.
- Puncture collecting system: pass guide wire; dilate tract, stone extracted by endoscopist.

Renal artery interventions: percutaneous transluminal angioplasty (PTA) and stent insertion

Indications:

- Renal artery stenosis.
- Three types of renal artery lesions are seen:
  (i) Atheroma at the artery origin, i.e. ostial lesion.
  (ii) Distal atheroma.
  (iii) Fibromuscular hyperplasia.
- Goals of treatment:
  (i) Normal blood pressure.
  (ii) Hypertension able to be controlled medically.
  (iii) Improved renal function.

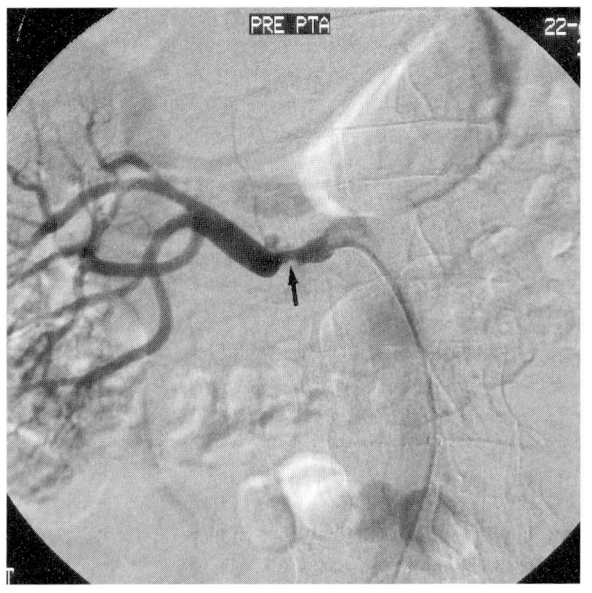 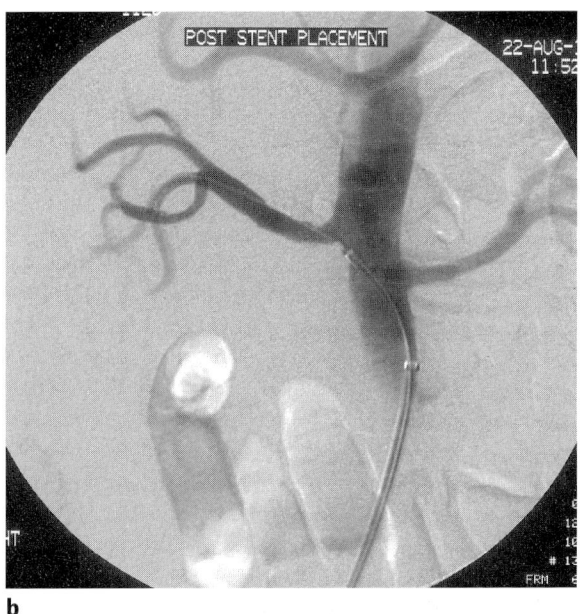

a   b

Figure 6.20 *Renal artery stent.*
(a) Angiogram shows a localised stenosis of the right renal artery (arrow). (b) Following stent deployment the stenosis is no longer seen.

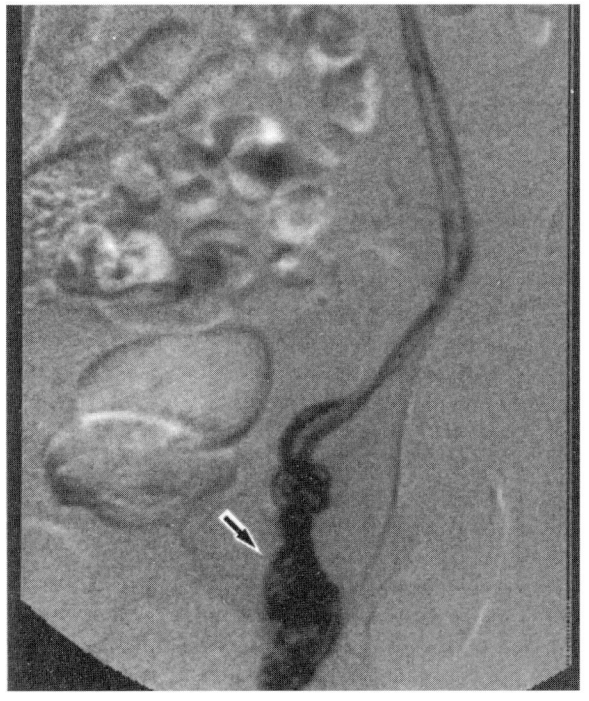 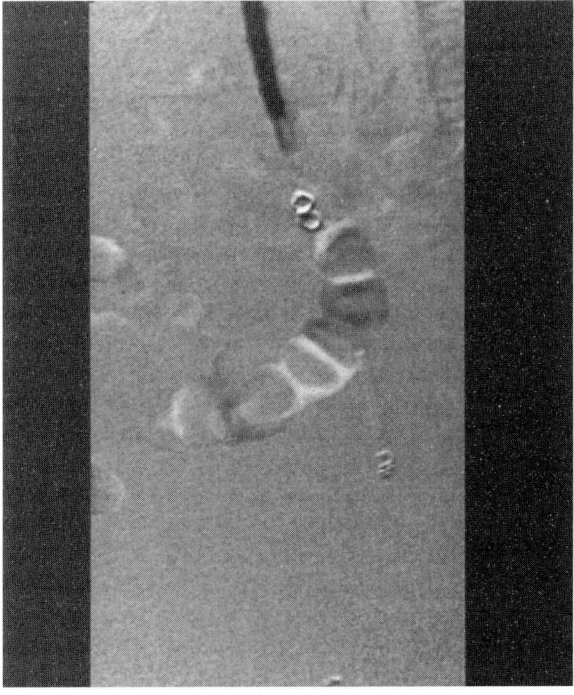

a   b

Figure 6.21 *Embolisation of varicocele.*
(a) Pre-embolisation. The varicocele is seen as a nest of tortuous dilated veins (arrow) filling from the left spermatic vein. (b) Post-embolisation. Good result with non-filling of the varicocele.

Technique:

- Most lesions are initially treated with PTA though stents are now being more frequently used, especially in the following situations:
  (i)   Ostial lesion.
  (ii) Early or late restenosis following PTA.
  (iii) Complicated PTA, e.g. arterial dissection (*Fig. 6.20*).

- Advantages of stents:
  (i)   Better technical results.
  (ii) Lower rate of restenosis, particularly in ostial/severe disease.

- Disadvantages of stents:
  (i)   More invasive complex procedure with a large arterial sheath required.
  (ii) Stent positioning is critical.
  (iii) Higher cost.

Renal artery embolisation

Indications:

- Control of bleeding, e.g. post-surgery, post-biopsy, trauma.

- Treatment of AVM and fistulae (most commonly seen post-biopsy, nephrostomy, etc.).

- Palliation/pre-operative reduction of renal tumour.

Testicular vein embolisation

Indications:

- Varicocele associated with infertility.

- Large varicocele with normal fertility.

Technique:

- Femoral vein puncture.

- Diagnostic venography of renal and testicular veins.

- Embolisation of testicular vein and collateral channels, usually with steel coils (*Fig. 6.21*).

Further Reading

1. Amis ES Jr. (ed.). Contemporary uroradiology. *Radiological Clinics of North America* 1991; **29**:3.

2. Korobkin M, Francis IR. Adrenal imaging. *Seminars in US, CT, and MRI* 1995; **16**: 317–330.

3. Lemaitre L, Claudon M, Dubrelle F, Mazeman E. Imaging of angiomyolipomas. *Seminars in US, CT, and MRI* 1997; **18**:100–114.

4. Pollack HM, Resnick MI. Prostate-specific antigen and screening for prostate cancer: much ado about something. *Radiology* 1993; **189**:353–356.

5. Rifkin MD, Dahnert W, Kurtz AB. State of the art: endorectal sonography of the prostate gland. *AJR* 1990; **154**:691–700.

7 Breast

Investigation of a breast lump

Mammography

- First investigation of choice in women over 30 years of age.

- Screening: non-palpable mass in asymptomatic woman.

- Diagnostic: palpable mass or mass found on a mammogram done for other reasons, e.g. nipple discharge, search for a primary tumour where metastases are found elsewhere.

- Two standard views: craniocaudad and lateral oblique.

- A range of further views may be used to delineate an abnormality seen on the two standard views; these include spot compression, magnification, craniocaudad angulated medially or laterally.

Mammography: features of a benign mass

- The two most common benign masses seen on mammography are simple cyst and fibroadenoma (*Fig. 7.1*).

- Round or oval in shape.

- Well circumscribed.

- Homogeneous; usually low or medium density, i.e. normal structures can be seen through the mass.

- 'Halo' – a lucent line around all or part of the boundary of a mass; may occasionally be seen with a malignant mass, so must be interpreted with caution.

- Radiological size equal to, or greater than, clinical size.

- Benign calcification of which many patterns may be seen:
  - (i) Cyst: thin rim peripherally; fluid layer due to precipitated calcium in cyst fluid (milk of calcium).
  - (ii) Fibroadenoma: calcify with involution after menopause; 'popcorn' calcification or well-defined peripheral calcification (*Fig. 7.2*).

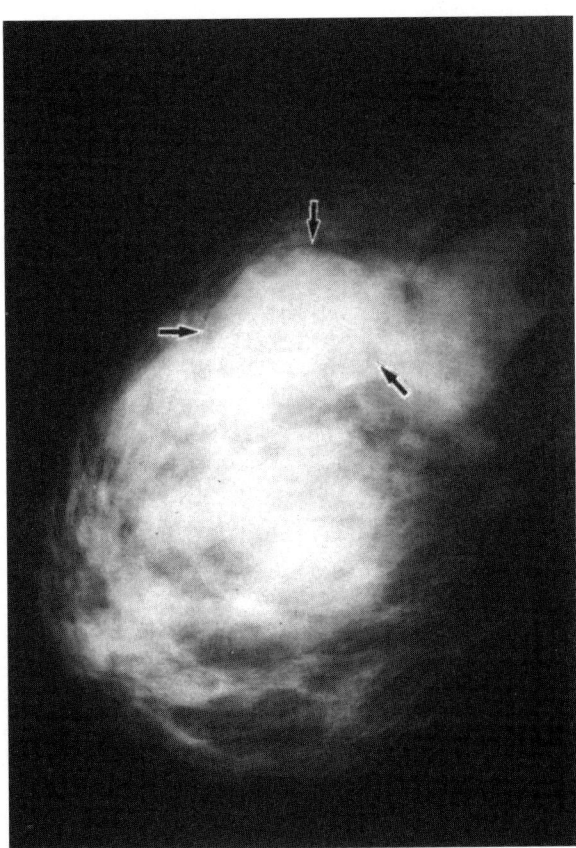

Figure 7.1 *Simple cysts.*
Multiple well circumscribed lesions. Note: lucent 'halo' around part of the upper cyst (arrows).

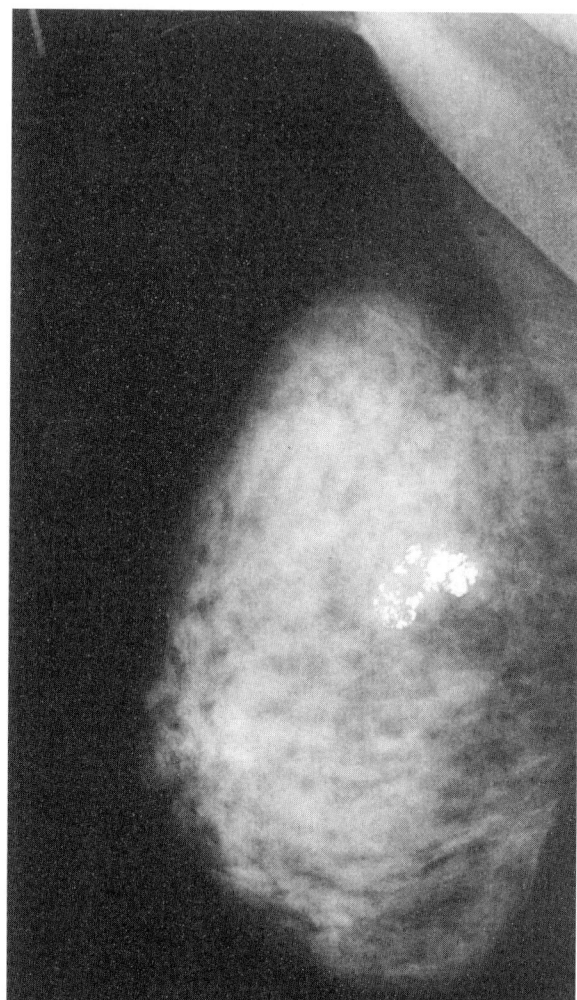

Figure 7.2 Benign calcification.
'Pop corn' type calcification in a fibroadenoma.

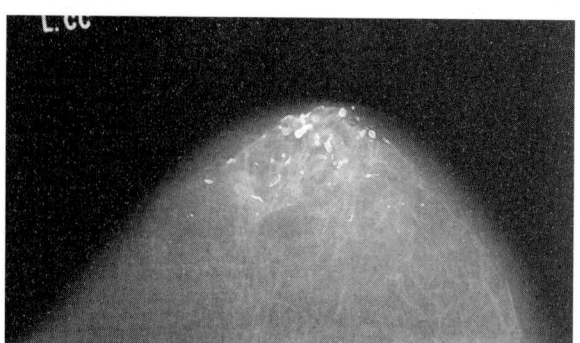

Figure 7.3 Benign calcification.
Dense calcification in dilated ducts near the nipple.
Pattern typical of periductal inflammatory disease.

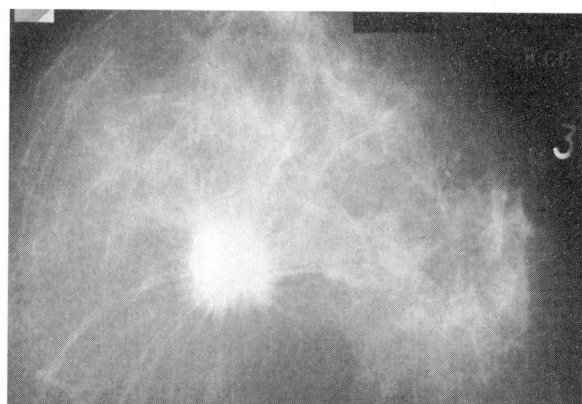

Figure 7.4 Carcinoma.
Typical appearance of a large carcinoma. Dense mass
with a spiculated, ill-defined margin.

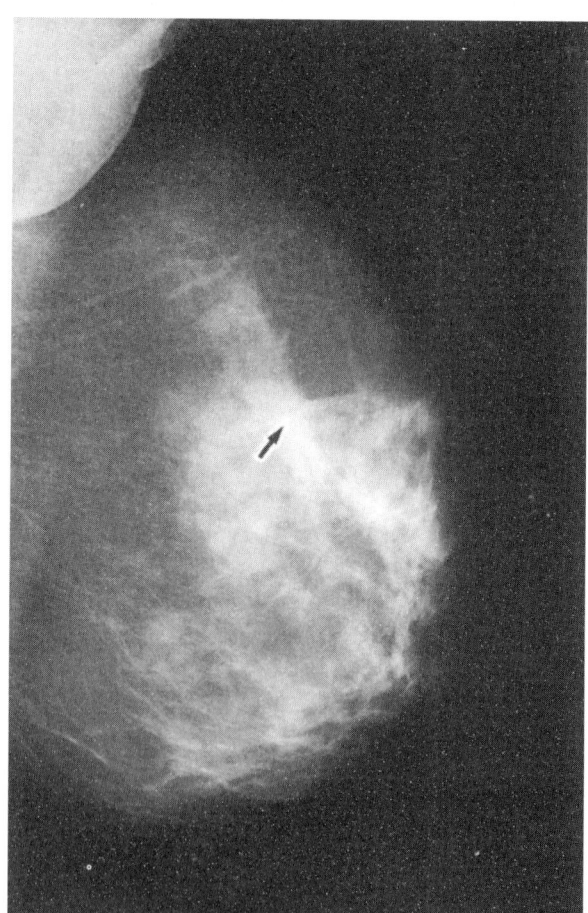

Figure 7.5 Carcinoma.
This is an example of distortion of breast architecture
caused by a small carcinoma (arrow).

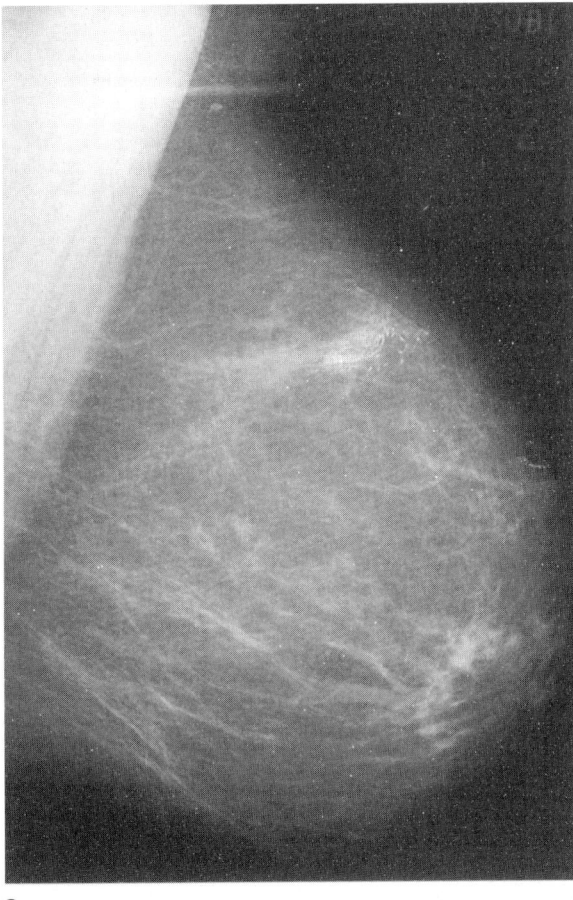

a

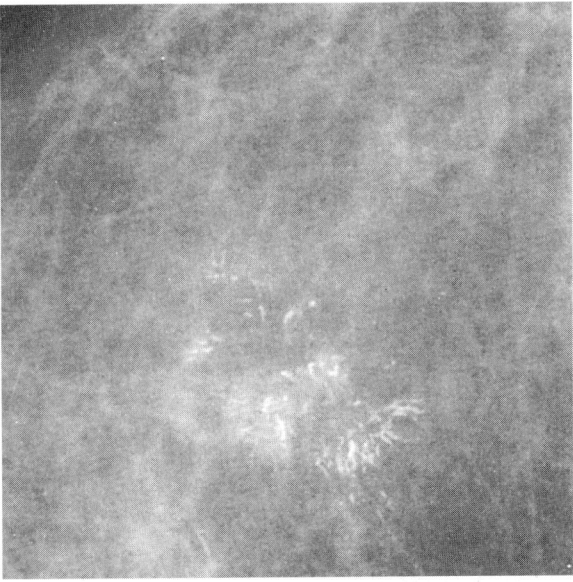

b

Figure 7.6 *Malignant calcification.*
Typical clusters of branching, ductal or 'casting' type classifications. Note that the calcification is irregular in outline and of variable shape and density.

(iii) Arterial calcification.

(iv) Duct ectasia (secretory disease): rod-like well-defined calcification in an obvious ductal orientation toward the nipple (*Fig. 7.3*).

(v) Cysts, adenosis, hyperplasia: multiple, tiny, pinpoint calcifications; milk of calcium in tiny cysts with multiple small fluid levels on the oblique view ('tea cupping').

Mammography: features of a malignant mass

- Irregular outline:

    (a) Spiculated (*Fig. 7.4*).

    (b) Indistinct.

    (c) Microlobulated.

- Often high density, i.e. normal structures cannot be seen through the mass.

- Non-homogeneous.

- Disruption of surrounding architecture: architectural distortion (*Fig. 7.5*).

- Radiological size less than clinical size.

- Secondary signs: increased vascularity, skin thickening, nipple retraction.

- Malignant microcalcification:

    (i) Irregular.

    (ii) Variable shape and size.

    (iii) Branching, ductal pattern, i.e. 'casting'.

    (iv) Grouped in clusters.

    (v) Variable density (*Fig. 7.6*).

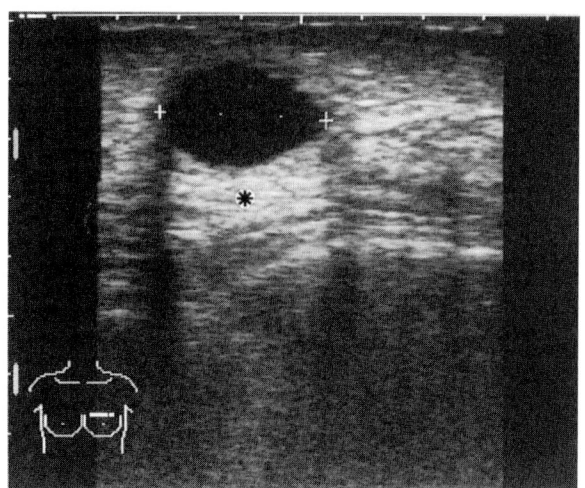

Figure 7.7 *Simple cyst – ultrasound. Anechoic lesion with sharply defined posterior wall. Note acoustic enhancement (*).*

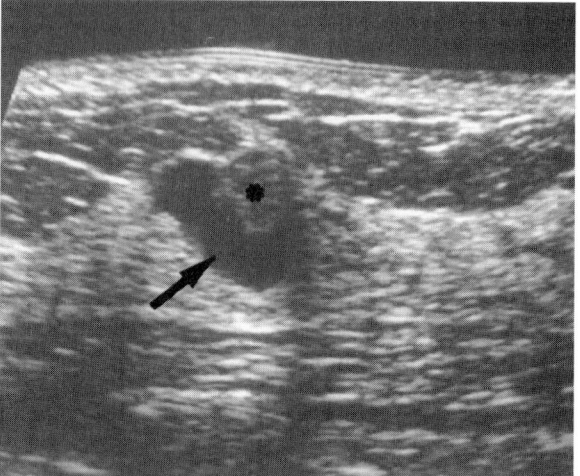

Figure 7.8 *Tumour in a cyst – US. Note the following features:*
- *anechoic cyst (arrow)*
- *small soft tissue mass in the wall of the cyst (*)*
- *small papilloma excised following fine needle aspiration biopsy.*

Ultrasound

- High resolution US now has multiple roles in breast imaging.

- First investigation of choice for a palpable breast lump in a woman under 30 years of age.

- The traditional role for US has been differentiating cystic from solid lesions seen on mammography or found on palpation.

- As well as diagnosing cysts, US is useful for providing further definition of solid masses.

- US is also useful for assessment of mammographically dense breasts where small masses or cysts may be obscured by overlying breast tissue.

- Guidance of cyst aspiration, needle biopsy, drainage placement.

- US is not used to assess microcalcification.

(a) US features of a simple cyst:

- Anechoic contents.

- Low-level internal echoes may be seen due to infection, haemorrhage, cellular or proteinaceous debris.

- Smooth walls.

- Sharp anterior and posterior borders.

- Posterior acoustic enhancement; may not be seen in deep cysts near the chest wall (*Fig. 7.7*).

(b) US features of an intracystic tumour (benign or malignant):

- Soft tissue mass (*Fig. 7.8*).

- Cyst wall thickening and irregularity.

- Soft tissue septum.

(c) US features of a carcinoma:

- Irregular infiltrative margin.

- Central hypoechoic or heterogeneous nidus.

- Surrounding hyperechoic halo.

- Acoustic shadow (*Fig. 7.9*).

(d) US features of a fibroadenoma:

- Well-defined, oval, lobulated mass.

- Mostly hypoechoic.

- Variable acoustic enhancement.

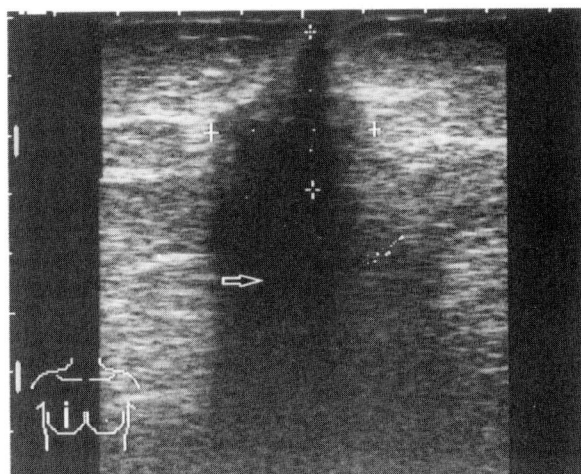

Figure 7.9 *Carcinoma – ultrasound.*
Hypoechoic lesion with an irregular margin. Note
acoustic shadow (arrow).

Breast biopsy

Fine-needle aspiration (FNA)

- Minimally invasive.

- 20–25 gauge needle.

- Quick, relatively inexpensive.

- Requires experienced cytopathologist.

- Often non-specific report such as 'no malignant cells seen'.

Core biopsy

- Best results obtained with 14 gauge core biopsy needle used with automated core biopsy 'gun'.

- When biopsying calcification, may combine with specimen radiography to confirm calcifications within the specimen.

- Definitive histological diagnosis usually obtained.

Mammotome

- Consists of a probe which is positioned in or near a breast mass or area of calcification.

- A vacuum pulls a small sample of breast tissue into the probe.

- This is cut off and transported back through the probe into a specimen chamber.

- Particularly useful for microcalcification.

- Performed under mammographic control.

Open surgical biopsy

- Non-palpable masses may be localised under US or mammographic control prior to surgery; suspicious microcalcifications may be localised under mammographic control.

- A needle containing a hook shaped wire is positioned in or near the breast lesion.

- Once correct positioning is attained, the needle is withdrawn leaving the wire in place.

- US or mammography of the excised specimen is performed to ensure that the mass or calcifications have been removed.

Imaging guidance

- The mammotome is positioned using stereotactic mammography.

- FNA or core needles may be positioned using US or mammography.

- For microcalcification, mammography will be used.

- For most masses, US is the quickest and most accurate method.

- With the 'freehand' technique, the US probe is held in one hand and the needle in the other; the needle is guided into the mass under direct US visualisation (*Fig. 7.10*).

Management of a cyst

Guided aspiration

If it is non-palpable, a cyst may be aspirated under ultrasound control; FNA of any soft tissue component may be performed at this time.

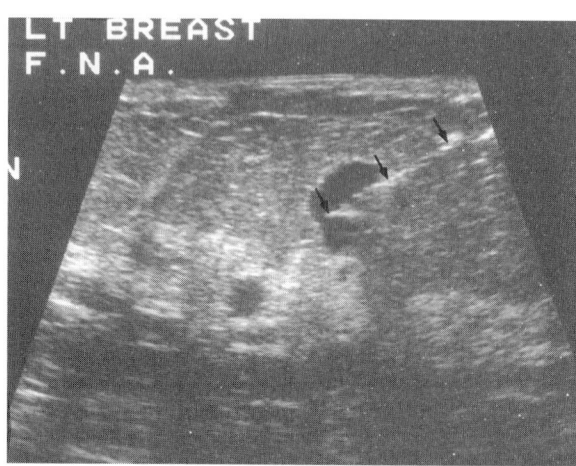

Figure 7.10 *Fine-needle aspiration – FNA.*
FNA of a breast cyst. The needle is well seen with its tip positioned in the cyst (arrows).

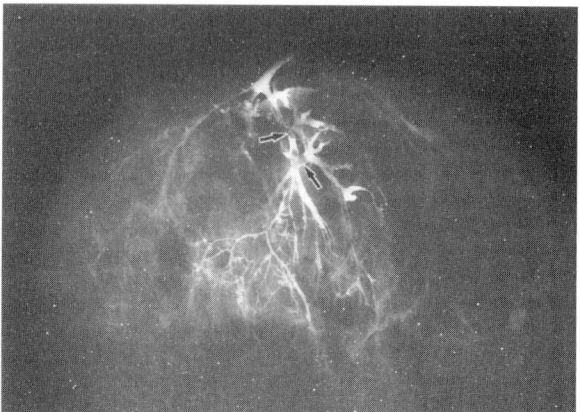

Figure 7.11 *Duct papillomas.*
The ducts show variable dilatation. The papillomas are seen as filling defects within the ducts.

Pneumocystography

- May be used in the assessment of a complicated cyst.
- After the cyst fluid is aspirated, an equal amount of air is injected into the cyst cavity.
- The procedure may be diagnostic or therapeutic.

(a) Diagnostic:

- After the air is injected, mammographic views are performed.
- A tumour in the wall of the cyst will show as a soft tissue mass projecting into the air-filled cyst.

(b) Therapeutic:

- There is a lower cyst recurrence rate following pneumocystography.

Investigation of nipple discharge

Radiological investigation is particularly useful if the discharge is either unilateral, from a single duct, or blood-stained.

Mammography

Galactography

- Duct orifice is gently cannulated and a small amount of contrast injected.
- A small amount of fluid can usually be 'milked' as a guide to which duct to inject; also, the offending duct is usually slightly dilated.
- Intraduct papilloma shows as a smooth or irregular filling defect; may be multiple (*Fig. 7.11*).
- Invasive carcinoma shows as an irregular duct narrowing with distal dilatation.

Brief notes on breast screening

- Mammographic screening is of benefit in reducing mortality in the over-50 age group. Recent literature would suggest a benefit also for the 40–49 age group.
- Aim to reduce mortality in the 55–69 age group.
- A dedicated team is essential, comprising radiographer, radiologist, surgeon, pathologist and counselling nurse.

- X-ray mammography is the initial screening test of choice and strict quality control over equipment, film processing, and training of personnel is essential to provide optimum images and maximise diagnostic efficiency.

- An abnormality on initial screening leads to recall and a second stage of investigation comprising:
  (i) Ultrasound.
  (ii) Further mammographic views including magnification.
  (iii) Clinical assessment.
  (iv) Fine-needle aspiration or core biopsy.
  (v) Radiological localisation and surgical biopsy where percutaneous techniques are unhelpful, especially areas of suspicious microcalcification.

- If, after this second stage, a lesion is found to be malignant, the patient is referred for surgery; if benign, she is brought back for routine screening. Indeterminate lesions would usually undergo open biopsy or be reassessed after one year.

Further Reading

1. Gordon PB, Goldenberg SL, Chan NHL. Solid breast lesions: diagnosis with US-guided fine-needle aspiration biopsy. *Radiology* 1993; **189**:573–580.

2. Jackson VP (ed.). Breast imaging. *Radiological Clinics of North America* 1995; **33**(6).

3. Jackson VP, Reynolds HE, Hawes DR. Sonography of the breast. *Seminars in US, CT, and MRI* 1996; **17**: 460–475.

8 Cardiovascular system

General investigation of cardiac disease

CXR

* The most common use of plain films in cardiac disease is in the assessment of cardiac failure and its treatment.
* CXR signs of cardiac failure include:
  (i)   *Cardiac enlargement:* cardiothoracic ratio is unreliable as a one-off measurement; of more significance is an increase in heart size on serial CXR, or a transverse diameter of greater than 15.5 cm in adult males or 14.5 cm in adult females.
  (ii) *Pulmonary venous hypertension:* upper lobe blood vessels larger than those in the lower lobes.
  (iii) *Interstitial oedema:* reticular (linear) pattern with Kerley-B lines, i.e. thin lines predominantly in the lower lobes extending 1–2 cm horizontally inwards from the pleural surface of the lung (*Fig. 8.1*).
  (iv) *Alveolar oedema:* fluffy, ill-defined areas of consolidation in a perihilar or 'bat's-wing' distribution (*Fig. 8.2*).
  (v)   *Pleural effusions:* right larger than left.

* Signs of specific chamber enlargement:
  (i)   *Right atrium:* bulging right heart border.
  (ii) *Left atrium:* prominent left auricle on the left heart border; double outline of the right heart border; splayed carina; bulge of the posterior heart border (*Fig. 8.3*).
  (iii) *Right ventricle:* elevated cardiac apex; bulging of anterior upper part of the heart border on the lateral view.
  (iv) *Left ventricle:* bulging lower left cardiac border with depressed cardiac apex.

* Valve calcification (*Fig. 8.4*).

* Changes of pulmonary vasculature:
  (i)   *Oligaemia,* i.e. decreased pulmonary blood flow as occurs in pulmonary hypertension and in right outflow tract obstruction, e.g. Fallot tetralogy, Ebstein anomaly, pulmonary atresia, tricuspid atresia.
  (ii) *Plethora,* i.e. increased pulmonary blood flow as occurs with left to right shunts such as ASD, VSD, and PDA.

* Rib notching: due to enlarged tortuous intercostal arteries associated with coarctation of the aorta (*Fig. 8.5*).

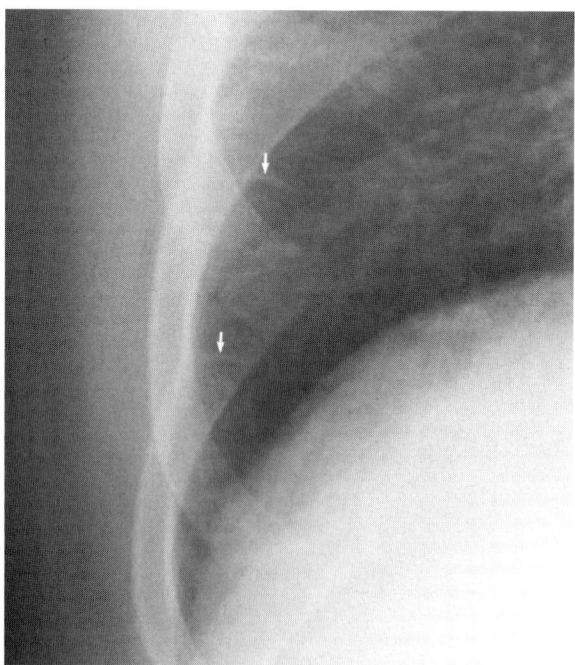

Figure 8.1 *Kerley-B lines – interstitial oedema. Short, horizontal lines extending to the pleural surface (arrows).*

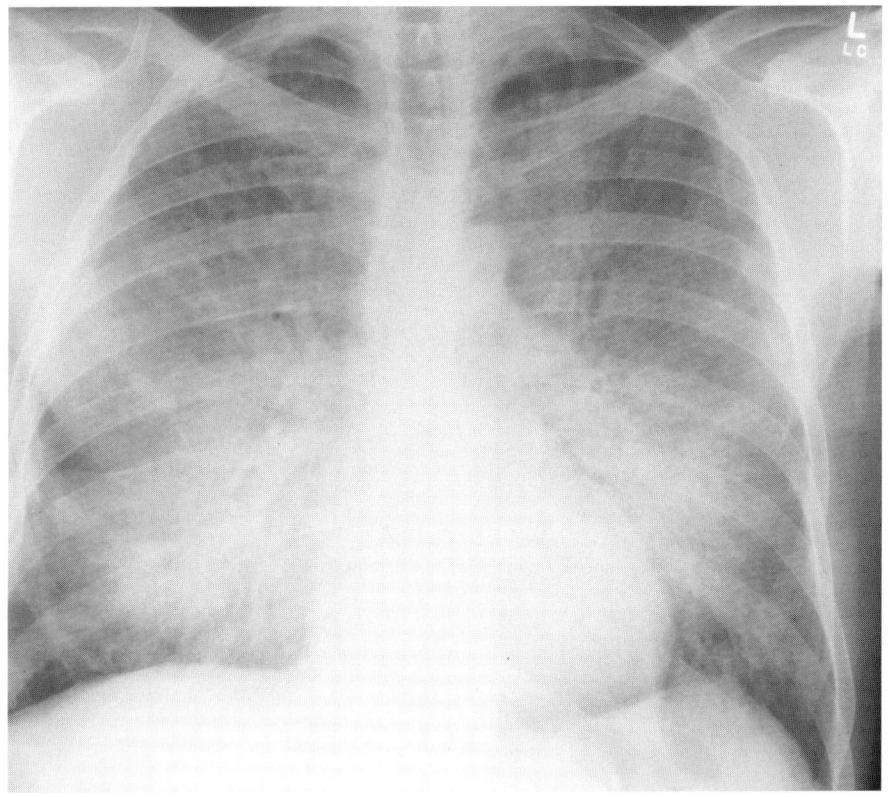

Figure 8.2 *Congestive cardiac failure. Note extensive bilateral alveolar shadowing in keeping with pulmonary oedema.*

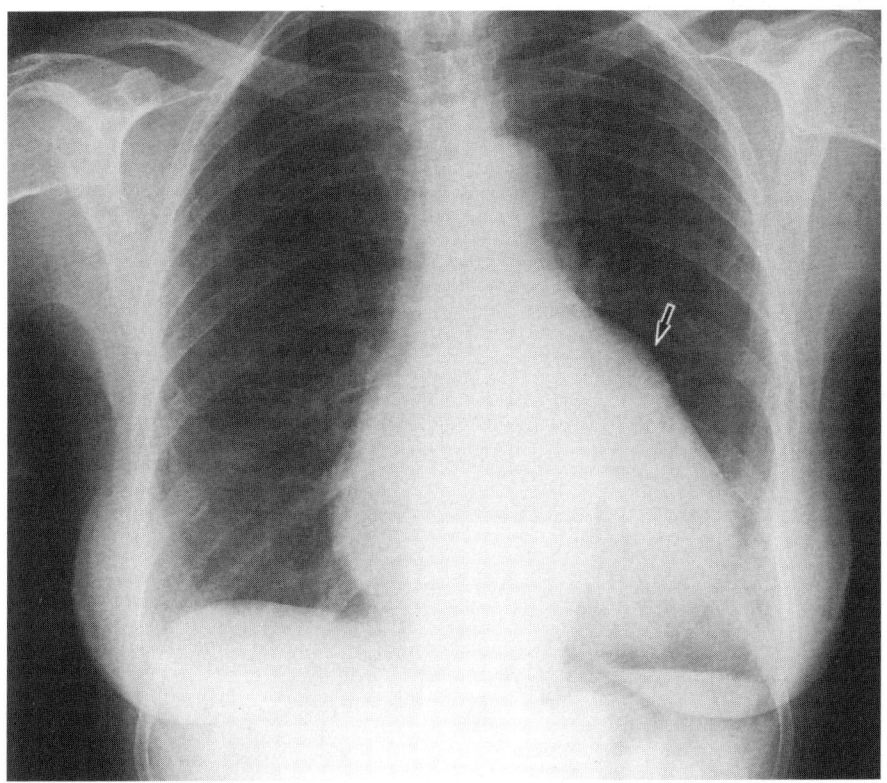

Figure 8.3 *Left atrial enlargement. Bulge of the upper left cardiac border (arrow) due to prominence of the left atrial appendage in a patient with mitral valve disease.*

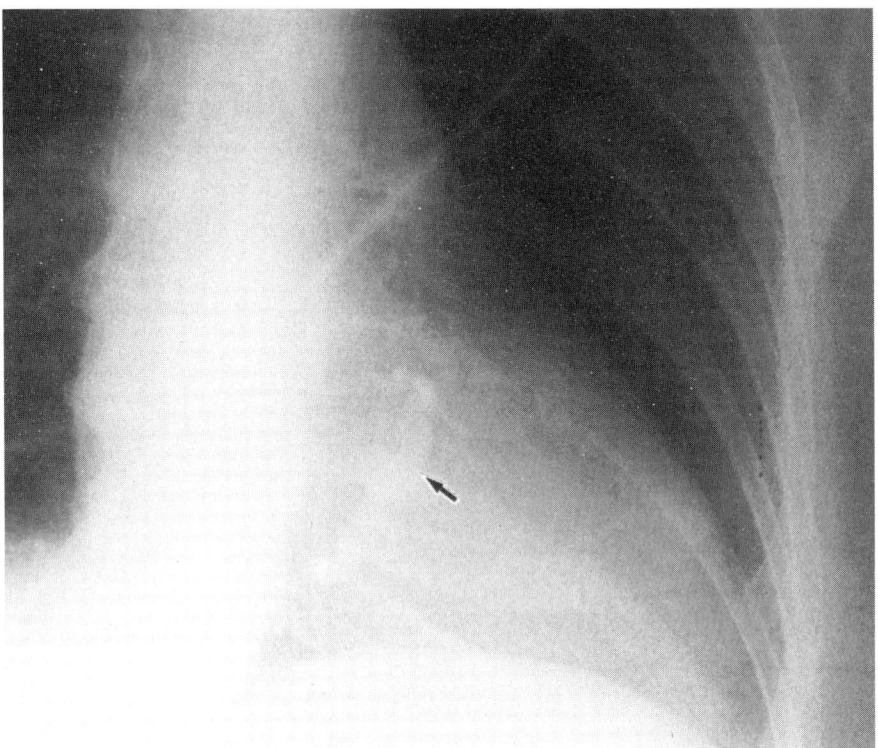

Figure 8.4 *Mitral valve annulus calcification. Dense calcification in the mitral valve (arrow).*

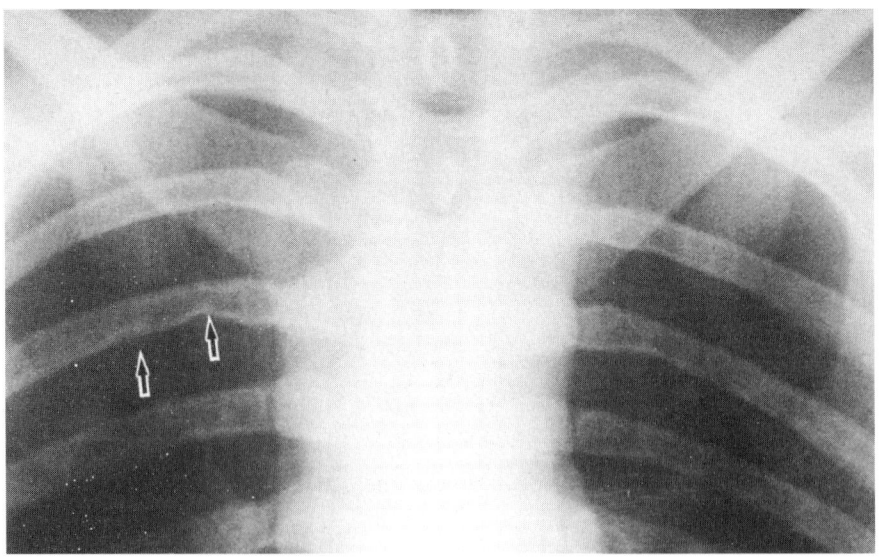

Figure 8.5 *Coarctation of the aorta.*
Rib notching (arrows) due to hypertrophy and tortuosity of the intercostal arteries.

Echocardiography

(a) M-Mode:

- Movement of valves.

- Chamber size.

- Ventricular wall thickness and motion.

(b) Two-dimensional imaging:

- Cardiac anatomy.

- Ventricular wall movement.

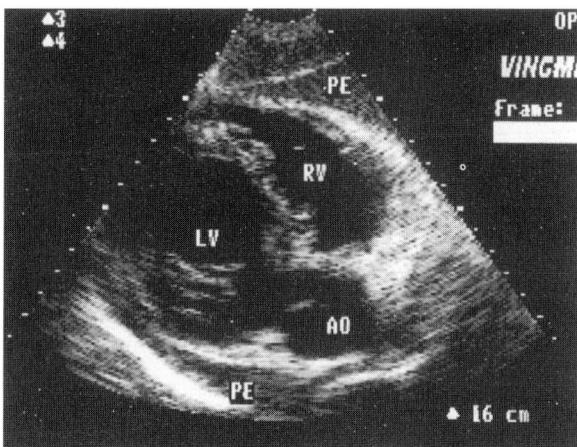

Figure 8.6 *Pericardial effusion – echocardiogram.*
Note the following:
- *pericardial effusion seen as a hypoechoic rim surrounding the heart (PE)*
- *right ventricle (RV)*
- *left ventricle (LV)*
- *aortic root (AO).*

- Valvular disease.
- Pericardial effusion (*Fig. 8.6*).
- Cardiac masses.

(c) Doppler studies including colour Doppler imaging:

- Valvular disease including quantitation of pressure gradients.
- Calculation of cardiac output.
- Congenital heart disease.
- Post-surgical (paravalvular/paraprosthetic leaks).

(d) Transesophageal echocardiography (TEE):

- The main problem with ultrasound techniques is interference from the bony thoracic cage and air-filled lung, especially in elderly or emphysematous patients.
- This problem is overcome by transesophageal probes which offer direct contact and excellent visualisation through the left atrium.
- Most useful applications include acute aortic dissection, endocarditis, congenital heart disease, and paraprosthetic leaks.

(e) Contrast agents:

- Contrast agents currently under development may allow echocardiographic differentiation of viable from non-viable myocardium.

MRI

Advantages:

- No radiation or iodinated contrast media.
- Good tissue characterisation.
- Multiplanar imaging.
- No interference from bone or air.

Applications:

- Cardiac function: calculation of ejection fraction, chamber volumes, stroke volumes and myocardial mass.
- Congenital heart disease: multiplanar imaging allows even very complex malformations to be imaged.
- Cardiomyopathies.
- Pericardial disease.
- Post-surgery: valve prosthesis assessment; bypass graft patency.
- Great vessel disease, e.g. aortic dissection, coarctation.
- Cardiac masses (*Fig. 8.7*).

Scintigraphy

Multiple-gated acquisition scan

- ^{99m}Tc-labelled red blood cells.
- Ejection fraction calculation.
- Regional wall motion analysis.
- Most common indications include:
  (i) Coronary artery disease.
  (ii) Drug-induced cardiomyopathy, most commonly doxorubicin (Adriamycin).
  (iii) Other cardiomyopathies.
  (iv) Chronic aortic regurgitation.

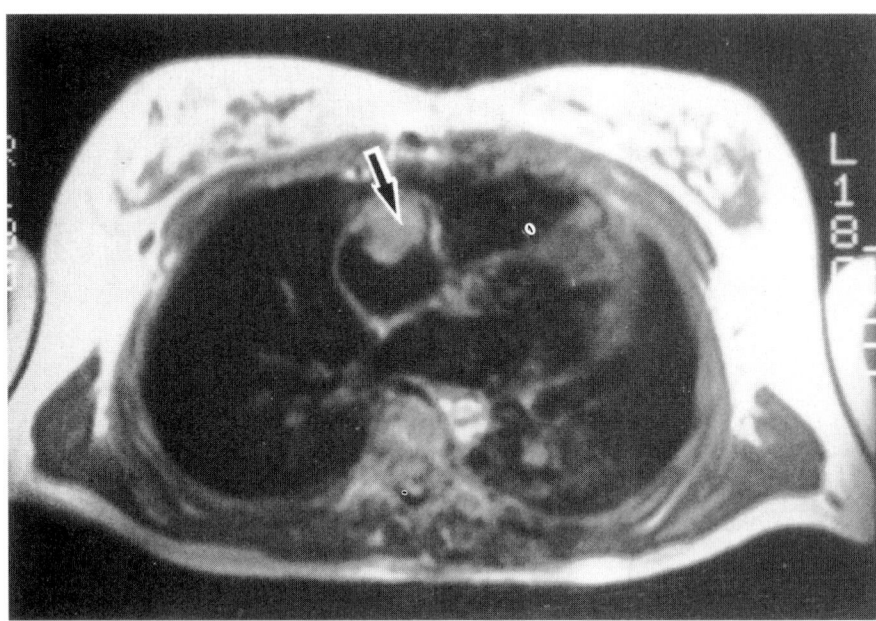

Figure 8.7 *Angiosarcoma of the right atrium – MRI. Transverse MRI scan through the heart. The tumour is seen as a soft tissue mass in the anterior wall of the right atrium (arrow).*

(v)   Pre-operative evaluation of patients with known coronary artery disease for whom major surgery is planned.

Myocardial perfusion scintigraphy

- Indications include:
  (i)   Chest pain.
  (ii)   Acute myocardial infarct.
  (iii)   Coronary artery stenosis seen at angiography.
  (iv)   Evaluation post-treatment of coronary artery disease, i.e. after angioplasty or CABG.
  (v)   Evaluation of patients at high risk of coronary artery disease, especially pre-operatively.

- Thallium-201 (^{201}Tl), ^{99m}Tc methoxyisobutylisonitrile (sestamibi).

- Areas of ischaemia or infarction show as areas of decreased or no uptake, i.e. 'cold' spots (*Fig. 8.8*).

- Ischaemia: 'cold' spot on exercise; normal after 4 hours.

- Infarct: 'cold' spot on exercise and after 4 hours of rest.

Infarct imaging

- ^{99m}Tc-labelled phosphates.

- Infarct shows as an area of increased uptake, i.e. 'hot' spot.

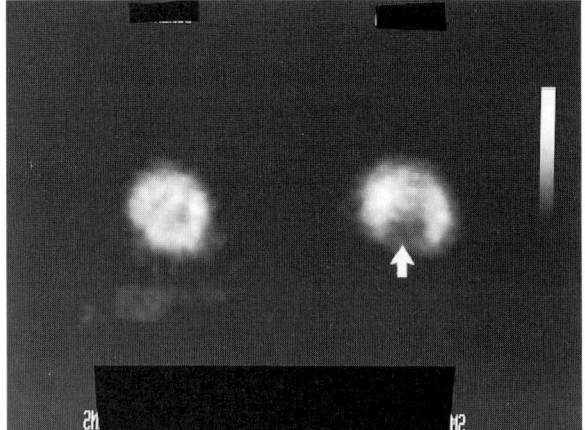

Figure 8.8 *Cardiac ischaemia – thallium scan. At rest (left) there is normal distribution of thallium. The exercise scan (right) shows a large defect at the cardiac apex indicating an area of ischaemia (arrow).*

Helical CT

- Coronary artery graft patency.

- Great vessel disease.

- Pericardial disease (*Fig. 8.9*).

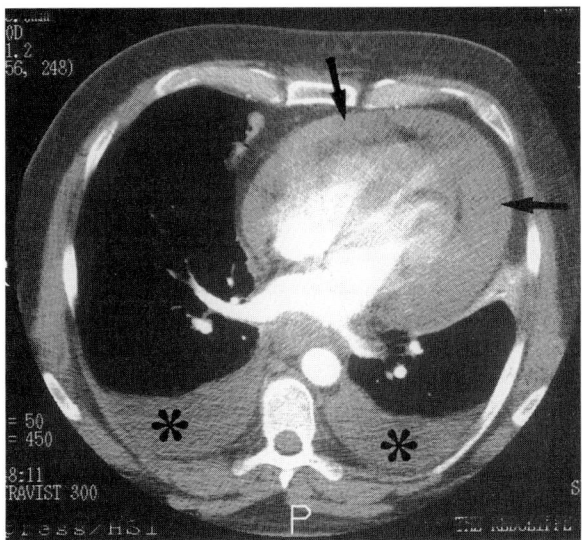

Figure 8.9 *Pericardial effusion – CT.*
Pericardial and pleural seeding from adenocarcinoma of
the colon. A large pericardial effusion is seen as a thick
rim of low attenuation fluid surrounding the heart
(arrows). There are also bilateral pleural effusions (*).

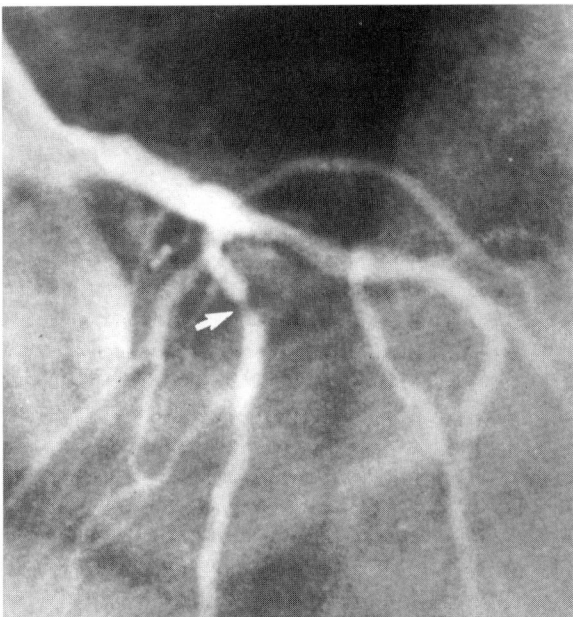

Figure 8.10 *Coronary artery stenosis.*
Left coronary angiogram shows a localised stenosis of
the anterior descending branch (arrow).

Ultrafast CT

- Not a widely used technique due to the high cost and limited availability of equipment.

- Where available, ultrafast CT is used for quantification of cardiac function including ejection fraction, chamber volumes, stroke volumes, and myocardial mass.

Angiocardiography

- Still investigation of choice for imaging coronary arteries (*Fig. 8.10*).

- Combined with angioplasty, stent placement, or streptokinase infusion.

- Indications for coronary artery angiography include:
  (i)   Angina, especially where risk factors such as cigarette smoking, positive family history, or hypercholesterolaemia are present.
  (ii) Following cardiac arrest
  (iii) Positive stress ECG or thallium scan.
  (iv) Occupation, e.g. airline pilot.

- To a large degree otherwise replaced by the other imaging modalities, though may be used in specific situations, especially to define complex congenital problems.

Abdominal aortic aneurysm (AAA)

CT

- Investigation of first choice for measurement, definition of anatomy, and diagnosis of complications such as leakage, hydronephrosis, etc.

- Anatomy of aneurysm:
  (i)   Shape.
  (ii) Size.
  (iii) Relationship to renal arteries and aortic bifurcation.
  (iv) Thrombus.
  (v)   Anatomical variants which may be important to know about pre-operatively, e.g. horseshoe kidney, post-aortic left renal vein.

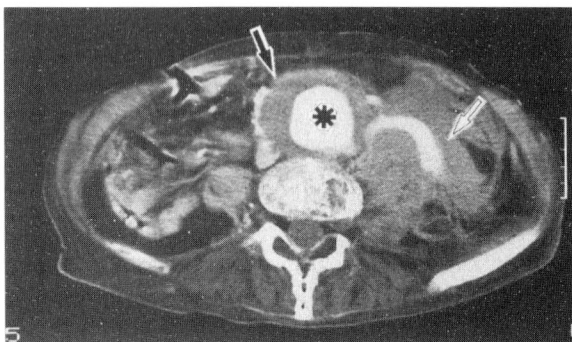

Figure 8.11 *Ruptured aortic aneurysm – CT. Contrast enhanced lumen (*). Encircling thrombus in dilated aorta (solid arrow). Large left retroperitoneal haematoma with central contrast indicating active bleeding at the time of the scan (hollow arrow).*

- Leakage:

  (a) Soft tissue surrounding the aneurysm.

  (b) Active leakage may demonstrate extravasation of contrast material (*Fig. 8.11*).

- Complicated cases, e.g. inflammatory aneurysm, retroperitoneal fibrosis.

- Post-operative: assessment of grafts (infection, blockage, leakage); aortoduodenal fistula; retroperitoneal fibrosis.

- Helical CT is particularly useful as the whole of the aorta may be scanned during peak contrast enhancement giving excellent definition.

- 2D and 3D reconstructions may be performed to further highlight the anatomy of the aneurysm. Three reconstruction techniques are commonly used:
  (i) Multiplanar reconstruction (MPR).
  (ii) Maximum intensity projection (MIP).
  (iii) Surface shading display (SSD) (*Fig. 8.12*).

Ultrasound

- Used where CT is unavailable or for follow-up measurement of a known asymptomatic aneurysm.

- May be difficult owing to bowel gas or obesity.

- Anatomy of aneurysm (i.e. shape, size, relations to renal arteries and aortic bifurcation).

- Thrombus.

- Leakage: US is not as reliable as CT for detection of leakage.

Abdomen X-ray

- AAA may be seen as an incidental finding on AXR or X-ray of the lumbar spine. Plain film signs of AAA may include:
  (i) Soft tissue mass.
  (ii) Curvilinear calcification especially on the lateral view (*Fig. 8.13*).
  (iii) Loss of retroperitoneal planes (i.e. psoas margins and renal outlines) with leakage.

Angiography

Angiography is rarely required prior to surgery for AAA as CT and US usually provide adequate information.

Aortic dissection

Depending on local availability and expertise transesophageal echocardiography and MRI are the investigations of choice for diagnosis and staging of aortic dissection. Where these modalities are not immediately available CT should be used.

Transesophageal echocardiography (TEE)

- Where available TEE is the investigation of choice for diagnosis and staging of aortic dissection (*Fig. 8.14*).

- Excellent spatial resolution makes TEE a highly sensitive technique.

- Potential errors include artefacts seen in the ascending aorta which may mimic dissection flaps; TEE must be performed and interpreted by experienced operators.

- As well as the dissection TEE will diagnose complications such as aortic insufficiency and pericardial fluid.

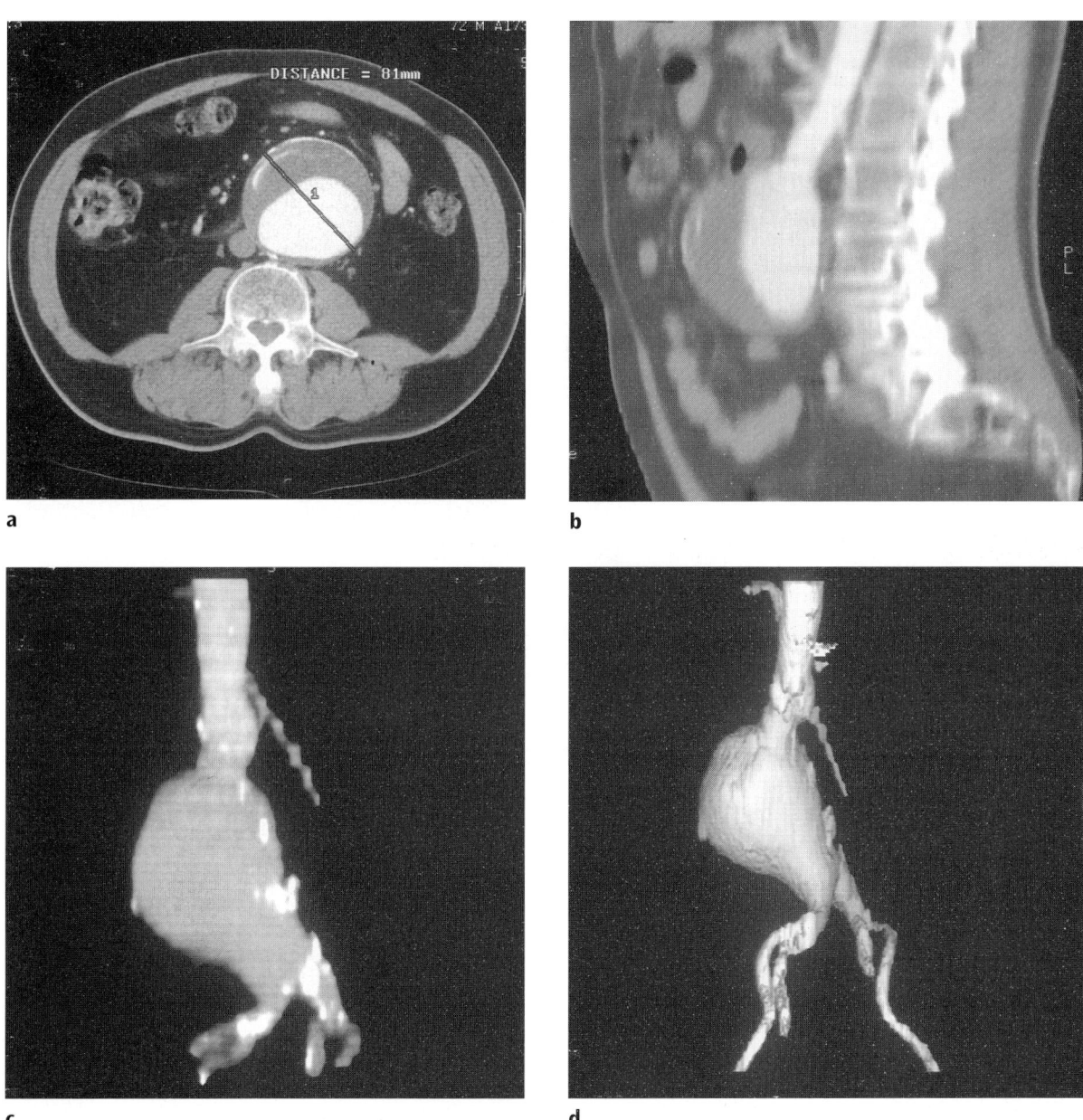

a

b

c

d

Figure 8.12 *Aortic aneurysm – helical CT and CT angiography.*
(a) Axial image. The diameter of the aneurysm is measured. Note the high attenuation lumen with thick lining thrombus anteriorly. (b) Multiplanar reconstruction (MPR). Following acquisition of data by helical CT reconstructions may be performed in any plane. A sagittal reconstruction shows the relationship of the aneurysm to the upper aorta. (c) Maximum intensity projection (MIP). MIP is a simple method of volume rendering which provides good differentiation of vascular structures and visualisation of mural calcifications. Its principal disadvantage is lack of information on vessel depth; furthermore extensive calcification may obscure the vessel lumen. (d) Shaded surface display (SSD). Also known as surface rendering. The outer surface of the contrast column is displayed as an opaque surface. The computer adds surface shading from an imaginary light source. This produces shades of grey on the surface and produces a striking 3D effect. Calcifications are not differentiated with SSD; overlapping vessels are better shown than with MIP. MIP and SSD should be regarded as complementary 3D reconstruction techniques.

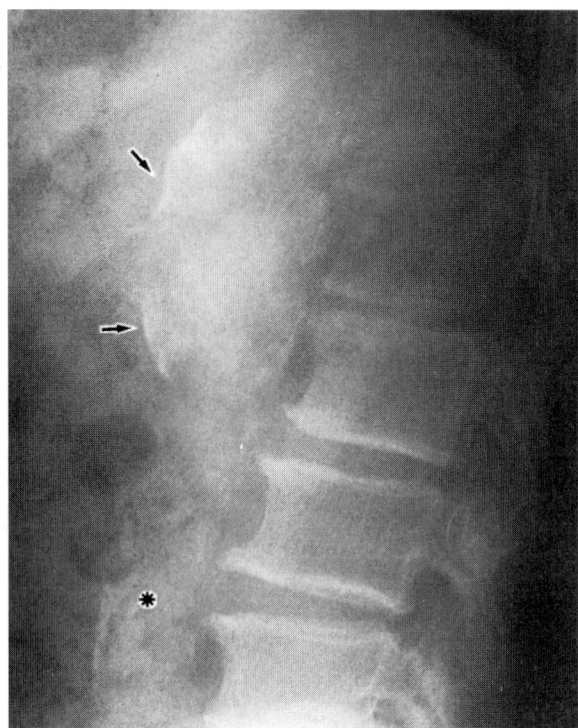

Figure 8.13 *Aortic aneurysm.*
Curvilinear calcification (arrows) marks the anterior wall of an aneurysm of the upper aorta. The lower aorta is calcified though not aneurysmal (*).

MRI

- Excellent contrast between flowing blood and soft tissue, plus the ability to image in sagittal as well as transverse planes, makes MRI an excellent modality for diagnosing and classifying aortic dissections.

- As MRI is very sensitive to flowing blood, the true and false lumens can usually be distinguished, though certainly not in all cases.

- MRI is more specific though slightly less sensitive than TEE.

CT

- Investigation of choice where TEE and MRI are unavailable or impractical (*Fig. 8.15*).

- Scans performed during the infusion of i.v. contrast may show the following:

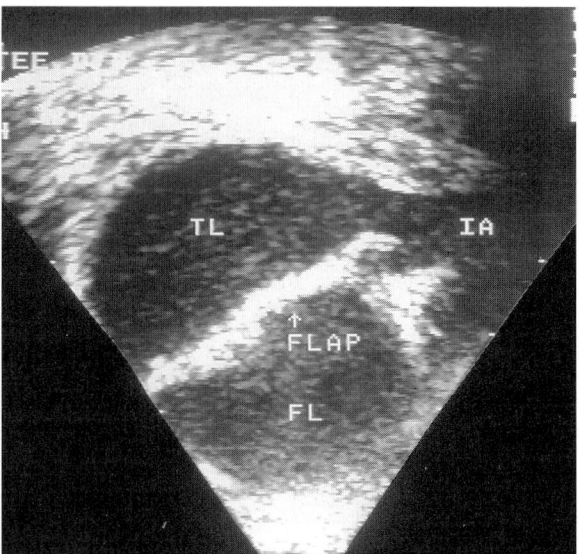

Figure 8.14 *Aortic dissection – transoesophageal echocardiogram (TEE).*
An intimal flap in the ascending aorta (arrow) is well shown with TEE. TL: true lumen; FL: false lumen; IA: innominate artery.

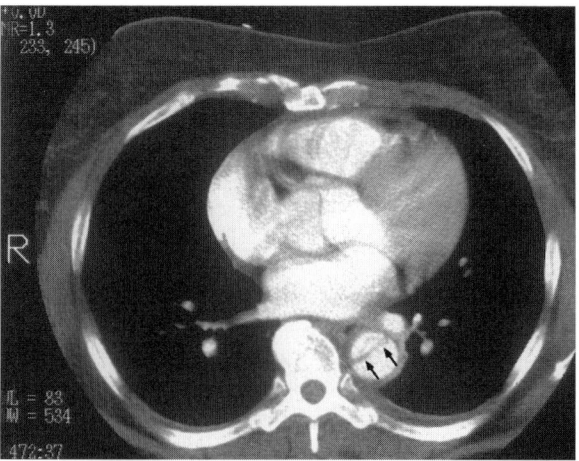

Figure 8.15 *Aortic dissection – CT.*
An intimal flap is well seen in the descending aorta (arrows).

(a) Visualisation of the intimal flap.

(b) Differentiation of true and false lumen.

(c) Extent of dissection.

(d) Rupture.

(e) Involvement of branch vessels and infarction of organs.

Angiography

Angiography may be required for better definition prior to surgery, though less so with the advent of TEE and MRI.

Chest X-ray

- Unreliable, i.e. CXR often normal.

- One may see any or all of the following signs:
  (i)   mediastinal widening;
  (ii) pleural fluid;
  (iii) separation of intimal calcification from the margin of the aortic outline;
  (iv) widening of the paravertebral stripe;
  (v)   depression of the left main bronchus.

- Regardless of findings on CXR more definitive imaging must be performed where a clinical suspicion of aortic dissection exists.

Peripheral vascular disease

Clinical signs and symptoms of peripheral vascular disease include:

- Intermittent claudication, i.e. muscle pain induced by exertion and relieved by rest.

- Rest pain.

- Tissue changes: ischaemic ulcers, gangrene.

Further assessment of limb ischaemia should combine physiological and anatomical information. The non-invasive vascular laboratory combines physiological tests with Doppler US imaging to define those patients requiring angiography and possible further treatment, either surgery or interventional radiology.

Physiological assessment

- Ankle–brachial index (ABI).

- Pulse volume recordings.

- Post-exercise ABI and pulse volume recordings.

Doppler US

- Signs of arterial stenosis:
  (i)   Narrowing of the vessel seen on 2D and colour images;
  (ii) Focal zone of increased flow velocity or turbulent flow;
  (iii) Altered arterial wave pattern distal to significant stenosis.

- Particularly useful to differentiate focal stenosis from diffuse disease and occlusion.

- Other arterial abnormalities such as aneurysm, pseudoaneurysm, and AVF are well seen on Doppler US.

- Doppler US is also useful for post-operative graft surveillance.

Digital subtraction angiography (DSA)

Digital subtraction is a process whereby a computer removes unwanted information from a radiographic image. It is particularly useful for angiography and the technique is referred to as DSA.

First, an image is taken of the relevant area prior to injection of contrast. This is called the 'mask'. Images are then taken with contrast in the blood vessels; the computer subtracts the 'mask' image leaving an image of the contrast-filled blood vessels unobscured by overlying structures (*Fig. 8.16*).

Most peripheral angiography is done via a femoral artery puncture. Occasionally, if the femoral route cannot be used due to previous surgery or extreme tortuosity of the iliac arterias, the axillary or brachial arteries may be punctured.

Method:

- The artery is punctured with a needle.

- A wire is threaded through the needle into the artery.

- The needle is removed leaving the wire in the artery.

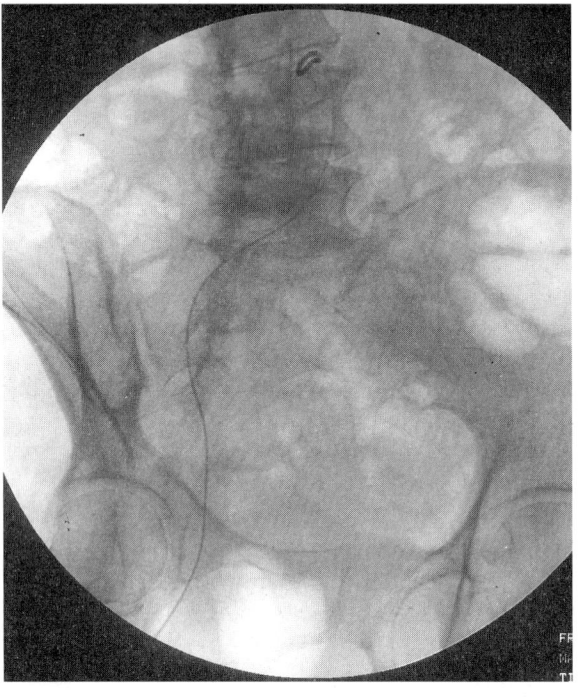

a

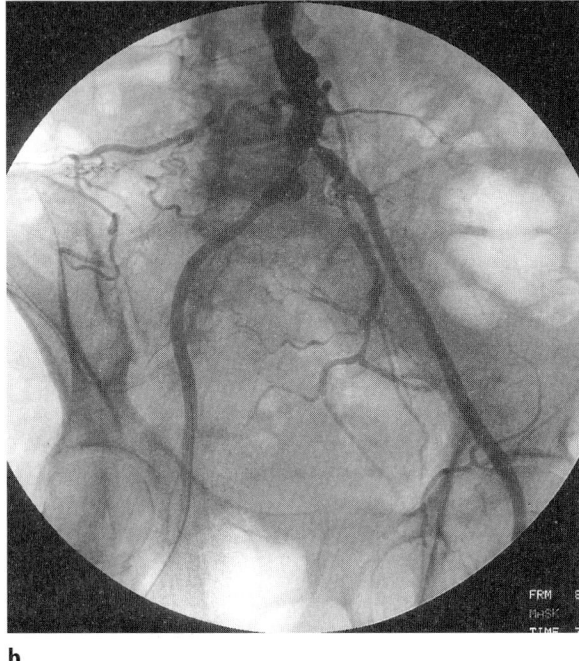

b

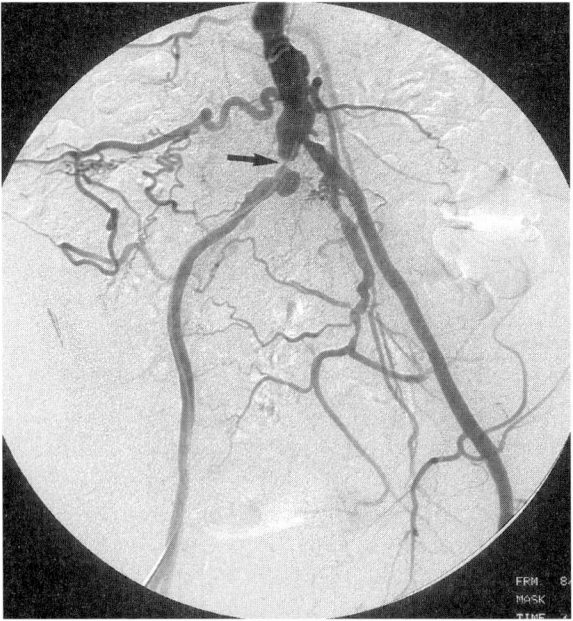

c

Figure 8.16 *Digital subtraction angiography.*
(a) Mask. Immediately prior to contrast injection a preliminary digitised image known as the 'mask' is performed. Note:
* *pelvic bones*
* *bowel gas*
* *arterial catheter.*
(b) Contrast image. Contrast is injected through the catheter producing opacification of the arteries. (c) Subtracted image. The computer subtracts the 'mask' from the contrast image leaving an image of contrast-filled blood vessels unobscured by overlying bone and bowel. Note a tight localized stenosis of the right common iliac artery (arrow).

* A catheter is inserted over the wire into the artery.

* Contrast is injected through the catheter and images obtained to document the following:

    (a) Site of stenosis.

    (b) Length of stenosis.

    (c) Status of distal run-off vessels.

Post-procedure care:

* Bed rest for several hours.

* Observe puncture site for bleeding/swelling.

Complications:

- Haematoma at the puncture site.

- False aneurysm formation.

- Damage to brachial plexus with axillary artery puncture.

- Arterial dissection.

- Embolism due to dislodgement of atheromatous plaques.

- Allergy to contrast material.

Magnetic resonance angiography (MRA)

- Uses sequences which show flowing blood as high signal (bright white) and stationary tissues as low signal (dark).

- Contrast material may also be used to enhance blood vessels and reduce scanning times.

- Problems include long examination times and flow related artefacts.

- These are being overcome and in centres where the technology is available, MRA has replaced diagnostic DSA in the assessment of patients with severe arterial disease. The development of interventional techniques however, particularly PTA and stent placement, has ensured a steady increase in the therapeutic role of DSA. These techniques are described below.

Venous insufficiency

For the patient with varicose veins for whom surgery is contemplated, US with Doppler is the imaging investigation of choice for assessment. The competence of a leg vein, deep or superficial, is determined with Doppler US using calf compression and release. A competent vein will show no or minor reflux (reversal of flow) on release of calf compression. Incompetence is defined as reflux of greater than 0.5 seconds in duration (*Fig. 8.17*).

The following information may be obtained with Doppler US:

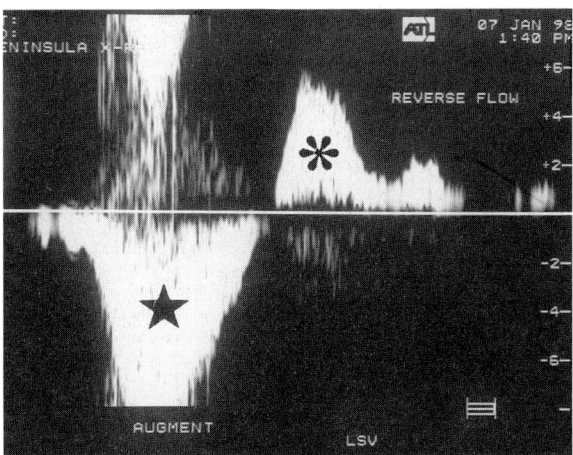

Figure 8.17 *Venous insufficiency – Doppler US. Wave forms for the long saphenous vein are displayed. There is good augmentation of flow with calf pressure (star). Following release of calf pressure there is reversed flow of 1.4 seconds duration (*). Reversed flow of greater than 0.5 seconds indicates venous insufficiency, also known as venous incompetence.*

- Patency and competence of the deep venous system from the common femoral vein to the lower calf.

- Competence and diameter of saphenofemoral junction.

- Competence and diameter of long saphenous vein.

- Duplications, tributaries, varices arising from the long saphenous vein.

- Competence and diameter of the saphenopopliteal junction.

- Document location of saphenopopliteal junction.

- Anatomical variants of the saphenopopliteal junction.

- Course and connections of superficial varicose veins.

- Incompetent perforator veins connecting deep system with superficial system.

  (a) Diameter.

  (b) Position in relation to anatomical landmarks such as groin crease, knee crease, medial malleolus.

(c) To assist further with surgical planning marks may be placed on the skin over incompetent perforating veins pre-operatively.

- For clarity, a diagram of the venous system based on the US examination is usually provided.

Deep venous thrombosis (DVT)

Doppler US

- In combination with colour Doppler imaging (CDI) ultrasound is the investigation of choice for DVT.

- Non-invasive and painless.

- Relatively inexpensive.

- Reliable for femoral and popliteal veins.

- Can also assess pelvic veins and IVC.

- Will detect conditions which may mimic DVT, e.g. ruptured Baker's cyst.

- With CDI can reliably image calf veins, so thrombus confined to the calf veins, as occurs in 10% of cases, should be detected.

- Signs Of DVT On US:
  (i) Non-compressibility of the vein (*Fig. 8.18*).
  (ii) Failure of venous distension in Valsalva's manoeuvre.
  (iii) Doppler signs: lack of normal venous Doppler signal; lack of increased signal with calf compression; lack of phasic nature of signal with respiration; loss of flow on colour images.
  (iv) Acute blood clot may be anechoic and hence not visible.
  (v) Chronic clot is usually hyperechoic and adherent to the vein wall.

- The main disadvantage of Doppler US is operator dependence.

The above comments assume a skilled operator using high quality equipment.

Venography

- With the advent of Doppler US, venography is no longer the investigation of choice for DVT.

- Venography may be performed where US is equivocal or unavailable.

- Signs of DVT include:
  (i) Filling defects within contrast-filled vessels.
  (ii) Non-filling of occluded deep veins.
  (iii) Collateral flow via the superficial system or cross-pelvic collaterals with iliac vein thrombosis.

Scintigraphy

- ^{125}I-labelled fibrinogen.

- Fibrinogen is incorporated with thrombus, so DVTs show as areas of increased uptake.

- A major disadvantage is that results are not available for 24–48 hours and this technique is rarely used.

Pulmonary embolism

Pulmonary embolism (PE) is a common cause of morbidity and mortality in post-operative patients, as well as in patients with other risk factors such as prolonged bed rest, malignancy and cardiac failure. Diagnosis of PE however remains problematical. Symptoms include: pleuritic chest pain, shortness of breath, cough, and haemoptysis, though a large number of pulmonary emboli are clinically silent. Clinical signs such as hypotension, tachycardia, reduced oxygen saturation, and ECG changes (S1 Q3 T3) are non-specific and often absent. Imaging studies are used to try to increase the accuracy of diagnosis. These include: chest X-ray, (CXR), ventilation/perfusion nuclear lung scan (V/Q scan), pulmonary angiography, and more recently helical CT pulmonary angiography.

CXR

- Signs of PE on CXR include:
  (a) pleural effusion;
  (b) localised area of consolidation contacting a pleural surface;

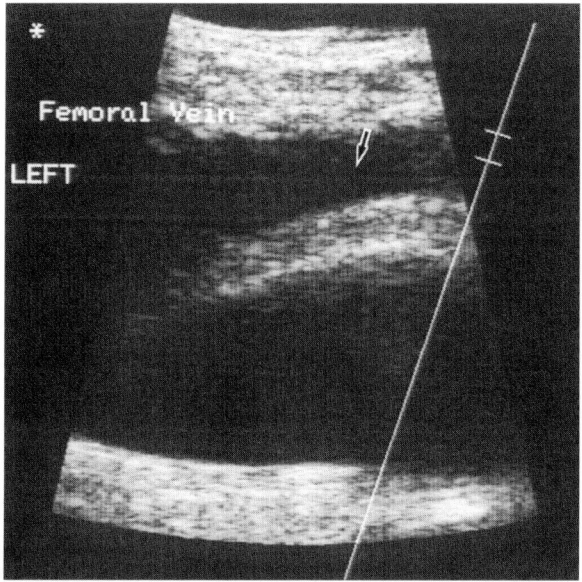

a

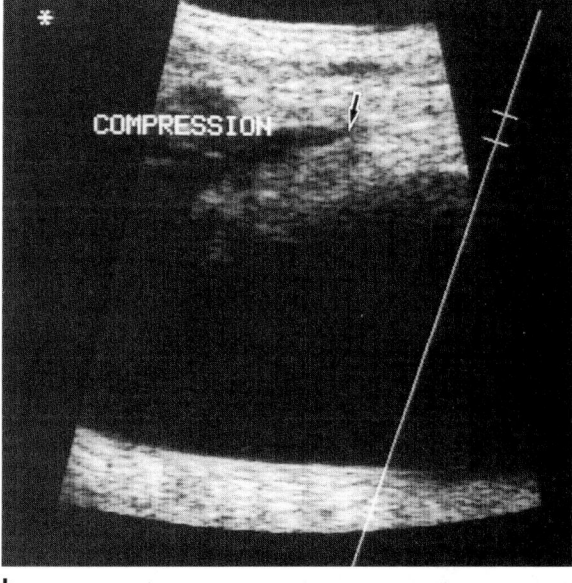

b

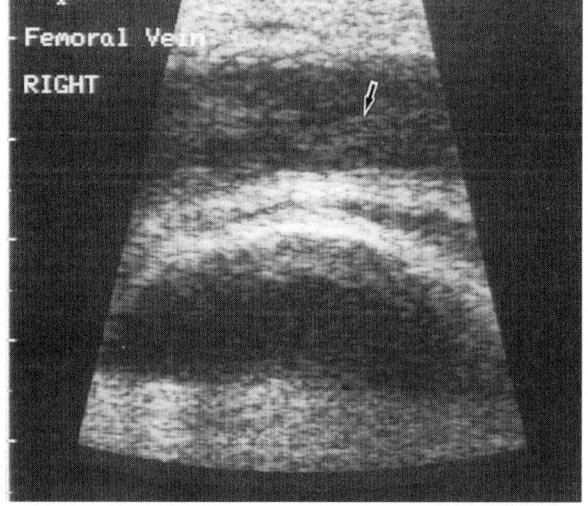

c

Figure 8.18 *Deep venous thrombosis (DVT).*
(a) Normal left femoral vein. The left femoral vein is seen in longitudinal section (arrow). (b) Compression. With only light pressure the normal femoral vein is easily compressed (arrow). (c) Thrombosed right femoral vein. The right femoral vein is distended and filled with echogenic thrombus (arrow). The vessel cannot be compressed.

(c) localised area of collapse.

- These signs are non-specific and often absent; the CXR in a patient with PE is often normal.

Scintigraphy V/Q scan

- In V/Q scans, a ventilation phase is first performed with the patient breathing a radioactive tracer ^{99m}Tc-labelled aerosol.

- Six images are performed using anterior, posterior, and oblique projections.

- This is followed by the perfusion phase in which images are obtained using an intravenous injection of ^{99m}Tc-labelled macroalbumen aggregates (MAA).

- These aggregates which have a mean diameter of 30–60 micrometres are trapped in the pulmonary microvasculature on first pass through the lungs.

- The same six projections are performed and the

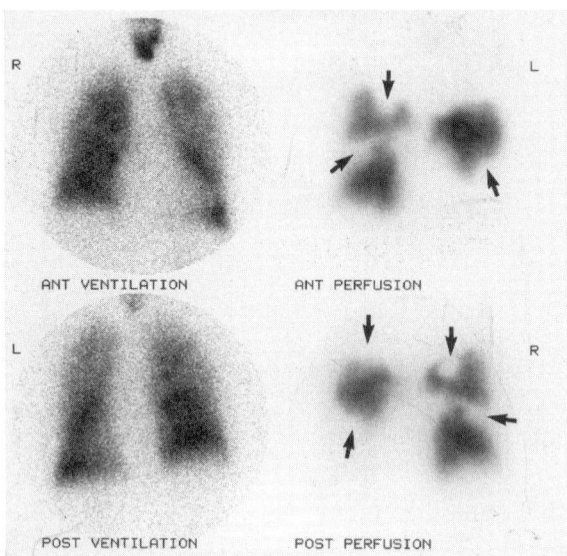

Figure 8.19 *Pulmonary embolism – scintigraphy. There are multiple wedge shaped defects seen on the perfusion phase (arrows). These are unmatched on the ventilation phase indicating multiple pulmonary emboli.*

perfusion phase compared with the ventilation phase.

- The diagnostic hallmark of PE is one or more regions of ventilation/perfusion mismatch, i.e. a region of lung where perfusion is reduced or absent and ventilation is preserved (*Fig. 8.19*).

- Lung scans after correlation with an accompanying CXR are graded as low, intermediate, or high probability of PE.

- Unfortunately a large proportion of patients (up to 75%) have an intermediate probability scan.

- The difficulty is compounded by 25–30% disagreement between experts in interpretation of low and intermediate probability scans.

Pulmonary angiography

- Pulmonary angiography has long been considered the gold standard for imaging of PE.

- A catheter is introduced usually via the femoral vein and passed through the right atrium and right ventricle and into the pulmonary arteries.

- Thrombo-emboli are seen as filling defects in the arteries with secondary signs such as non-filling of peripheral vessels.

- As the performance of pulmonary angiography requires highly skilled operators, expensive angiography equipment, and adequate patient monitoring, it is performed only in large multimodality institutions and even then only rarely.

- Pulmonary angiography is also performed for selective urokinase infusion where this is clinically indicated.

CT pulmonary angiography (CTPA)

- The recent advent of helical CT has added a further dimension to the imaging of PE.

- Helical CT is much faster than conventional CT and allows imaging of the thorax in a single breath hold.

- This in turn allows imaging of the entire pulmonary vascular bed during optimum peak contrast enhancement.

- Pulmonary emboli are seen on CTPA as filling defects within contrast-filled blood vessels (*Fig. 8.20*).

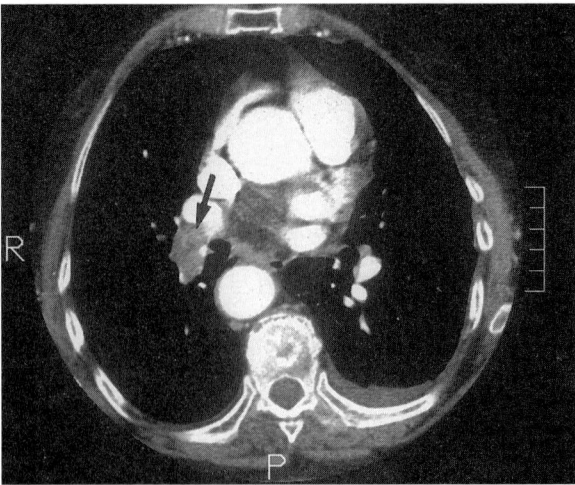

Figure 8.20 *Pulmonary embolism – helical CT. Pulmonary embolus is seen as a low attenuation filling defect in the right pulmonary artery (arrow). Note dense enhancement of aorta, SVC, main pulmonary artery, and branches of the left pulmonary artery.*

- Recent literature has shown that helical CT demonstrates thrombo-emboli in central pulmonary arteries, i.e. main, lobar and segmental arteries, with greater than 90% sensitivity and specificity.

- CTPA is less accurate is depicting PE confined to smaller subsegmental arteries. The clinical importance of such small subsegmental emboli is yet to be firmly established. If as many believe these are not clinically important, then CTPA may well be the imaging modality of choice for diagnosis of PE. However, if subsegmental PE is shown to be clinically important, either as an indicator of larger thrombo-emboli to come, or as a cause of death in patients with severe pre-existing cardiopulmonary disease, then CTPA alone may not be adequate.

Suggested protocol

Given the current state of knowledge and availability of technology, the following protocol for investigation of PE is suggested. Clinical suspicion of PE in a high-risk patient should be first investigated with CTPA. If this is positive, i.e. thrombus is shown in the first three divisions of the pulmonary artery, treatment is commenced. If negative, the patient may be observed or, where there is a persisting high level of clinical suspicion, perform a V/Q lung scan. If this is positive, treatment is commenced; if negative or equivocal, either the patient is observed or, in the occasional difficult case, go on to pulmonary angiography.

Interventional radiology of the peripheral vascular system

Percutaneous transluminal angioplasty (PTA)

Indications:

- Short segment arterial stenosis with associated clinical evidence of limb ischaemia.

Technique:

- Arterial puncture.

(a)   Femoral: ipsilateral/contralateral.

(b)   Brachial/axillary.

(c)   Popliteal.

- Wire passed across stenosis.

- Balloon catheter passed over wire and balloon positioned in the stenosis; balloon dilated.

- Pressure readings proximal and distal to the stenosis pre- and post-dilatation may be performed.

- Post-dilatation angiogram also performed (*Fig. 8.21*).

Post-procedure care:

- Haemostasis and bed rest as for angiography.

- Low-dose aspirin.

- Heparin following complicated procedure.

Complications:

- Complications of angiography.

- Arterial occlusion due to dissection.

- Arterial rupture and haemorrhage.

- Distal embolisation.

Stent placement

Arterial stents are of two types:

(a) Balloon-expandable (Palmaz):

- Stent–balloon assembly passed to the stenosis over a guide wire and within a protected sheath.

- Sheath withdrawn and stent deployed by balloon inflation.

- Balloon catheter removed leaving stent in place.

(b) Self-expanding (Wallstent):

- Delivered to stenosis on a catheter over a guide wire.

- When stent properly positioned, catheter withdrawn leaving stent in place.

- Stent consists of stainless steel spring filaments woven into a flexible self-expanding band.

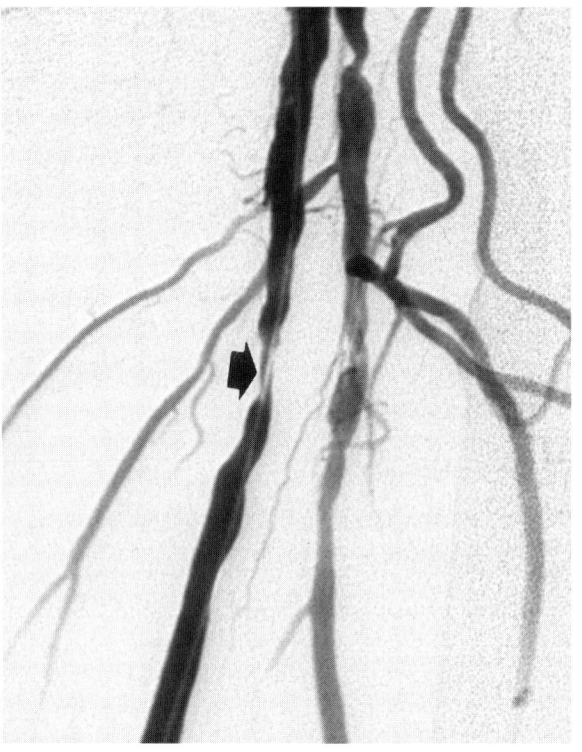
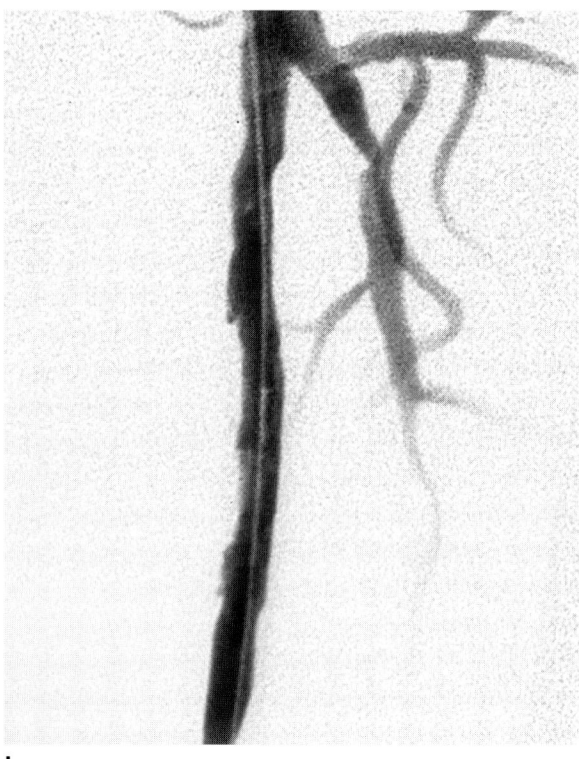

a   b

Figure 8.21 *Percutaneous transluminal angioplasty (PTA).*
(a). Pre-angioplasty. There is a localised stenosis of the left superficial femoral artery (arrow). Note that a wire has been passed across the stenosis. (b) Post-angioplasty. Following PTA there is good resolution of the stenosis with restoration of normal vessel calibre.

Indications:

- Stents are being used more often by interventional radiologists in the management of stenotic and occlusive vessel disease.

- Severe/calcified iliac stenosis/occlusion.

- Acute failure of PTA due to recoil of the vessel wall.

- PTA complicated by arterial dissection.

- Late failure of PTA due to restenosis.

Thrombolysis

Indications:

- Acute or acute on chronic arterial ischaemia.

- Arterial thrombosis post-angioplasty.

- Graft thrombosis.

- Acute upper limb DVT.
    (i)   Central venous catheters.
    (ii) Underlying venous stenosis.
    (iii) Mediastinal tumour/radiotherapy.

Technique:

- Arterial puncture.
    May be performed under US control when the artery is occluded.

- Position catheter in or just proximal to thrombosis.

- Infusion of thrombolytic agent, e.g. urokinase by continuous or pulsed spray infusion.

- Regular follow-up angiograms to ensure dissolution of thrombus with repositioning of catheter as required.

- PTA/stent for any underlying stenosis.

- Anticoagulation following thrombolysis.

Contraindications:

- Bleeding diathesis.
- Active/recent bleeding from any source.
- Anticoagulation therapy.
- Recent surgery, pregnancy, trauma.

Complications:

- Complications of angiography, especially haematoma.
- Distal embolisation of partly lysed thrombus.
- Systemic bleeding: GIT, cerebral, haematuria, epistaxis.

IVC filtration

Indications:

- PE/DVT where anticoagulation therapy is contra-indicated.
- Recurrent PE despite anticoagulation.
- During surgery in high-risk patients.

Technique:

- Inferior cavogram to check IVC patency, exclude anatomical anomalies, measure IVC diameter, and document position of renal veins.
- Filter type depends upon approach to be used, i.e. via femoral or jugular vein.

Complications (rare):

- Femoral vein/IVC thrombosis.
- IVC perforation.
- Filter migration.

Embolisation

Indications:

- Systemic arterio-venous malformation.
  - (i)   Definitive treatment.
  - (ii) Pre-operative.
  - (iii) Palliative.

- Trauma.
  - (i) MVA, especially with pelvic/lower limb fracture/ dislocation.
  - (ii) Penetrating injuries, e.g. gunshot wounds.
- Tumours.
  - (i)   Palliative: embolic agents labelled with cytotoxics, radioactive isotopes, or monoclonal antibodies.
  - (ii) Definitive treatment for tumours of vascular origin, e.g. aneurysmal bone cysts.
  - (iii) Pre-operative to decrease vascularity or deliver chemotherapy.

Complications:

- Complications of angiography.
- Inadvertent embolisation of normal structures.
- Pain.
- Post-embolisation syndrome, i.e. fever, malaise, leucocytosis 3–5 days post-embolisation.

Further Reading

1. Goodman LR, Lipchik RJ. Diagnosis of acute pulmonary embolism: time for a new approach. *Radiology* 1996; **199**:25–27.
2. Greaves SM, Hart EM, Aberle DR. CT of pulmonary thromboembolism. *Seminars in US, CT, and MRI* 1997; **18**:323–337.
3. Kopecky KK, Gokhale HS, Hawes DR. Spiral CT angiography of the aorta. *Seminars in US, CT, and MRI* 1996; **17**:304–315.
4. Link KM, Lesko NM. (eds.). Cardiac imaging. *Radiological Clinics of North America* 1994; **32**:3.
5. McGrath BP, Clarke K. Renal artery stenosis: current diagnosis and treatment. *MJA* 1993; **158**:343–345.
6. Remy-Jardin M, Remy J, Dechildre F *et al*. Diagnosis of pulmonary embolism with spiral CT: comparison with pulmonary angiography and scintigraphy. *Radiology* 1996; **200**:699–706.
7. Semba CP, Rubin GD, Dake MD. Three-dimensional spiral CT angiography of the abdomen. *Seminars in US, CT, and MRI* 1994; **15**:133–138.
8. Shively BK. Transesophageal echocardiography in the diagnosis of aortic disease. *Seminars in US, CT, and MRI* 1993; **14**:106–116.

9. Spies JB, Bakal CW, Burke DR *et al.* Standard for diagnostic arteriography in adults. *JVIR* 1993; **4**:385–395.

10. Stein PD, Henry JW. Prevalence of acute pulmonary embolism in central and subsegmental pulmonary arteries and relation to probability interpretation of ventilation/perfusion lung scans. *Chest* 1997; **111**:1246–1248.

9   Neck and head topics

Investigation of a neck mass

Roles of imaging

- Localisation of the mass: thyroid or non-thyroid.

- Features of the mass:, e.g. cystic/solid; calcification.

- Anatomical relations:
  (a) Position relative to the great vessels, thyroid gland, laryngeal cartilages.
  (b) Retrosternal extension.

- Evidence of malignancy:
  (i) Invasion of surrounding structures.
  (ii) Lymphadenopathy.

Ultrasound

- Accurate non-invasive screening test for initial localisation and characterisation of a neck mass.

- Will usually differentiate cystic from solid lesions, although branchial and thyroglossal cysts may appear solid owing to infection and haemorrhage.

CT

- CT is the investigation of choice for assessment of neck masses.

- Good localisation and definition of anatomical relations.

- Complications such as invasion/displacement of surrounding structures and lymphadenopathy are well seen.

MRI

- MRI is an excellent technique for neck masses and

in centres where it is freely available it may replace CT.

- The principal advantages of MRI in imaging masses of the neck are:
  (i) No iodinated contrast is needed to delineate blood vessels.
  (ii) Multiplanar imaging allows easy assessment (e.g. retrosternal spread of a thyroid mass well seen in the sagittal plane).

Common neck masses

Abscess:

- Usually closely related to airway.

- *CT*: low-attenuation mass; thick enhancing wall; obliteration of surrounding soft tissue planes; may compress/deform airway; CT may be used to guide aspiration and drainage (*Fig. 9.1*).

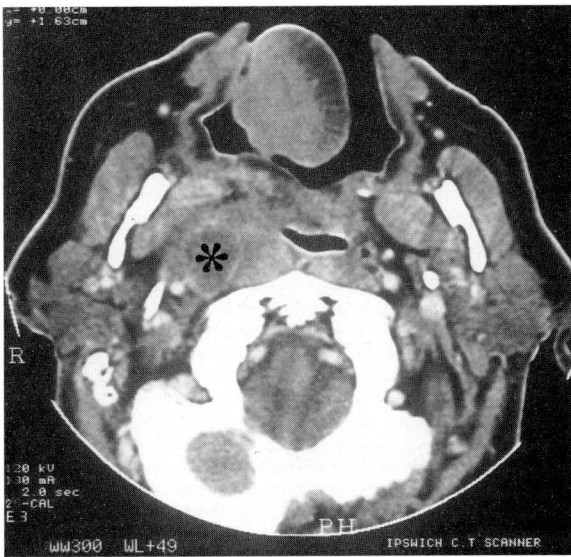

Figure 9.1 *Parapharyngeal abscess – CT. The abscess is seen as a low attenuation mass (*) to the right of the oropharynx. Note the enhancing wall.*

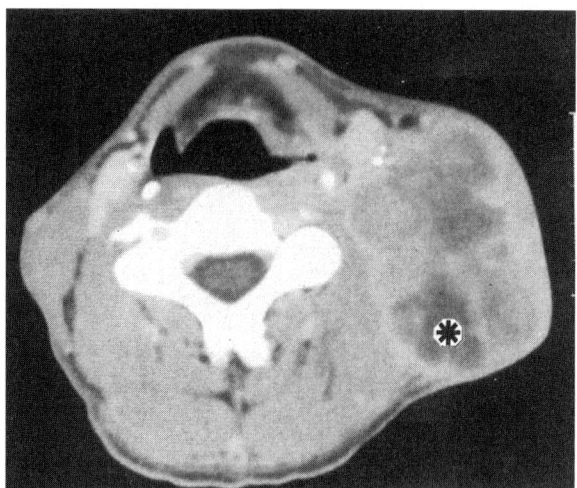

Figure 9.2 *Cervical lymph node mass – CT.*
Large mass in the left side of the neck. Central area of
low attenuation due to necrosis (*).

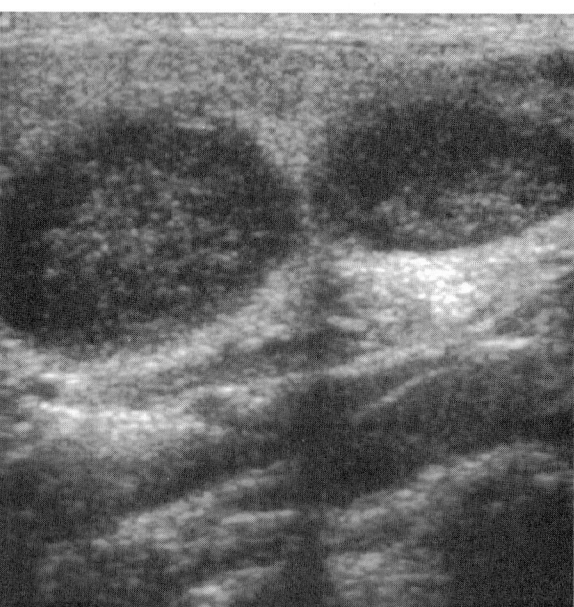

Figure 9.3 *Cervical lymphadenopathy – US.*
Enlarged cervical lymph nodes in a patient with
lymphoma. The lymph nodes are seen as well defined,
round, hypoechoic masses.

Malignant lymphadenopathy:

- Malignant cervical lymphadenopathy may be seen
  in lymphoma or secondary to other head and neck
  tumours (*Figs 9.2 and 9.3*).

- *CT:* soft tissue masses; central low-attenuation due
  to necrosis may be a prominent feature.

Second branchial cleft cyst:

- Young adults.

- Most commonly located in the upper neck anterior
  to the sternomastoid muscle (*Fig. 9.4*).

- *CT:* usually a thin-walled low-attenuation cyst; with
  inflammation may see thickening of the cyst wall
  and increased density of the cyst contents.

Thyroglossal duct cyst:

- Arise from remnants of the thyroglossal duct
  anywhere from the base of the tongue to the
  pyramidal lobe of the thyroid.

- Usually located anteriorly in the midline; occasionally lie posterior to the hyoid bone.

- *CT:* well-defined low-attenuation cyst; may contain
  internal septations; often have peripheral enhancement (*Fig. 9.5*).

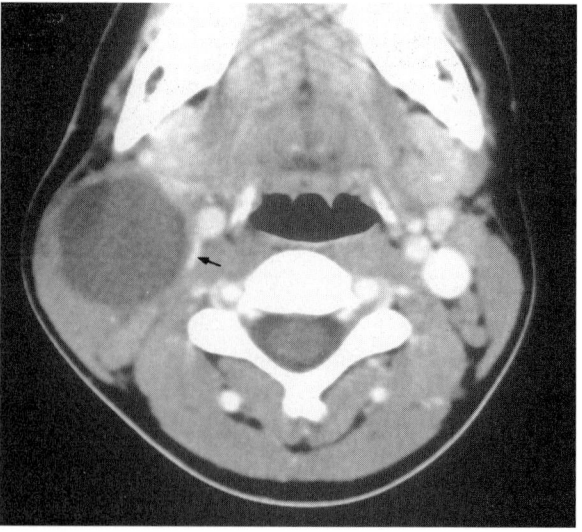

Figure 9.4 *Second branchial cleft cyst – CT.*
Well defined low attenuation cyst anterior and deep to
the right sternomastoid muscle. Note compression of the
right internal jugular vein (arrow).

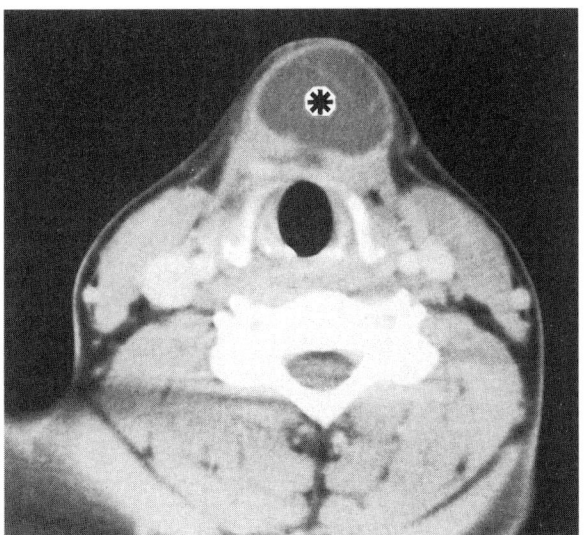

Figure 9.5 *Thyroglossal cyst – CT.*
Cystic lesion (*) anterior to the larynx.

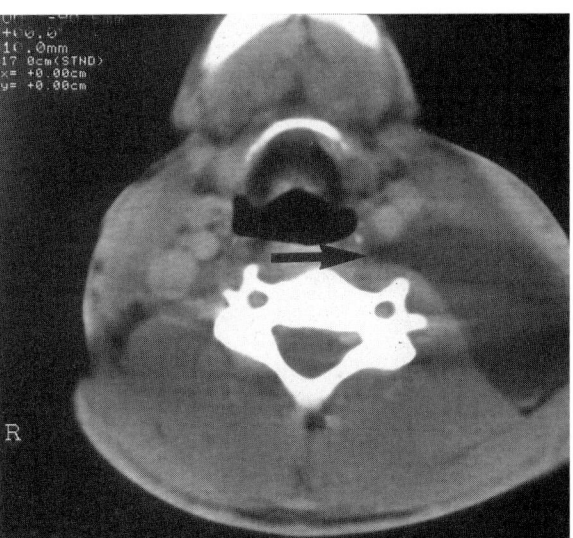

Figure 9.6 *Cystic hygroma – CT.*
Fluid-filled structure in the lower neck, posterior to the left sternomastoid muscle. Its medial extent lies posterior to the great vessels (arrow).

Cystic hygroma:

- Children under 2 years; high association with Turner syndrome.

- Usually located in the lower neck posterior to the sternomastoid muscle.

- *CT:* thin-walled, low-attenuation mass; may infiltrate into surrounding tissue planes and between the great vessels of the neck; may extend into the superior mediastinum (*Fig. 9.6*).

Dermoid cyst:

- Occur in the midline in the floor of the mouth.

- *CT:* well-defined mass; low-attenuation fat content; fluid levels.

Carotid body tumour:

- Paraganglioma located in the carotid bifurcation.

- *CT:* well-defined mass showing dense contrast enhancement lying between the internal and external carotid arteries (*Fig. 9.7*).

Lipoma:

- Usually occur in the superficial tissues though may be seen in virtually any anatomical location.

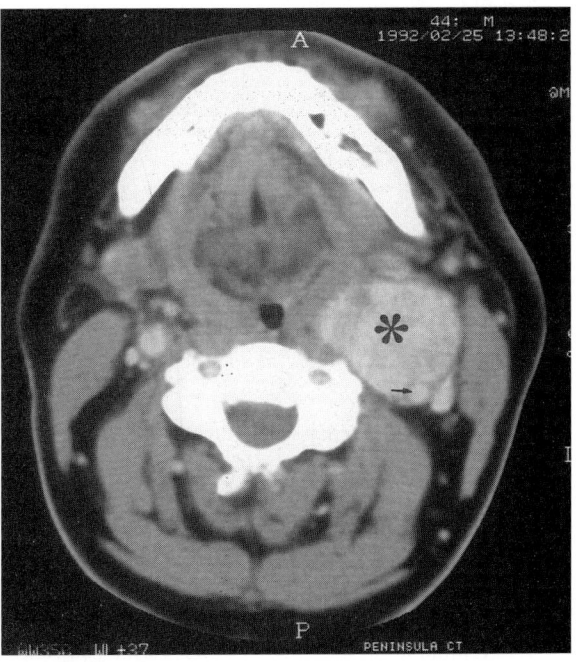

Figure 9.7 *Carotid body tumour – CT.*
Densely enhancing mass (*) lying directly anterior to the left internal carotid artery (arrow) and deep to the sternomastoid muscle.

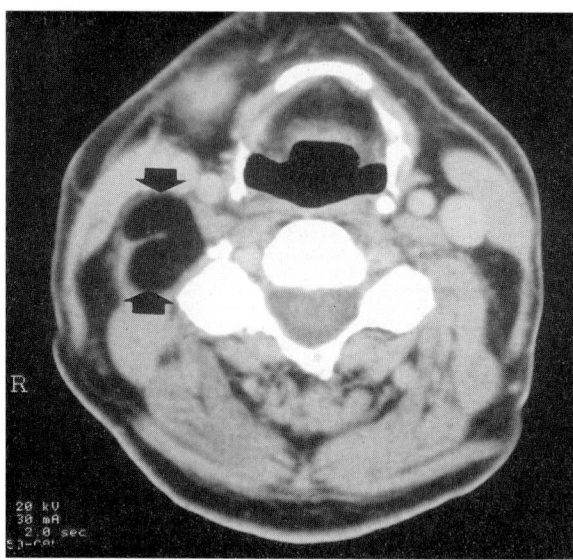

Figure 9.8 *Lipoma – CT.*
Well defined mass in the right scalene muscles (arrows).
The dark low attenuation contents are typical of the CT
appearance of fat. Note the similar density of fat planes
elsewhere in the neck.

- *US:* well-defined hypoechoic mass.
- *CT:* well-defined low-attenuation mass (*Fig. 9.8*).

Thyroid imaging

- With the development of high resolution US, fine-needle aspiration (FNA) techniques, and accurate laboratory tests including cytopathology, the diagnostic evaluation of thyroid disease has evolved over the past few years.

- Diffuse thyroid disease, e.g. Graves' disease, Hashimoto's and subacute thyroiditis, multinodular goitre:
    (i) Diagnosis often achieved by clinical history and examination plus laboratory tests for thyroid function and antibodies.
    (ii) These may be complemented by thyroid scintigraphy and US including colour Doppler.
    (iii) CT may be required for intrathoracic goitre to show its location and extent, and to distinguish it from other causes of superior mediastinal mass (*Fig. 9.9*).

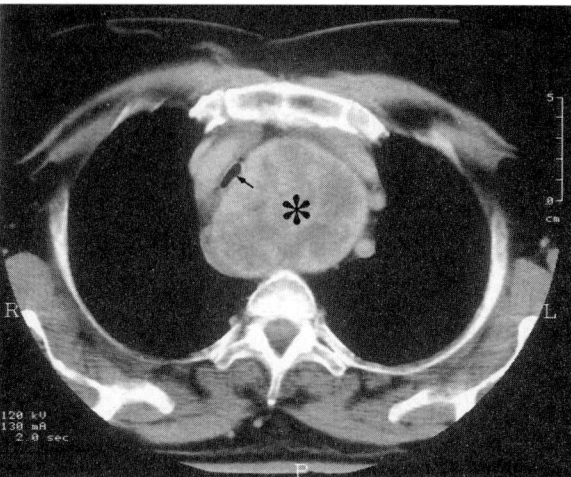

Figure 9.9 *Retrosternal goitre – CT.*
Retrosternal goitre seen as a large heterogeneous mass
(*) in the superior mediastinum posterior to the
sternum. Note compression of the trachea to the right
(arrow).

Thyroid nodules and masses

- FNA under direct palpation is often the first and only diagnostic procedure performed for a palpable thyroid nodule.

- US and scintigraphy may be used for further characterisation of a thyroid nodule and US-guided FNA has several advantages over palpation-directed FNA.

- CT is usually reserved for staging of thyroid carcinomas and for assessment of large multinodular goitre as above.

- The most common thyroid nodules are benign colloid nodules usually seen as partly cystic thyroid masses.

- Follicular adenoma is a true benign neoplasm of the thyroid gland.

- Thyroid carcinoma is usually of epithelial origin and is classified into papillary, follicular, medullary, and anaplastic.
    (a) Papillary carcinoma is the most common type (60%).
    (b) High incidence of spread to regional cervical lymph nodes.

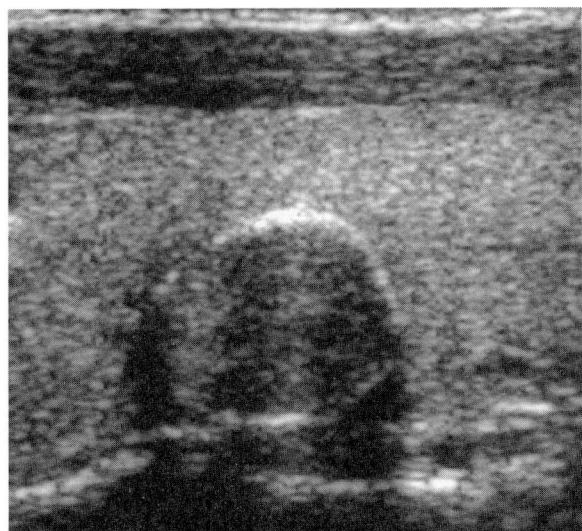

Figure 9.10 *Benign thyroid nodule – US.*
Well defined hypoechoic nodule. Peripheral hyperechoic
rim due to 'egg-shell' calcification. Note homogeneous
hyperechoic texture of surrounding normal thyroid
tissue.

(c) Pulmonary and bone metastases are also common.
(d) For further notes on staging of thyroid carcinoma *see* Chapter 12.

Ultrasound

- Roles of US in assessment of thyroid nodules:
  (i) Differentiate thyroid mass from non-thyroid mass or cyst (see above).
  (ii) Characterise nodule.
  (iii) Diagnose multiple nodules.
  (iv) FNA guidance.

- Highly sensitive for nodules of 2 mm or greater.

- Features of a benign thyroid nodule:
  (i) Hypoechoic with well-defined margins.
  (ii) Cystic components; malignant cysts are exceedingly rare.
  (iii) Most thyroid cysts have some wall irregularity and contain echogenic debris.
  (iv) The majority of thyroid cysts are due to necrosis or haemorrhage complicating a colloid nodule; simple epithelial cysts of the thyroid are rare.

(v) Peripheral 'egg shell' calcification (*Fig. 9.10*).
(vi) Hyperechoic nodules, though rare, are usually benign.

- Features of a malignant mass:
  (i) Hypoechoic.
  (ii) Ill defined margins.
  (iii) Fine internal calcifications.
  (iv) Heterogeneity due to haemorrhage and necrosis.

- There is considerable overlap in the US appearances of benign and malignant nodules so FNA is often required for diagnosis.

Ultrasound-guided FNA

- US-guided FNA has several advantages over palpation directed FNA:
  (i) With high resolution US the needle can be selectively directed into cystic and solid components.
  (ii) With colour Doppler the needle is directed away from blood vessels; a highly blood stained specimen is a common cause of non-diagnostic FNA.
  (iii) Small, non-palpable nodules may also be aspirated.

- Technique:
  (i) 22 to 25 gauge needle attached to a 10 ml syringe.
  (ii) 'Free hand' method is quick, easy, and safe: US probe is held in one hand and the syringe in the other.
  (iii) Under direct US visualisation the needle tip is directed into the nodule.
  (iv) Gentle suction is applied while the needle is rapidly moved in and out through the area of interest.

- FNA should be reported by the cytopathologist in one of four ways:
  (i) Benign, i.e. no malignant cells seen.
  (ii) Malignant.
  (iii) Suspicious or equivocal.
  (iv) Non-diagnostic, usually due to a heavily blood-stained specimen.

- Repeat FNA may be performed for cases reported as suspicious or non-diagnostic.

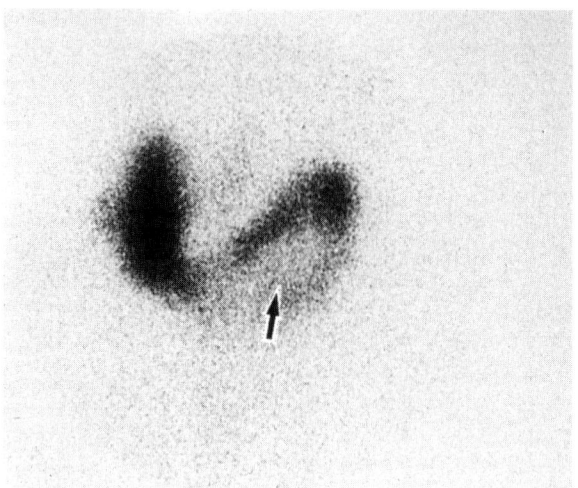

Figure 9.11 *'Cold' thyroid nodule.*
Area of decreased uptake in the left lobe of the thyroid, i.e. a 'cold' nodule (arrow) in this case due to a cyst. Other causes of this appearance include non-functioning thyroid adenoma and thyroid carcinoma.

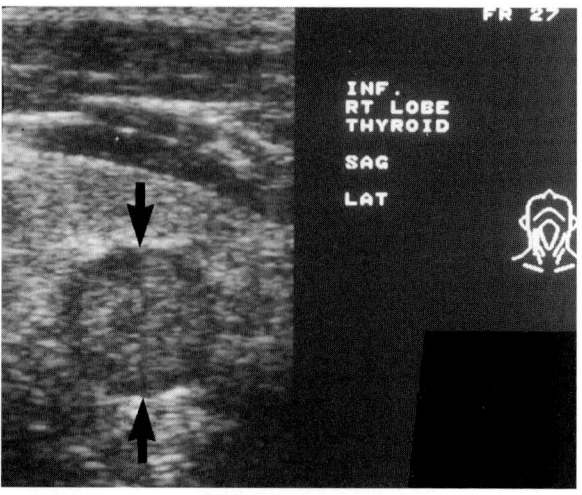

Figure 9.12 *Parathyroid adenoma – US.*
Adenoma of the right inferior parathyroid gland. Well defined hypoechoic mass (arrows) deep to the inferior pole of the right lobe of the thyroid.

Scintigraphy

- ^{99m}Tc pertechnetate.

- Reduced role in the assessment of thyroid nodules with widespread use of US and FNA.

- Not sensitive for nodules of 5 mm or less.

- Nodules are described according to their level of uptake of isotope as 'hot', 'warm', or 'cold'.

- Only 1% of 'hot' nodules are malignant.

- 'Warm' nodules, i.e. those with a similar level of uptake to the surrounding thyroid gland, are usually benign though up to 10% may be malignant.

- Approximately 20% of 'cold' nodules are malignant (*Fig. 9.11*).

Primary hyperparathyroidism

- Primary hyperparathyroidism is the most common indication for imaging of the parathyroid glands.

- Causes of primary hyperparathyroidism are as follows:

(i)   Solitary parathyroid adenoma: 80%.
(ii) Multiple parathyroid adenoma: 7%.
(iii) Parathyroid hyperplasia: 10%.
(iv) Parathyroid carcinoma: 3%.

- Pre-operative imaging for localisation of parathyroid adenoma is not always performed, as in some centres it is felt unlikely to improve the rate of surgical success.

- However, where pre-operative localisation is required by the surgeon, US is the investigation of first choice.

- US with high resolution equipment has a high sensitivity (80–90%) in detection of parathyroid adenoma.

- US appearance of parathyroid adenoma:

- Well defined hypoechoic mass usually of around 1.0–1.5 cm in diameter (*Fig. 9.12*).

- The principal cause of a false-negative US is ectopic adenoma as may be present in up to 10% of cases.

- Where US is negative further imaging may be performed, i.e. scintigraphy, CT and MRI.

- The imaging technique chosen will reflect local expertise and availability.

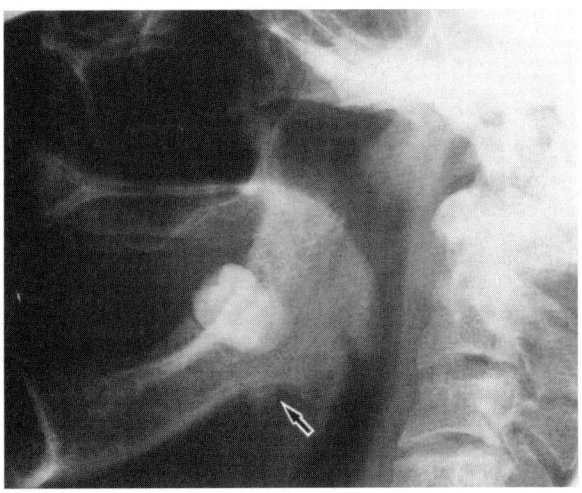
a

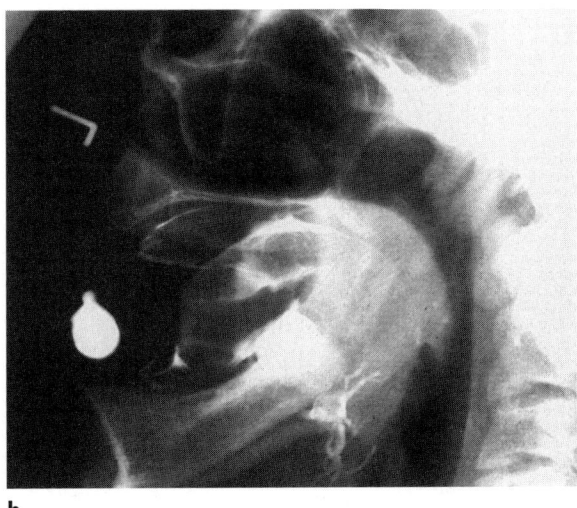
b

Figure 9.13 *Salivary gland calculus.*
(a) Plain film. Calcified opacity beneath the angle of the mandible (arrow). (b) Sialogram. The calculus now shows as a filling defect within the contrast-filled duct system of the submandibular gland.

- CT and MRI:
  Particularly useful for ectopic adenoma located in the mediastinum.

- Scintigraphy:
  (i) ^{99m}Tc-sestamibi.
  (ii) High rate of uptake in parathyroid adenoma.
  (iii) Especially useful for ectopic or multiple adenomas.

- Post-operative imaging for recurrent or persistent hyperparathyroidism is best performed with US complemented by sestamibi scintigraphy.

Investigation of a salivary gland calculus

Plain films

- Most salivary calculi are radio-opaque and therefore visible on plain films.

- Specific views are used for the gland of interest.

Sialography

- Oil-based or water-soluble contrast media.

- Used to investigate parotid and submandibular ducts and glands.

- Calculus appears as a filling defect within a localised expansion of the duct, and the proximal duct may be dilated (*Fig. 9.13*).

- Other findings may be seen:
  (a) Strictures.
  (b) Sialectasis, i.e. dilated ducts and cavities within the gland, some of which may contain calculi.

Investigation of a salivary gland mass

- Common salivary gland tumours include:
  (i) Pleomorphic adenoma: benign; 70% of all parotid tumours.
  (ii) Adenolymphoma (Warthin's tumour): second most common benign parotid tumour; 10% bilateral.

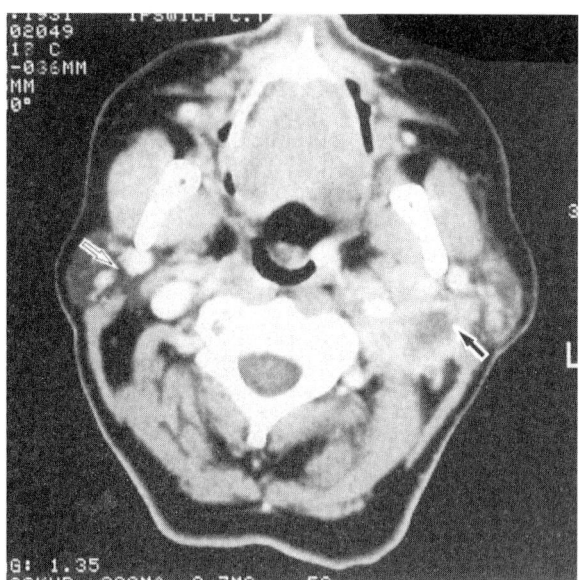

Figure 9.14 *Pleomorphic adenoma of the parotid gland – CT.*
Mass of mixed attenuation occupying mainly the deep lobe of the left parotid gland (solid arrow). Note the appearance of the normal right parotid gland for comparison (hollow arrow). (Courtesy of Dr W Lun, Brisbane.)

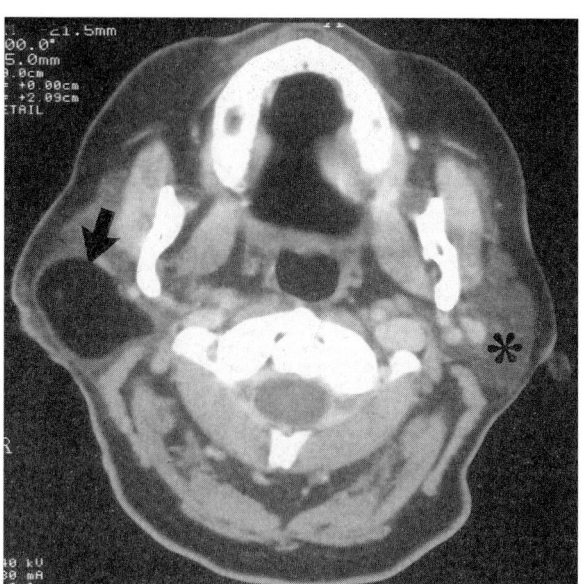

Figure 9.15 *Lipoma of the parotid gland – CT.*
Lipoma in the superficial lobe of the right parotid gland (arrow). Note the CT features of a lipoma:
- *homogeneous fat density contents*
- *well defined margins.*
Compare with the normal appearance of the left parotid gland (*).

   (iii) Adenoid cystic carcinoma (cylindroma): malignant; usually arise in minor salivary glands.
   (iv) Mucoepidermoid carcinoma: most common malignant tumour of the parotid gland.
   (v) Other soft tissue tumours may occur in the parotid gland: lipoma, neuroma, melanoma.

- Cross-sectional imaging with ultrasound and CT or MRI is usually sufficient prior to surgery.

- Sialography and scintigraphy are used only in a few difficult or uncertain cases.

CT

- Define the extent of tumour.

- Relationship to facial nerve (parotid tumours).

- Benign tumours tend to be well defined; malignant tumours often have irregular, ill defined margins (*Figs 9.14 and 9.15*).

- Complicating factors, e.g. lymphadenopathy, invasion of deep structures.

MRI

- MRI is useful for imaging tumours of the parotid gland because the facial nerve can be seen in the gland and hence a tumour's relationship to it can be demonstrated.

- Multiplanar imaging is also useful in this regard.

- As with other modalities a specific histological diagnosis cannot be made, with the possible exception of adenolymphoma which may appear as a multiloculated cystic mass.

Ultrasound

- US is of limited use, other than for defining if a lesion is cystic or solid.

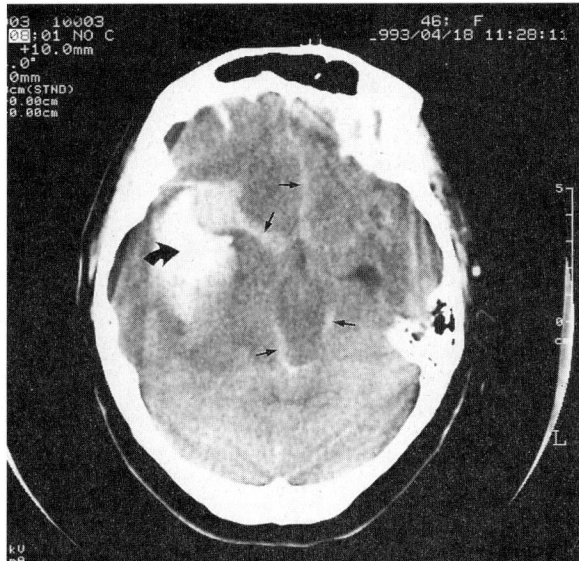

Figure 9.16 *Subarachnoid haemorrhage – CT. Subarachnoid blood is seen as high-attenuation material in the interhemispheric fissure, Sylvian fissures and in the basal cisterns around the brain stem (straight arrows). Note also the large intracerebral haematoma in the right temporal lobe (curved arrow). Haemorrhage, in this case, was caused by rupture of an aneurysm of the right middle cerebral artery.*

Sialography

- Masses show as filling defects in the gland surrounded by displaced ducts.

- Malignant masses may be more irregular with distortion of intraglandular ducts.

Scintigraphy

- Most masses show as a photon-deficient ('cold') filling defect, the exception being adenolymphoma which may accumulate isotope.

Subarachnoid haemorrhage

CT

- Subarachnoid blood shows as high attenuation material in the basal cisterns, Sylvian fissures, cerebral sulci and ventricles (*Fig. 9.16*).

- A normal CT does not exclude a small subarachnoid bleed; 5% of patients with a proven subarachnoid haemorrhage have a normal CT.

- In such cases diagnostic lumbar puncture *must* be performed.

- With aneurysms, which account for 75% of nontraumatic subarachnoid haemorrhage, CT can often predict the vessel of origin by the most concentrated site of bleeding, e.g. Sylvian fissure: middle cerebral artery; septum pellucidum: anterior communicating artery.

- Associated CT findings:
  (i) Large aneurysms show as well-defined areas of high attenuation with dense contrast enhancement.
  (ii) Hydrocephalus is commonly seen, often within hours of the haemorrhage.
  (iii) Areas of low-attenuation due to ischaemia and infarction secondary to vasospasm may also be present.

- Arteriovenous malformation (AVM) accounts for 5% of subarachnoid bleeds.

- CT signs of AVM:
  (i) poorly-defined, irregular areas of mixed attenuation, often with calcification;
  (ii) enhancement with contrast;
  (iii) large feeding arteries;
  (iv) large tortuous draining veins.

Angiography

- The timing of angiography varies from centre to centre.

- The aims of angiography are:
  (i) Show the aneurysm (*Fig. 9.17*).
  (ii) Demonstrate the relationship of its neck to the vessel of origin.
  (iii) Diagnose multiple aneurysms if present (10% of cases).

- In the case of multiple aneurysms, the one responsible for the bleed may be predicted by the CT as above, may be associated with local vasospasm, and is usually the largest.

- Bleeding seen at angiogram by actively leaking contrast is very rare, bears a poor prognosis, and necessitates immediate cessation of the procedure.

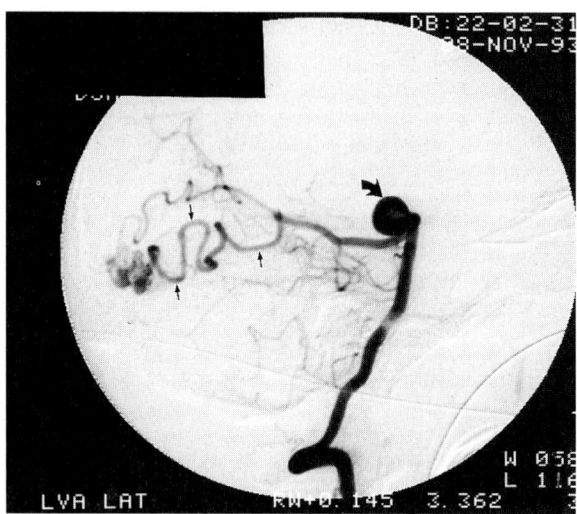

Figure 9.17 *Aneurysm and AVM – angiogram.*
Note:

- *aneurysm arising from the tip of the basilar artery (curved arrow)*
- *large artery supplying a posterior AVM (straight arrows).*

- Negative angiograms occur in up to 15% and may be due to clotting of the aneurysm or non-filling due to severe local vasospasm; in these cases a repeat angiogram may be worthwhile.

- If the repeat angiogram is negative, a spinal site of bleeding should be considered and MRI of the spine performed.

- MRI will usually show any spinal vascular lesions and act as a guide for spinal angiography.

- MRI will also occasionally turn up an unexpected finding such as a spinal tumour which may rarely present with a subarachnoid haemorrhage.

- Other intracranial vascular lesions, most commonly AVMs, will also be shown by angiography and may be amenable to embolisation.

- Large aneurysms unsuitable for surgery may also be amenable to embolisation techniques.

Helical CT angiography (CTA) and magnetic resonance angiography (MRA)

- CTA and MRA may be used to image the cerebral vessels.

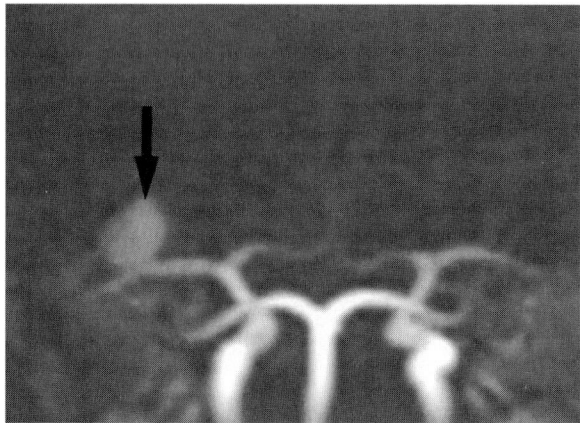

Figure 9.18 *MRA – berry aneurysm.*
Magnetic resonance angiography of the intracranial circulation shows an aneurysm of the right middle cerebral artery (arrow).

- Both techniques are of comparable sensitivity to conventional angiography for displaying aneurysms of 3 mm or greater; below this size CTA and MRA are significantly less sensitive than angiography.

- Conventional angiography remains the technique of choice for acute subarachnoid haemorrhage though this may change in the future.

- CTA and MRA may be used for screening purposes or for specific clinical problems.

- Indications include:
  (i) Screening in 'at risk' patients: family history of aneurysm and/or subarachnoid haemorrhage, coarctation of the aorta, autosomal dominant polycystic kidney disease.
  (ii) Isolated third cranial nerve palsy to exclude aneurysm of the posterior communicating artery.
  (iii) Assess possible aneurysm seen on conventional CT or MRI.

- CTA and MRA each have relative advantages and disadvantages which influence selection of technique in individual patients.

- MRA (*Fig. 9.18*):
  (i) Non-invasive.
  (ii) Contrast material not required.
  (iii) Relatively long scan times: problem in restless or claustrophobic patients.
  (iv) Contraindicated by pacemakers, ferromagnetic clips and implants, ocular metal foreign bodies.

- CTA:
    - (i)   Short scan times (30–40 seconds), therefore better tolerated in restless patients.
    - (ii) Claustrophobia less of a problem.
    - (iii) Requires use of iodinated contrast material.

Further Reading

1. Hopkins CR, Reading CC. Thyroid and parathyroid imaging. *Seminars in US, CT, and MRI* 1995; **16**:279–295.

2. Katz DA, Marks MP, Napel SA *et al*. Circle of Willis: Evaluation with spiral CT angiography, MR angiography, and conventional angiography. *Radiology* 1995: **195**:445–449.

3. McBiles M, Lambert AT, Cote MG, Kim SY. Sestamibi parathyroid imaging. *Seminars in Nuclear Medicine* 1995; **25**:221–234.

4. Schwartz RB Helical (Spiral) CT in neuroradiologic diagnosis. *Radiological Clinics of North America* 1995; **33**:981–995.

10 Transplantation

Kidney transplantation

Pre-operative investigation of a kidney donor

Ultrasound or CT

- To identify contraindications to nephrectomy.
- Congenital anomalies (e.g. hypoplasia/agenesis; horseshoe kidney).
- Acquired disease (e.g. tumour, chronic pyelonephritis).

Arteriogram

- To demonstrate number and configuration of renal arteries.
- To demonstrate length of renal artery.
- Diagnose vascular anomalies, particularly unrecognised renal artery stenosis.

Scintigraphy

- ^{99m}Tc-DTPA.
- Demonstrate quantitative function.

Post-operative complications of renal transplantation

The two most commonly performed imaging techniques post-renal transplant are ultrasound with Doppler and renal scintigraphy. These techniques will diagnose the vast majority of post-transplantation complications. For both methods, early post-operative assessment is essential to establish a baseline and to diagnose early problems. The more common complications with their imaging findings are outlined below.

Ultrasound and scintigraphy

1. Fluid collection

- Perinephric fluid collections are seen in up to 50% of renal transplantations.
- Most common are small crescent-shaped perinephric fluid collections seen in the immediate post-operative period: these are presumably small haematomas or seromas.
- Urinomas and haematomas usually occur in the early post-operative period.
- Lymphoceles usually occur later, i.e. 4–8 weeks post-operatively.
- *Ultrasound:*
  - (i)   Fluid appearance is often non-specific.
  - (ii) Haematoma may contain visible septations.
  - (iii) Abscesses usually have an irregular wall and may contain echogenic debris.
  - (iv) Ultrasound useful to guide aspiration and drainage.
- *Scintigraphy:*
  Most fluid collections appear as photopenic areas, i.e. 'cold' spots, the exception being urinoma which will show as a photopenic area on early scans which fills with tracer on later scans (*Fig. 10.1*).

2. Rejection

- Ultrasound findings are unreliable and include:
  - (i)   Swelling.
  - (ii) Altered (increased or decreased) cortical echogenicity.
  - (iii) Swollen pyramids.
  - (iv) Loss of corticomedullary differentiation.
- Rejection is not excluded by a normal ultrasound appearance.
- *Duplex ultrasound:*
  - (i)   Elevated resistive index (RI) above 0.8 has in the past been considered indicative of rejection.

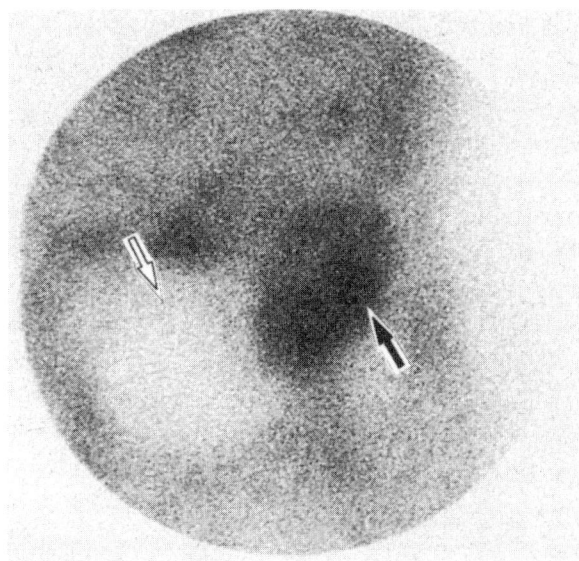

Figure 10.1 *Haematoma – scintigraphy.*
The transplant shows good tracer uptake (solid arrow).
The haematoma is seen as a large photon deficient or
'cold' area (hollow arrow). (Courtesy of Dr J Reasbeck,
Brisbane.)

(ii)   RI = peak systolic velocity – end-diastolic
       velocity/peak systolic velocity.
(iii) Recent literature has shown inconsistent
       results and elevated RI is now considered a
       non-specific indicator of graft dysfunction.

* Scintigraphy may show decreased perfusion as well
  as poor uptake and excretion of tracer.

* Biopsy is usually required for diagnosis; this is best
  performed under ultrasound guidance.

3. Hydronephrosis

* Mild transient hydronephrosis is common in the
  immediate post-operative period.

* More severe hydronephrosis may be due to anastomosis stricture, renal calculus, or ureteric blood
  clot.

* *Ultrasound:*
  (i)   Dilatation of collecting system.
  (ii) Hyperechoic foci within the collecting system
        may be due to pyonephrosis, gas-forming
        organisms, blood, or fungus balls.
  (iii) Useful for guidance of percutaneous nephros-
        tomy placement.

* *Scintigraphy:*
  (i)   Diuretic renography is performed to differenti-
        ate obstructive from non-obstructive
        hydronephrosis.
  (ii) Furosemide (0.4 mg/kg) is injected i.v. 20
        minutes after ^{99m}Tc-MAG3 injection.
  (iii) Non-obstructive dilatation shows rapid 'wash-
        out' of tracer.
  (iv) Obstruction shows increased accumulation of
        tracer in a dilated system.
  (v)   Observed changes may be quantitated by
        plotting a time–activity graph.
  (vi) Clearance half-time is calculated, i.e. time
        taken to clear 50% of activity after furosemide
        injection:
        (a)   < 10 minutes = normal.
        (b)   10–20 minutes = equivocal.
        (c)   > 20 minutes = abnormal.

4. Renal artery stenosis

* Most common post-transplantation vascular complication.

* Presents with graft dysfunction or hypertension.

* Most common site is the anastomosis.

* *Ultrasound:*
  (i)   Renal artery narrowing on colour Doppler.
  (ii) Velocity increase (> 200 cm/sec) with associated
        turbulence.

* *Scintigraphy:*
  (i)   Decreased perfusion.
  (ii) Decreased function.

5. Renal vein thrombosis

* Ultrasound shows lack of flow on colour and
  duplex examination.

6. Arteriovenous fistula (AVF)/pseudoaneurysm

* Most commonly seen as a complication of percutaneous biopsy.

* Biopsy is best performed under ultrasound control:
  (i)   Needle tip directly visualised.
  (ii) Intrarenal vessels visualised with colour
        Doppler.
  (iii) Needle tip directed into cortex away from
        intrarenal vessels will reduce the incidence of
        AVF and pseudoaneurysm.

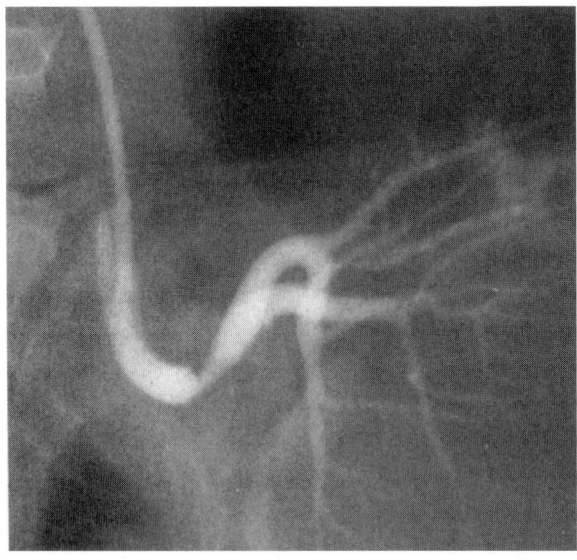 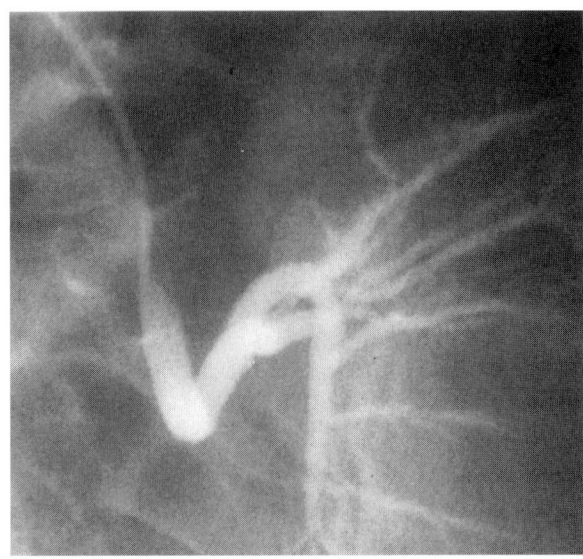

a   b

Figure 10.2 *Transplant artery stenosis.*
(a) Pre-angioplasty. Localised tight stenosis of the transplant artery. (b) Post-angioplasty. Following angioplasty the artery is of normal calibre.

- AVF and pseudoaneurysm are well seen on colour Doppler.

Further investigations and radiological techniques are used as indicated by the results of ultrasound and MAG3 scans, or where these methods are equivocal.

Arteriography

- Used to confirm or exclude transplant artery stenosis as suggested by ultrasound.

- Transplant artery stenoses are of two types: either commonly a short-segment stenosis at the anastomosis site, or rarely a long-segment stenosis distal to the anastomosis (*Fig. 10.2*).

CT

- Good for diagnosing and defining fluid collections and for guiding aspiration and drainage procedures.

- Investigation of choice for suspected abscess or post-transplant malignancy.

- Cannot differentiate acute tubular necrosis (ATN) from rejection.

MRI

Anatomical changes (i.e. hydronephrosis, fluid collections) are well seen, though with no particular advantage over ultrasound. The kidney shows altered signal in both ATN and rejection, though no consistent signs have been identified to allow differentiation.

Interventional radiology

- Ultrasound guided percutaneous biopsy.

- Ultrasound or CT-guided aspiration/drainage of fluid collections.

- Ultrasound or CT-guided percutaneous nephrostomy:
  (i) Relief of obstructive hydronephrosis.
  (ii) Balloon dilatation of ureteric strictures may obviate the need for surgical revision.
  (iii) Diversion for urine leak +/– placement of ureteric stent.

- Percutaneous transluminal angioplasty for transplant artery stenosis.

- Transcatheter embolisation for AVF/pseudoaneurysm.

- Treatment of renal calculi:
  (i) Extracorporeal shockwave lithotripsy (ESWL).
  (ii) Basket removal.

Liver transplantation

Pre-operative assessment of a liver recipient

The purpose of imaging the pre-operative candidate is exclusion of surgical or oncological contraindications to transplantation.

Full clinical work-up for the liver disease in question

Specific pre-operative tests

- Confirm patency of the portal vein: ultrasound with Doppler, and arteriography in doubtful cases.

- Measure liver volume: CT.

- Confirm patency and demonstrate anatomy of IVC: Doppler US and cavogram in doubtful cases.

- Identify cirrhosis and sequelae of portal hypertension: Doppler US and CT.

- Diagnose intra- or extrahepatic malignancy: CT.

Post-operative complications of liver transplantation

The two most commonly used imaging techniques in the early post-transplantation period are duplex ultrasound and T-tube cholangiography as follows:

(a) Duplex ultrasound:

- Daily screening for 1–2 weeks, less frequently thereafter.

- Hepatic parenchymal abnormalities.

- Perihepatic fluid collections.

- Biliary dilatation.

- Vascular thrombosis/stenosis, i.e. hepatic artery, portal vein, hepatic veins, inferior vena cava.

(b) T-tube cholangiography:

- Anastomotic stricture.

- Bile leak.

1. *Hepatic artery thrombosis*

- Most common vascular complication; more common in children than adults.

- Hepatic artery thrombosis leads to bile duct ischaemia and necrosis with bile leak.

- Presents with hepatic necrosis, bile leak, recurrent bacteraemia.

- *Duplex ultrasound:*
  (i) Absent flow in hepatic artery and its major branches.
  (ii) Collaterals may occasionally be seen.
  (iii) May confirm diagnosis with angiography.
  (iv) Retransplantation is usually required.

- Percutaneous drainage of biloma may prolong graft life prior to retransplantation.

2. *Hepatic artery stenosis*

- Usually occurs at the anastomosis.

- Presents with graft dysfunction or bile leak.

- *Duplex ultrasound:*
  Focal velocity increase with turbulent flow.

- May treat with balloon angioplasty.

3. *Hepatic artery pseudoaneurysm and arteriovenous fistula*

- Rare though potentially fatal complication.

- Either anastomotic or secondary to percutaneous biopsy.

- Particularly well seen with colour Doppler.

- Surgical reconstruction, embolisation or arterial stent placement.

4. *Portal vein thrombosis*

- Presents with graft dysfunction, ascites, other signs of portal hypertension.

- *Duplex ultrasound:*
  (i) Decreased or absent flow.

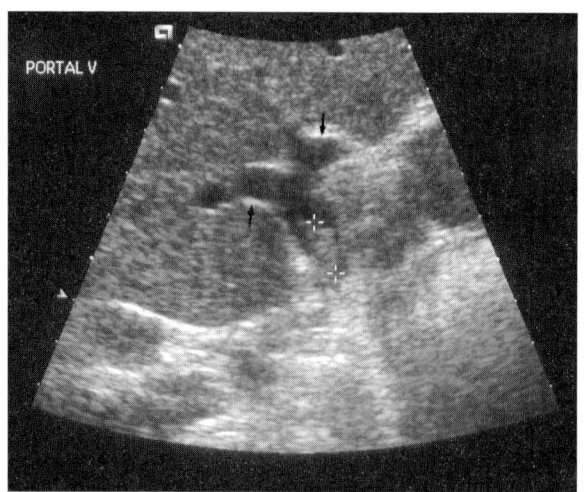

Figure 10.3 *Portal vein thrombosis – US.*
US examination in a paediatric patient following liver transplantation for biliary atresia. Thrombus is seen as echogenic material in the lumen of the portal vein. Note that the right and left branches of the portal vein are clear (arrows).

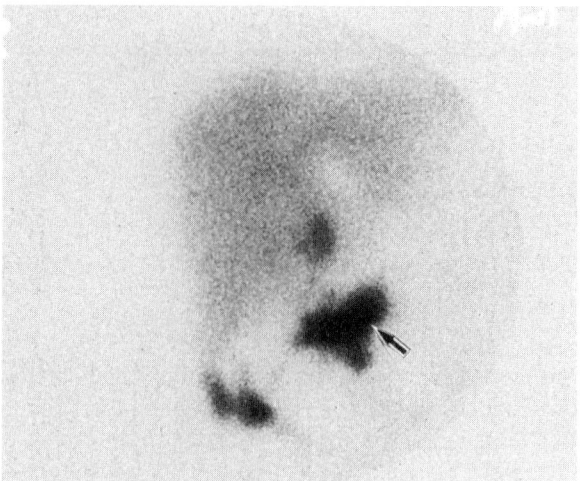

Figure 10.4 *Bile duct leak following liver transplant –*
^{99m}Tc HIDA scan.
The bile collection is seen as a persistent angular region of increased activity (arrow) in the subhepatic region. (Courtesy of Dr J Reasbeck, Brisbane.)

(ii) Direct visualisation of echogenic thrombus within the portal vein (*Fig. 10.3*).

• May be amenable to transhepatic percutaneous thrombolysis or require surgical thrombectomy, vein graft, or retransplantation.

5. IVC thrombosis and stenosis

• Usually occurs at the site of surgical anastomosis, either subhepatic or suprahepatic.

• *Duplex ultrasound:*
(i) Direct visualisation of echogenic thrombus.
(ii) Narrowing of the IVC.
(iii) Focal velocity increase and turbulence.
(iv) Loss of phasicity of waveform proximal to stenosis.

• Treat with angioplasty and stent placement.

6. Bile leak

• Occurs most commonly at T-tube site; non-anastomotic bile leaks are usually associated with hepatic artery thrombosis or stricture.

• *Ultrasound:*
(i) Anechoic fluid collection.
(ii) Signs of hepatic artery thrombosis.

• Scintigraphy (^{99m}Tc-IDA):
Leakage of tracer (*Fig. 10.4*).

• *Interventional radiology:*
(i) Percutaneous drainage of biloma.
(ii) Biliary decompression.

7. Bile duct stricture and obstruction

• Ultrasound demonstrates dilated proximal ducts, though is not as sensitive in transplant livers, so cholangiography is performed more often than in non-transplant patients.

• *Cholangiography:*
Via T-tube if present; ERCP; PTC (*Fig. 10.5*).

• *Scintigraphy (^{99m}Tc-IDA):*
(i) Dilated proximal ducts
(ii) Delayed or non-passage of tracer into bowel.

• *Interventional radiology:*
(i) Percutaneous biliary drainage.
(ii) Stent insertion.
(iii) Dilatation of strictures by angioplasty balloon.
(iv) Basket removal of calculi.

8. Fluid collections

• Small, transient haematomas and seromas in the

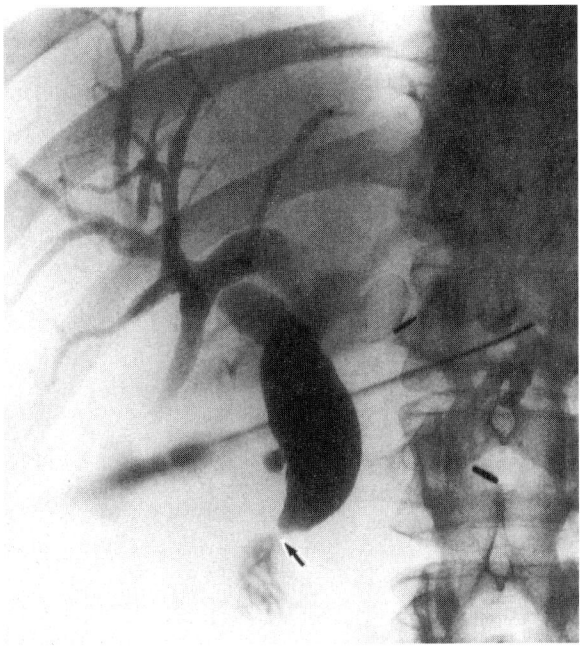

a

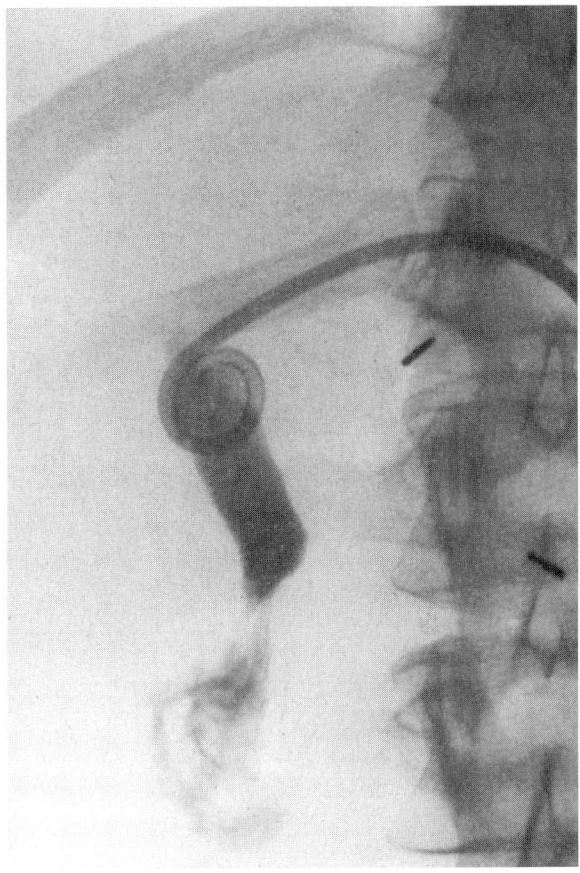

b

Figure 10.5 *Bile duct stricture following liver transplant.*
(a) PTC. The bile ducts are dilated. There is a localised stricture at the anastomosis of the common bile duct and the bowel (arrow). (b) Percutaneous drainage. Percutaneous drainage catheter in-situ with decreased calibre of the common bile duct. (Courtesy of Dr J Reasbeck, Brisbane.)

subhepatic space are common in the immediate post-operative period.

- Differential diagnosis of large fluid collections seen on ultrasound includes:
  (i)   Haematoma.
  (ii) Biloma.
  (iii) Abscess.

- Cholangiography and/or ^{99m}Tc-IDA scintigraphy are used to confirm bile duct leak and biloma.

- Ultrasound may be used to guide aspiration of fluid collections and drainage placement.

9. Rejection

- No consistent specific imaging findings have been identified as yet.

- Imaging does contribute to the diagnosis of rejection by:
  (a) Exclusion of other causes of liver dysfunction as above.
  (b) Guidance of percutaneous biopsy.

Heart and lung transplantation

Terms and abbreviations used in this section:

- OCT: orthotopic cardiac transplant.

- HCT: heterotopic cardiac transplant (new heart positioned to the right of the native heart).

- SLT: single lung transplant.

- DLT: double lung transplant.

- HLT: heart and lung transplant.

CXR will obviously be the predominant imaging investigation in the assessment of complications following heart, lung, and heart–lung transplants with other imaging such as CT performed as indicated. The more common complications are outlined below.

1. Miscellaneous acute sequelae

- Re-implantation response following SLT, DLT, or HLT.
  - (i) Transient non-cardiogenic pulmonary oedema occurring up to day 3 post-transplant and resolving over several days.
  - (ii) Diagnosis or exclusion of cardiac failure, acute rejection, and fluid overload.

- Pleural effusion.
  Usually transient.

- Pneumothorax.

- Airway dehiscence.

- Infection.
  - (a) Early: bacteria, fungi.
  - (b) Late: cytomegalovirus, *Pneumocystis carinii*.

2. Cardiac rejection

- Non-specific imaging findings.

- Signs of cardiac failure and cardiomegaly.

- Biopsy required for definitive diagnosis.

3. Acute lung rejection

- Usually occurs at least 5 days post-transplant.

- CXR may be normal or may show ground-glass opacity progressing to more focal areas of consolidation.

4. Graft coronary artery disease

- 'Accelerated atheroma' may occur in the coronary arteries.

- Usually presents with cardiac failure; angina does not occur due to denervation of the transplanted heart.

- Screen with annual coronary angiogram.

5. Bronchiolitis obliterans

- Commonest long-term complication in lung transplantation.

- CXR often normal or may show a subtle decrease of pulmonary vascularity.

- CT shows bronchial dilatation and decreased attenuation of lung parenchyma.

6. Post-transplantation lymphoproliferative disorders (PLPD)

- Spectrum of disorders ranging from benign, asymptomatic proliferations of lymphoid tissue to non-Hodgkin's lymphoma.

- Incidence varies with organ transplanted; more common following heart and lung transplants than with kidney and liver transplants.

- High association with the Epstein–Barr virus.

- May occur from one month to several years following surgery.

- Involve lymph nodes, lungs, gastrointestinal tract, CNS.

- Subset of PLPD seen in association with cyclosporine:
  - (a) Rapid onset: 4–6 months post-transplant.
  - (b) Sparing of the CNS.
  - (c) Regression or resolution following reduction of cyclosporine dose.

Pancreas transplantation

The two major indications for pancreas transplantation are:

1. Severely complicated diabetes.

2. Total pancreatectomy for carcinoma.

The majority of operations are simultaneous pancreas–kidney transplants:

- Higher rate of graft survival.

- Exocrine pancreatic secretions are drained into the

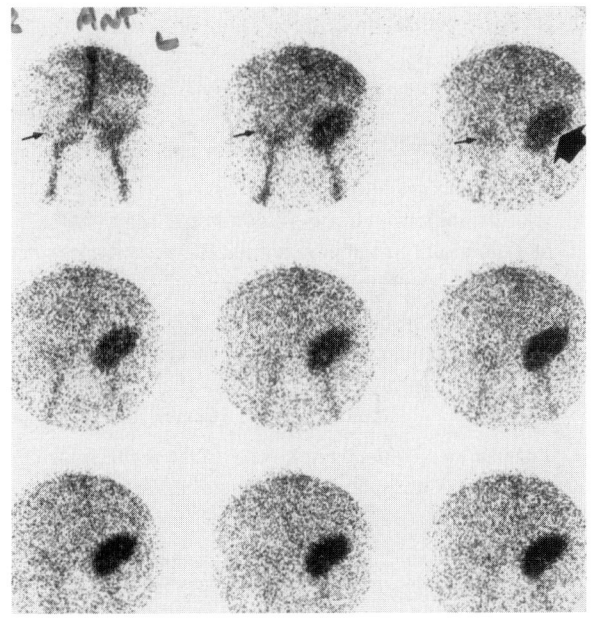
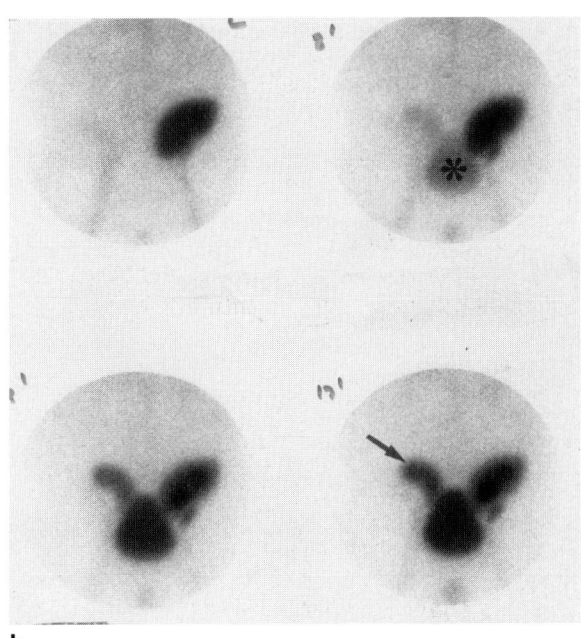

a   b

Figure 10.6 *Normal pancreas transplant – scintigraphy.*
(a) Early scans. Scans performed immediately after injection show tracer in the aorta and iliac arteries. The renal transplant shows good perfusion (large arrow). The faint blush of activity on the right (small arrows) indicates good perfusion of the pancreas transplant. (b) Late scans. Later scans show filling of the bladder with tracer (*) followed by filling of the duodenal loop (straight arrow). There is no evidence of leakage on this normal study. Note normal continued activity in the renal transplant.

bladder via a duodenal segment, both ends of which are stapled closed.

Pre-operatively the recipient will undergo ophthalmological, neurological, cardiological, and psychological assessment.

Pre-operative imaging includes:

- Thallium stress test.

- Barium meal.

- Angiogram of aorta and iliac arteries.

- MCU.

The most commonly performed imaging investigations following pancreas transplantation are:

- Duplex US: assess vasculature.

- CT: fluid collection and pancreatitis.

- Scintigraphy: viability of graft; anastomotic leak (*Fig. 10.6*).

The more common complications are described below.

1. Pancreatitis

- Mild pancreatitis in the immediate post-operative period is very common and usually transitory.

- More severe pancreatitis occurring later in the post-operative period is usually due to urinary reflux.

- CT used to define extent of inflammatory changes, ascites, and fluid collections.

2. Vascular thrombosis

- Assess with Duplex US and confirm with angiography.

3. Anastomotic leak

- Leak may occur from:
  (i)   duodenum–bladder anastomosis;
  (ii) lateral duodenal staple line;
  (iii) perforated duodenal ulcers.

- Assess with CT and scintigraphy to define source and extent of leak.

- CT-guided aspiration of fluid collections.

4. Infection

- US or CT guided aspiration and drainage of abscesses.

5. Urological complications

- Haematuria.
  If severe assess with cystoscopy.

- Urinary tract infection.
  Imaging usually not required.

- Urethral stricture.
  Urethrogram.

6. Rejection

- Most common form of graft failure.

- No specific imaging findings.

Further Reading

1. Bowen A, Hungate RG, Kaye RD *et al*. Imaging in liver transplantation. *Radiological Clinics of North America* 1996; **34**:757–778.

2. Garg K, Zamora MR, Tuder R *et al*. Lung transplantation: indications, donor and recipient selection, and imaging of complications. *RadioGraphics* 1996; **16**:355–367.

3. Harris KM, Schwartz ML, Slasky BS *et al*. Posttransplantation cyclosporine-induced lymphoproliferative disorders: clinical and radiological manifestations. *Radiology* 1987; **162**:697–700.

4. Pozniak MA, Propeck PA, Kelcz F, Sollinger H. Imaging of pancreas transplants. *Radiological Clinics of North America* 1995; **33**:581–594.

5. Rees JIS, Evans C. Imaging after renal transplantation. *Clinical Radiology* 1991; **43**:4–7.

11 Paediatrics

Investigation of an abdominal mass

The overall roles of imaging for an abdominal mass are:

- Diagnosis of a mass.

- Define organ of origin.

- Characterise mass:
  (a) Margins.
  (b) Calcification, necrosis, cyst formation, fat.

- Diagnose complications and evidence of malignancy:
  (a) Metastases.
  (b) Lymphadenopathy.
  (c) Invasion of surrounding structures.
  (d) Vascular invasion.

- Pre-treatment planning.

- Guidance of percutaneous biopsy or other interventional procedures, e.g. nephrostomy.

- Follow-up: response to therapy, recurrent tumour.

US is the first investigation of choice in a child with a suspected abdominal mass. CT is then used to further define the mass and to diagnose complications as above. Plain films of the abdomen and chest are usually also performed in the initial work-up. Other imaging modalities such as scintigraphy, MRI, and angiography are occasionally used in certain instances.

Ultrasound

- US is the first investigation for assessing the site of origin of a mass and as a guidance for further investigations.

- Excellent screening tool in children where lack of mesenteric and retroperitoneal fat allows good definition of organs and blood vessels.

Plain films

- AXR and CXR usually performed in initial work-up.

- *AXR:* calcification, displacement of bowel loops, bone destruction in vertebral invasion.

- *CXR:*
  (i) Lymphadenopathy, mediastinal and paravertebral.
  (ii) Pulmonary metastases.
  (iii) Although chest CT is more accurate an initial CXR is important to establish a baseline prior to treatment and follow-up.

CT

- Helical CT with fast scanning times is particularly advantageous in children.

- Accurate characterisation of an abdominal mass and its organ of origin.

- Highly sensitive for calcification and fat.

- Sensitive for evidence of malignancy:
  (i) Invasion of surrounding structures.
  (ii) Lymphadenopathy.
  (iii) Liver metastases.
  (iv) Vascular encasement/invasion.

MRI

- MRI has several advantages in children:
  (i) No radiation.
  (ii) No iodinated contrast media.
  (iii) Multiplanar scanning, e.g. coronal scanning may be useful in hydronephrosis for detecting the level of obstruction; coronal images also demonstrate liver, adrenal and renal tumours very well.
  (iv) Imaging of blood vessels, e.g. renal vein invasion by nephroblastoma can be detected without the use of iodinated contrast media.

- Disadvantages of MRI include cost, lack of availability in some areas, and the relative difficulties in administering anaesthesia to uncooperative patients.

- MRI is generally used for difficult cases to define specific clinical problems, e.g. spinal invasion by neuroblastoma.

Scintigraphy

- Renal scintigraphy complements US in the assessment of benign renal conditions which may present as an abdominal mass, i.e. hydronephrosis, multicystic dysplastic kidney, and polycystic conditions:
  (i) ^{99m}Tc-DTPA or ^{99m}Tc-MAG3.
  (ii) MAG3 (mercaptoacetyltriglycine) is a newer agent with more efficient renal extraction than DTPA; it is gaining wide acceptance in renal imaging, particularly in paediatric and transplant patients where in some centres it has replaced DTPA.
  (iii) Physiological information, e.g. differential renal function, diuretic 'wash-out'.
  (iv) Anatomical information, e.g. level of obstruction.

- Bone scintigraphy (^{99m}Tc-MDP) for suspected metastases.

- ^{131}I-MIBG for neuroblastoma.

Other modalities

- Micturating cystourethrogram (MCU) in hydronephrosis.

- Angiography: done rarely as a surgical 'road map', especially in liver tumours.

- Cavography: sometimes required to assess the IVC where US and CT are equivocal for the diagnosis of tumour invasion.

Common paediatric abdominal masses: imaging findings

Hydronephrosis

- The more common causes of hydronephrosis in children are:

  (i)   PUJ obstruction.
  (ii) Vesicoureteric reflux.
  (iii) Primary megaloureter.
  (iv) Duplex kidney with upper pole ureterocele.

- Hydronephrosis may present as a palpable abdominal mass, with urinary tract infection (see below), or may be detected on prenatal screening US.

- PUJ obstruction and multicystic dysplastic kidney are the most common benign renal conditions which present as an abdominal mass.

- The advent of virtually universal screening prenatal US has lead to a marked increase in the early diagnosis of hydronephrosis.

- The roles of imaging of hydronephrosis in the neonate are:
  (i)   Document severity of urinary tract dilatation.
  (ii) Define level of obstruction.
  (iii) Differentiate obstructive from non-obstructive causes.
  (iv) Diagnose underlying anatomical anomalies.

(a) *US:*

- Dilated renal pelvis and calyces.

- Round, markedly dilated renal pelvis in PUJ obstruction (*Fig. 11.1*).

- Thinned renal cortex.

- Underlying anomalies, e.g. ureterocele, Duplex collecting system (*Fig. 11.2*), dilated posterior urethra with urethral valves.

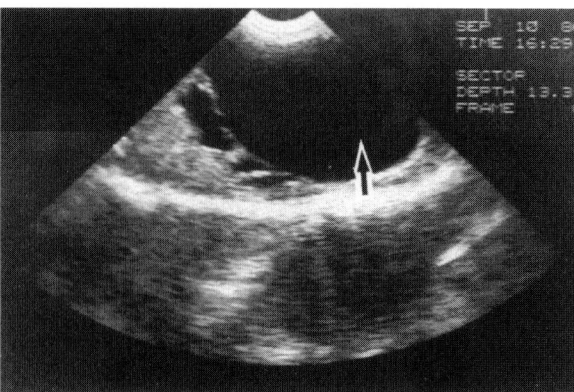

Figure 11.1 *Pelvi-uretic junction (PUJ) obstruction – ultrasound.*
Gross dilation of the renal pelvis (arrow). (Courtesy of Dr J Ratcliffe, Brisbane.)

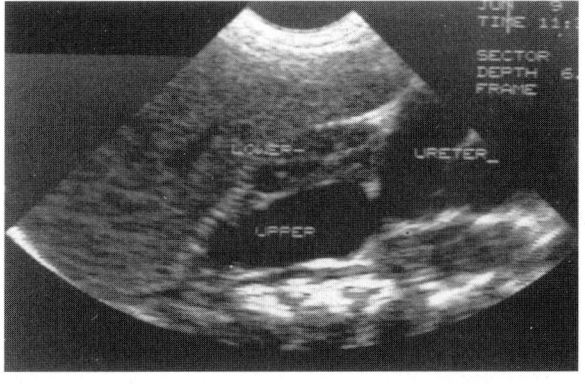

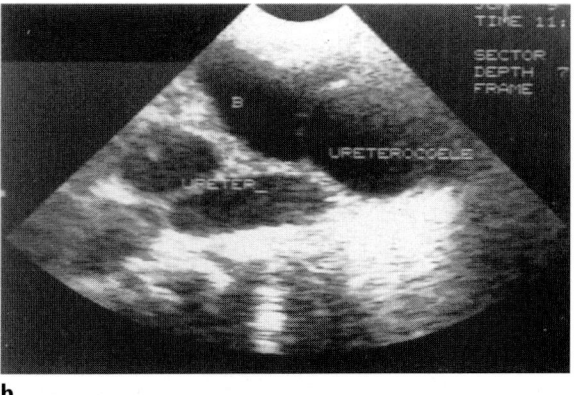

a   b

Figure 11.2 *(a) Duplex kidney with ectopic ureterocele. Normal lower moiety. Dilated collecting system of upper moiety. Dilated tortuous ureter. (b) Ectopic ureterocele – US. The ureterocele is well seen projecting into the bladder (b). Note the dilated tortuous ureter posterior to the bladder.*

- Poor sensitivity for diagnosis of vesicoureteric reflux.

(b) *Scintigraphy:*

- ^{99m}Tc-MAG3 or ^{99m}Tc-DTPA.

- Dilated collecting system.

- Diuretic scintigraphy to differentiate mechanical obstruction from other causes of hydronephrosis; furosemide injected after filling of the collecting system with isotope; measure rate of 'washout' of isotope.

- With mechanical obstruction, e.g. PUJ obstruction, isotope continues to accumulate in the collecting system following diuretic injection.

Micturating cystourethrogram (MCU):

- To document reflux and diagnose underlying anomalies, e.g. posterior urethral valves.

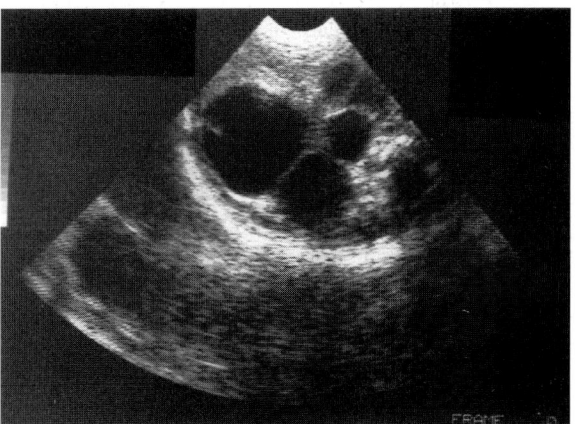

Figure 11.3 *Multicystic dysplastic kidney – ultrasound. The kidney is replaced by a large number of cysts of varying size. There is no recognisable renal tissue and no obvious communication between the cysts is demonstrated. (Courtesy of Dr J Ratcliffe, Brisbane.)*

Multicystic dysplastic kidney (MCDK)

(a) *US:*

- Kidney replaced by a lobulated collection of variably sized non-communicating cysts (*Fig. 11.3*).

- Anomalies in contralateral kidney in 15%, most commonly PUJ obstruction.

(b) *Scintigraphy:*

- ^{99m}Tc-MAG3/DTPA.

- Non-function on early scans (*Fig. 11.4*).

- Later may see minor peripheral activity with no evidence of central migration of isotope.

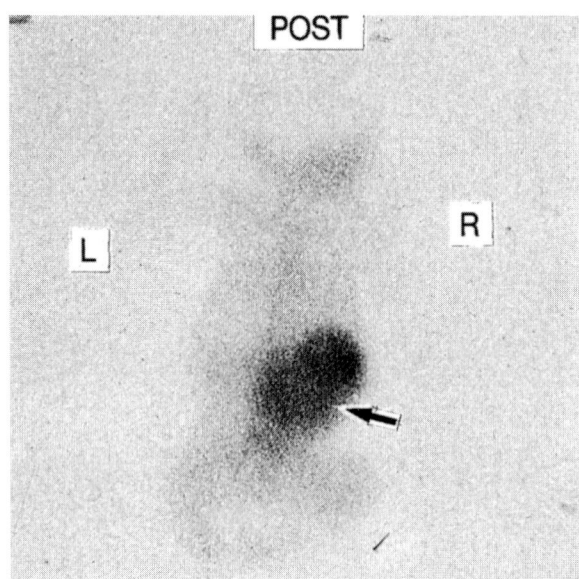

Figure 11.4 *Right PUJ obstruction and left multicystic dysplastic kidney (MCDK) – scintigraphy.*

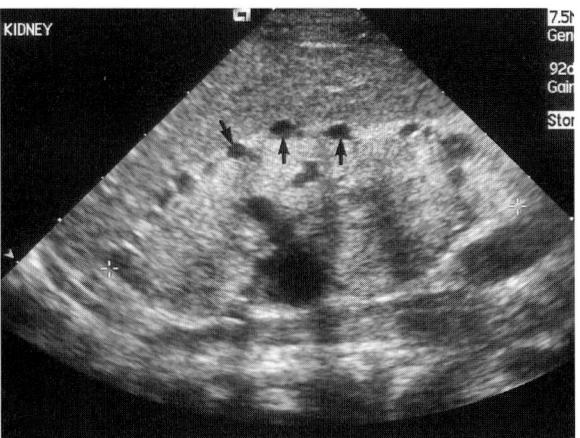

Figure 11.5 *Autosomal recessive polycystic kidney disease – US.*
Note that the kidney is enlarged and hyperechoic. The increased echogenicity is due to innumerable tiny cysts, too small to be seen on US. Note that some small peripheral cysts are just large enough to be seen individually (arrows).

Polycystic conditions

- Polycystic renal conditions are classified according to genetic inheritance, pathological findings, and clinical presentation.

1. Autosomal recessive polycystic kidney disease (ARPKD)

- Infantile and juvenile forms.

- Spectrum of disorders with associated liver disease.

- In infantile cases, the renal disease tends to be more severe with less hepatic involvement; in older children the liver disease is the dominant feature.

    US:
    - Symmetrically enlarged kidneys which are markedly hyperechoic (*Fig. 11.5*).

2. Autosomal dominant polycystic kidney disease (ADPKD)

- Rarely presents in childhood.

- Bilateral enlarged kidneys which may be asymmetrical.

    US:
    - Kidneys are of increased echogenicity due to multiple cysts which are too tiny to be seen

individually; occasionally separate small anechoic cysts are seen.

3. Glomerulocystic kidney disease

- Rare, non-genetic condition.

- Multiple glomerular cysts of around 2–3 mm diameter.

4. Hereditary syndromes associated with renal cysts

- Tuberous sclerosis.

- von Hippel–Lindau disease.

Nephroblastoma (Wilms' tumour)

- Most common solid intra-abdominal tumour in childhood.

- 15% have associated congenital anomalies, e.g. non-familial aniridia, congenital hemihypertrophy, Weidemann–Beckwith syndrome.

(a) *US:*
- Hyperechoic mass; hypoechoic areas due to necrosis.

- Replace renal parenchyma with progressive enlargement and distortion of the kidney.

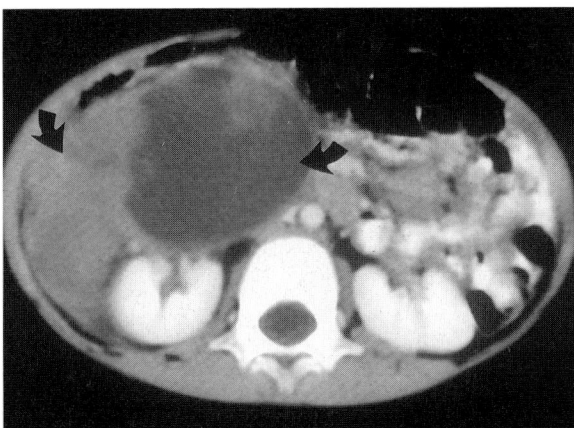

Figure 11.6 *Nephroblastoma (Wilms' tumour) – CT. A large heterogeneous mass is seen arising from the right kidney (arrows).*

- May be bilateral, therefore must always image the contralateral kidney.

- Complications: lymphadenopathy, invasion of renal vein/IVC, liver metastases.

(b) *CT:*

- Renal mass with distortion of kidney.

- Mass of equal or reduced attenuation compared with renal parenchyma and shows less enhancement than functioning renal tissue (*Fig. 11.6*).

- Invasion of surrounding structures.

- Vascular invasion: dilated renal vein with non-enhancement or peripheral enhancement around a filling defect which may extend into the right atrium.

(c) *Chest CT:*

- Chest CT is more accurate than CXR for the initial diagnosis of pulmonary metastases.

(d) *CXR:*

- Although less accurate than CT in initial diagnosis, a CXR should always be performed to establish a baseline for follow-up examinations.

Uncommon renal tumours

- Mesoblastic nephroma.

(a) *US*: large central hypoechoic area surrounded by a hyperechoic layer surrounded in turn by a thin hypoechoic rim giving a concentric pattern or 'ring sign'.

(b) *CT:* inhomogeneous renal mass.

- Multilocular cystic nephroma.

  (a) *US:* well-circumscribed mass containing multiple non-communicating cysts separated by soft tissue septa.

  (b) *CT:* multiple low-attenuation cysts.

Neuroblastoma

- Malignant childhood tumour arising from primitive sympathetic neuroblasts of the embryonic neural crest.

- 60% occur in the abdomen; of these two-thirds arise in the adrenal gland.

- Other abdominal sites are the periaortic sympathetic ganglia and ganglia at the aortic bifurcation.

- The peak age of incidence is two with most occurring below five.

- A less common subgroup is congenital neuroblastoma in infants; this tumour has a better prognosis due to its tendency to spontaneous regression.

(a) *US:*

- Homogeneous hyperechoic mass or heterogeneous texture due to areas of necrosis, haemorrhage and calcification.

- Tend to spread across midline to encase/displace major blood vessels (*Fig. 11.7*).

(b) *CT:*

- Heterogeneous mass with displacement or invasion of the kidney (*Fig. 11.8*).

- Calcification is seen in most cases on CT.

- Invasion of surrounding structures including vertebral invasion.

- Lymphadenopathy; liver metastases.

- Pulmonary metastases.

(c) *AXR:*

- Soft tissue mass with displacement of bowel loops and loss of retroperitoneal fat planes (*Fig. 11.9*).

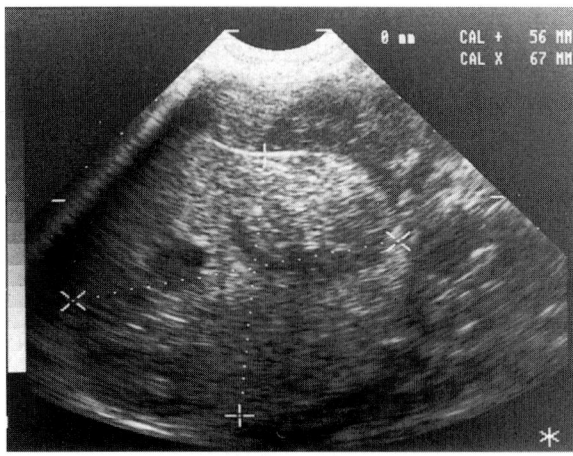

Figure 11.7 *Neuroblastoma – ultrasound.*
A large, mainly hyperechoic mass above the left kidney.
(Courtesy of Dr J Ratcliffe, Brisbane.)

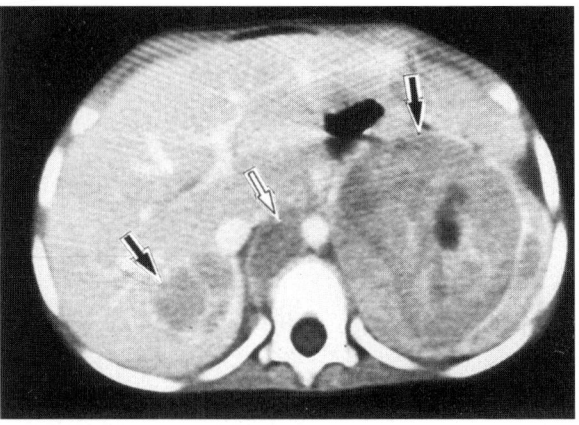

Figure 11.8 *Neuroblastoma – CT.*
In this case there are bilateral adrenal masses (solid arrows). Note:
*   low attenuation due to necrosis*
*   mass between the aorta and IVC due to retrocrural lymphadenopathy (hollow arrow).*
(Courtesy of Dr J Ratcliffe, Brisbane.)

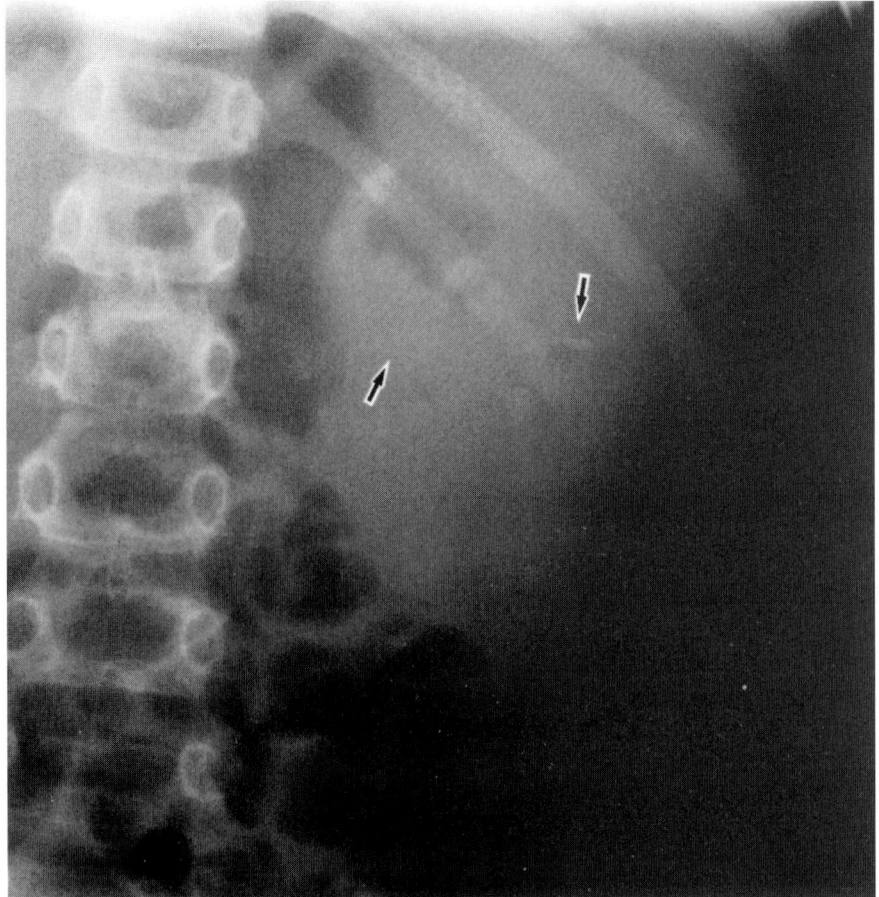

Figure 11.9
Neuroblastoma.
Left flank mass with displacement of surrounding bowel loops. Note areas of dense calcification (arrows). (Courtesy of Dr J Ratcliffe, Brisbane.)

- Calcification seen in 70%.

(d) *Bone scintigraphy:*

- ^{99m}Tc-MDP.

- More accurate than plain films in detection of skeletal metastases.

(e) *MIBG scintigraphy:*

- ^{131}I-MIBG (metaiodobenzylguanidine).

- Localisation of non-adrenal primary tumour.

- Staging: more sensitive than bone scintigraphy for detection of metastases.

- Monitoring response to therapy.

Hepatoblastoma

- Most common hepatic tumour in children.

- Increased incidence in Weidemann–Beckwith syndrome; not associated with cirrhosis.

(a) *US:*

- Well-circumscribed mass of higher echogenicity than surrounding liver.

- Hypoechoic areas due to necrosis.

- Invasion of portal vein or IVC.

(b) *CT:*

- Mass of equal or reduced attenuation compared with adjacent liver tissue.

- Less enhancement than liver (*Fig. 11.10*).

- Areas of necrosis, calcification, and occasionally fat.

- Vascular invasion: filling defect within an enlarged non-enhancing portal vein or IVC.

Angiography:

- Still often used for accurate demonstration of vascular anatomy prior to surgical resection.

- Full angiographic assessment includes anatomical localisation of the tumour, visualisation of the portal vein, hepatic artery, and in doubtful cases, the IVC.

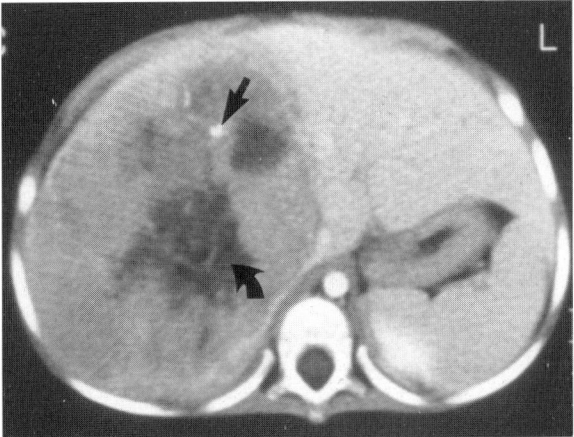

Figure 11.10 *Hepatoblastoma – CT. There is a large heterogeneous mass replacing the right lobe of the liver. As is often the case with hepatoblastoma there are areas of calcification (straight arrow) and necrosis (curved arrow).*

Hepatocellular carcinoma

- High incidence in chronic liver diseases, e.g. biliary atresia, tyrosinaemia.

(a) *US:*

- Ill-defined hypoechoic mass.

(b) *CT:*

- Multiple confluent low-attenuation masses.

Haemangioendothelioma

- Benign multicentric tumour which may be associated with cutaneous haemangiomas.

- May present with hepatomegaly, cardiac failure, or acute haemorrhage.

(a) *US:*

- Multiple discrete hyperechoic masses in the liver.

(b) *CT:*

- Multiple low-attenuation masses with occasional calcification.

(c) *Angiography:*

- Enlarged tortuous arteries, early filling of large draining veins, and pooling of contrast.

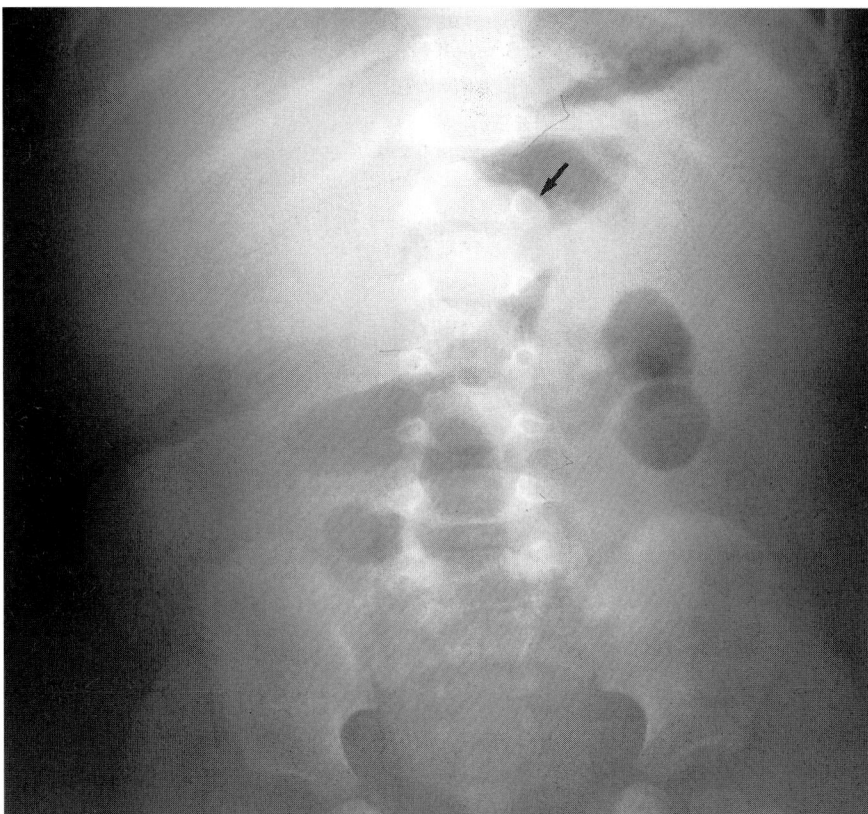

Figure 11.11
*Intussusception – AXR.
Note the curved 'meniscus'
in the transverse colon
(arrow). This is the outline
of the intussusceptum. There
is also the subtle impression
of a mass in the right upper
quadrant.*

Intussusception

- Common signs and symptoms of intussusception include vomiting, blood stained stool, colicky abdominal pain, listlessness and palpable abdominal mass.

- Imaging consists of an abdomen X-ray followed by US. Contrast enema should no longer be required for diagnosis of intussusception.

- Confirmation of intussusception is followed in suitable cases by radiological reduction.

AXR

- 'Target' lesion in right upper quadrant due to swollen hepatic flexure seen end-on with layers of peritoneal fat within and surrounding the intussusception.

- Meniscus sign due to air outlining intussusceptum (*Fig. 11.11*).

- Relatively gasless right side of abdomen.

- Small bowel obstruction.

- Free air with perforation.

Ultrasound

- Characteristic appearance with kidney-shaped mass longitudinally and 'target' lesion in cross-section (*Fig. 11.12*).

- Hypoechoic rim surrounding hyperechoic concentric rings due to layers of oedematous bowel wall and mesentery.

- May occasionally see a lead point such as lymphoma or duplication cyst though in the majority of cases in children no lead point is seen.

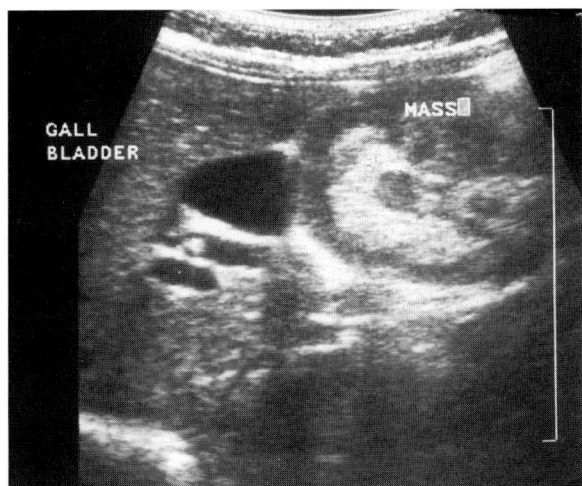

Figure 11.12 *Intussusception – US.*
Same case as Figure 11.11. The intussusception is well seen as a heterogeneous mass in the right upper abdomen, lying just to the left of the gallbladder. Note that the mass shows alternating hypoechoic and hyperechoic layers due to layers of oedematous bowel wall, mucosa and mesenteric fat.

Treatment of intussusception

- Early involvement of radiological and surgical teams.

- Contraindications to radiological reduction:
  (i) Shock: the child *must* be adequately hydrated.
  (ii) Perforation, i.e. signs of peritonism and/or free air on AXR.
  (iii) Small bowel obstruction and duration of greater than 12 hours make reduction more difficult and so decrease the likelihood of success, but are not of themselves absolute contraindications.

- *Reduction:*
  (i) X-ray screening: various operators use a variety of contrast agents including barium, water-soluble contrast and gas (*Fig. 11.13*).
  (ii) Gas reduction is now widely used and has several advantages:
    (a) Quick and clean.
    (b) If perforation occurs it is safer than with barium.
  (iii) Ultrasound: Some centres use US-guided liquid reduction.

- *Follow-up:*
  (i) A post-evacuation film is performed to exclude early recurrence.
  (ii) Recurrences occur in 3.5–10% of cases and should lead to repeat enema reduction.
  (iii) With multiple recurrences or a suspected pathological lead point, surgical intervention is mandatory.

Hypertrophic pyloric stenosis

- Palpation of a pyloric muscular mass in the right upper quadrant of an infant with a typical clinical history, i.e. forceful non-bile stained vomiting leading to dehydration and hypokalaemic alkalosis is diagnostic of hypertrophic pyloric stenosis and imaging is not required in such cases.

- Imaging is useful in infants with equivocal symptomatology or with typical symptoms where a mass cannot be palpated.

Ultrasound

- Very accurate and has replaced X-ray imaging.

- Thickened pylorus seen as a target lesion in cross-section; hypoechoic thickened muscle with hyperechoic centre.

- Positive measurements:
  (a) Total pyloric diameter > 13 mm.
  (b) Pyloric muscle thickness > 3 mm.
  (c) Pyloric length > 17 mm (*Fig. 11.14*).

- Distended stomach.

Barium meal

- Rarely used since implementation of ultrasound.

- Main role is in the post-operative patient to diagnose incomplete pyloromyotomy or to diagnose gastro-oesophageal reflux as a cause of persistent vomiting.

- Persistent thickened pyloric muscle gives a long narrow pyloric canal with rounded margins associated with delayed gastric emptying.

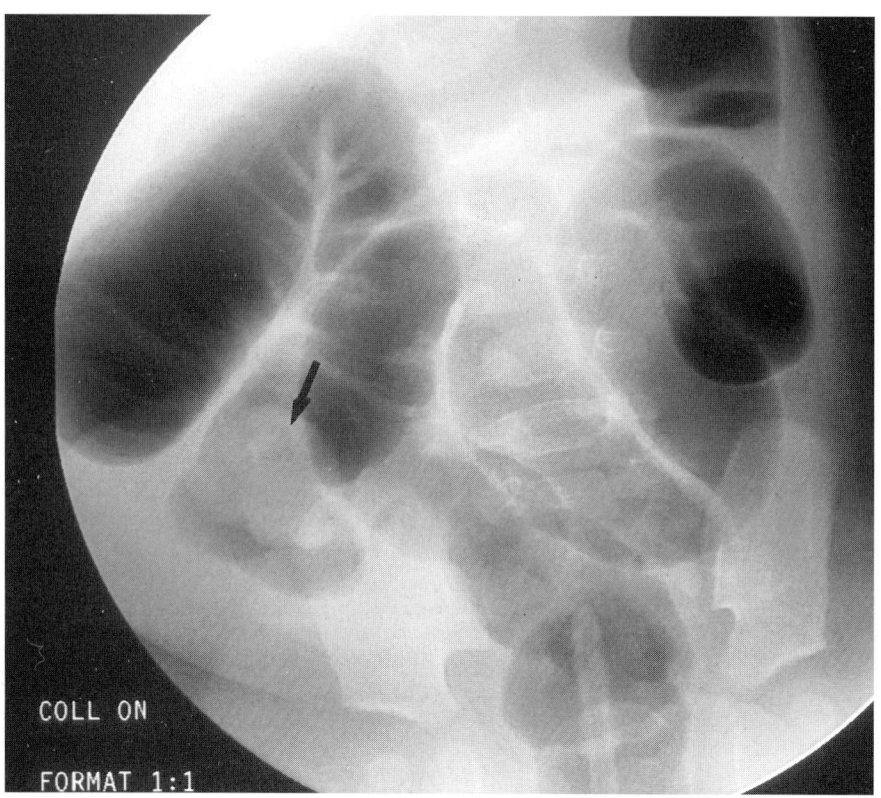

a

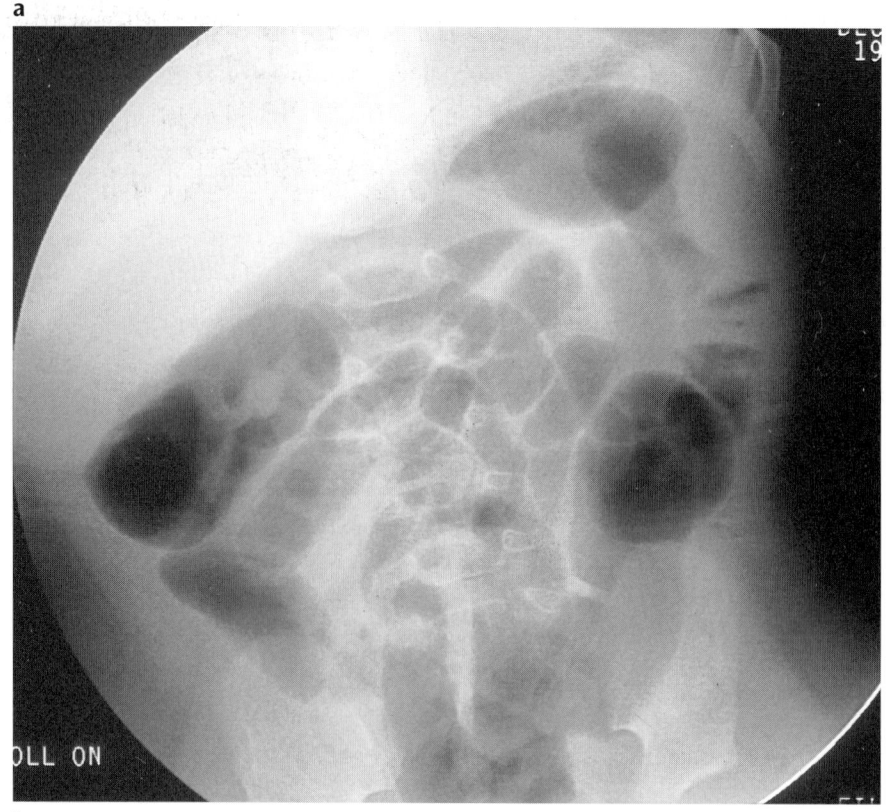

b

Figure 11.13
Intussusception – gas reduction.
(a) Same case as Figs 11.11 and 11.12. Note the following features:
* *catheter in the rectum*
* *large bowel distended with gas*
* *The intussusception has been reduced to the ileocaecal valve where a persistent soft tissue mass is seen (arrow).*
(b) Reduction of the intussusception is now complete. Complete reduction is signalled by gas filling of small bowel loops with the mass at the ileocaecal valve no longer seen.

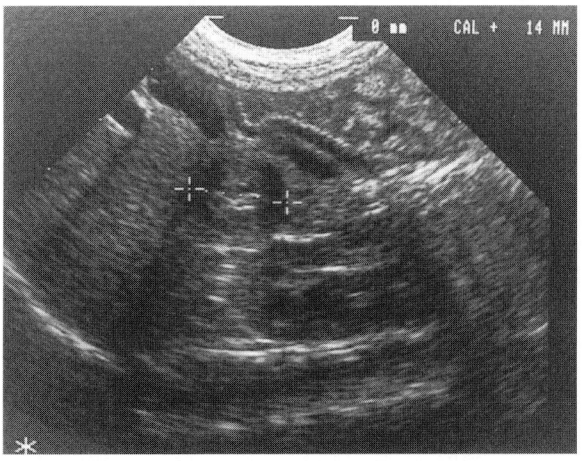

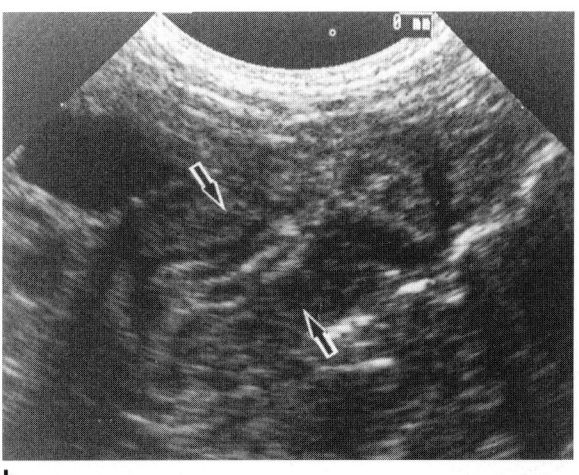

a b

Figure 11.14 (a) Pyloric stenosis – ultrasound. In transverse section pyloric stenosis appears as a 'target' lesion with an outer thick hypoechoic rim due to hypertrophied pyloric muscle, and a hyperechoic centre. (b) Pyloric stenosis – ultrasound. Longitudinal section of the pyloric canal showing the hypertrophied muscle wall (arrows).

Vesico-ureteric reflux (VUR)

All children with urinary tract infection should be investigated. The precise nature and sequence of investigations depends on local availability and expertise. The purposes of the investigations are to:

* diagnose underlying anatomical abnormalities;

* diagnose and grade severity of VUR;

* document renal damage;

* establish a baseline for subsequent evaluation of renal growth;

* establish the prognosis.

Initial investigations

* Ultrasound:
  (i) Renal tract anomalies.
  (ii) Renal cortical scarring.
  (iii) Calculi.
  (iv) US is not sensitive for the diagnosis of reflux.

* AXR: opaque calculi.

* Micturating cystourethrogram (MCU):
  (i) Document site of insertion of ureter.

(ii) Diagnose underlying anomalies, e.g. posterior urethral valves.
(iii) Diagnose VUR and grade severity as below (*Fig. 11.15*).
  (a) Grade I: Reflux into non-dilated ureter.
  (b) Grade II: Reflux into non-dilated collecting system.
  (c) Grade III: Reflux into mildly dilated collecting system.
  (d) Grade IV: Reflux into moderately dilated collecting system.
  (e) Grade V: Reflux into grossly dilated collecting system with dilated, tortuous ureter.

* When moderate to severe reflux is diagnosed, or in the presence of underlying anomalies, further imaging studies may be required.

Functional study by scintigraphy

* ^{99m}Tc-MAG3 or ^{99m}Tc-DTPA.

* Information on renal structure.

* Quantitate differential function.

* Differentiate obstructive from non-obstructive hydronephrosis.

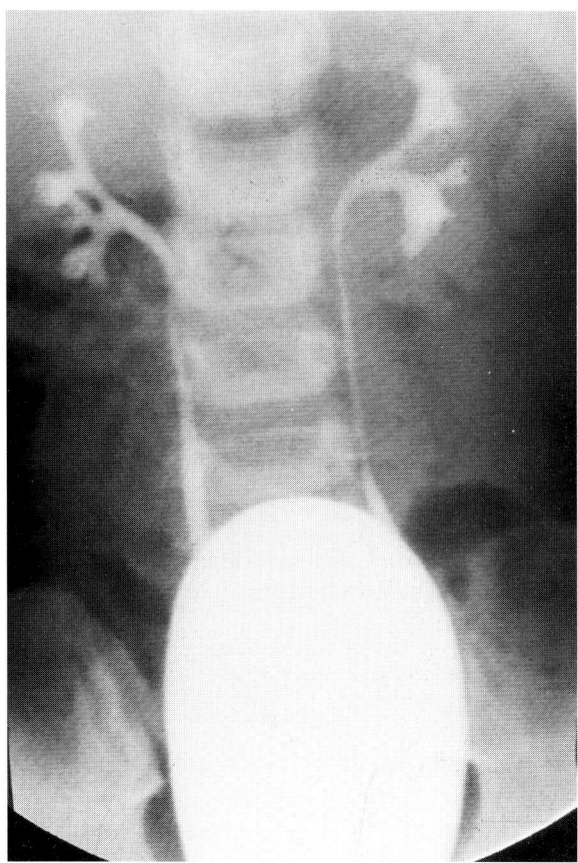

Figure 11.15 *Vesico-ureteric reflux – MCU.*
The bladder is well filled. There is bilateral vesico-ureteric reflux with mild dilatation of the collecting systems i.e. Grade III VUR.

Documentation of renal scars

- Scintigraphy :^{99m}Tc DMSA.

- DMSA is taken up by cells of proximal convoluted tubule and so outlines the renal cortex.

- More sensitive than US for documentation of renal scars (*Fig. 11.16*).

Scintigraphic reflux studies

- Once the diagnosis of VUR is established scintigraphic reflux studies may be performed for follow-up (*Fig. 11.17*).

- Main advantage is less radiation dose than with X-ray MCU.

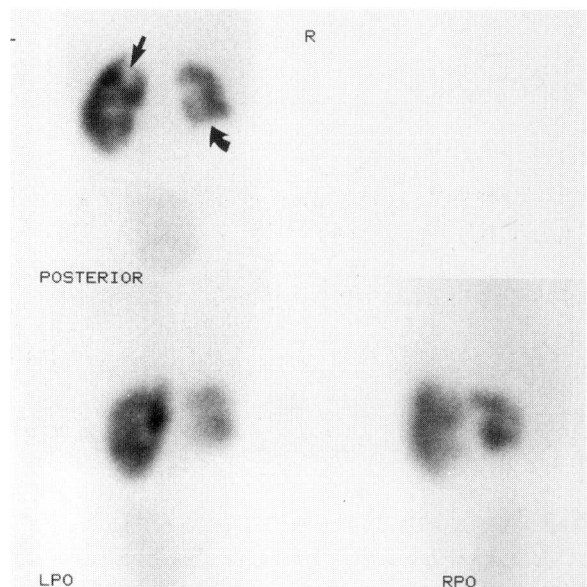

Figure 11.16 *Renal scars – DMSA scan.*
There is extensive scarring of the right kidney. The right kidney is much smaller than the left and in particular there is marked loss of cortex from its lower pole (curved arrow). There is also a scar in the upper pole of the left kidney (straight arrow).

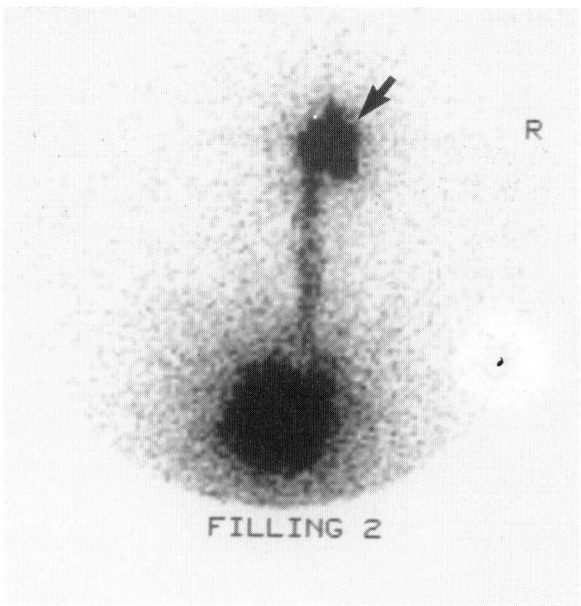

Figure 11.17 *Vesico-ureteric reflux – scintigraphic MCU.*
During bladder filling there is reflux into the right ureter and kidney (arrow). There is no evidence of reflux on the left.

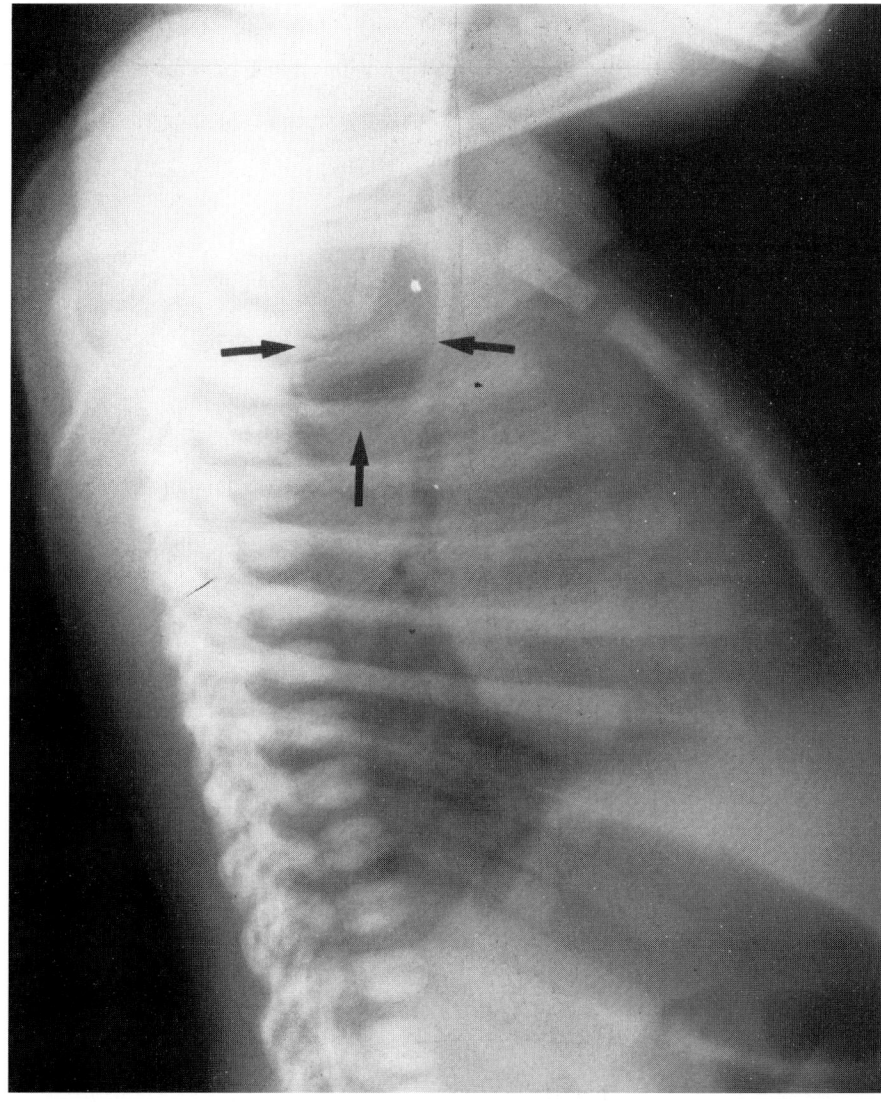

Figure 11.18 *Oesophageal atresia.*
The atretic oesophagus is well seen as a distended air filled pouch posterior to the trachea (arrows). Note the nasogastric tube. Contrast is not required in this situation. Note that there is gas in the stomach and small bowel indicating the presence of a tracheo-oesophageal fistula.

- Principal disadvantage is lack of anatomical resolution; for this reason MCU should always be used for initial assessment as above.

Oesophageal atresia with or without tracheo-oesophageal fistula (TOF)

- *Classification:*
  - (i)   Oesophageal atresia with distal TOF: 85%.
  - (ii) Oesophageal atresia without TOF: 10%.
  - (iii) TOF without oesophageal atresia ('H-type' fistula): 5%.
  - (iv) Oesophageal atresia with proximal TOF: very rare.

Plain films: CXR and AXR

- Air in upper oesophageal pouch posterior to trachea (*Fig. 11.18*)

- Nasogastric tube curled in pouch.

- Contrast studies not needed except as below.

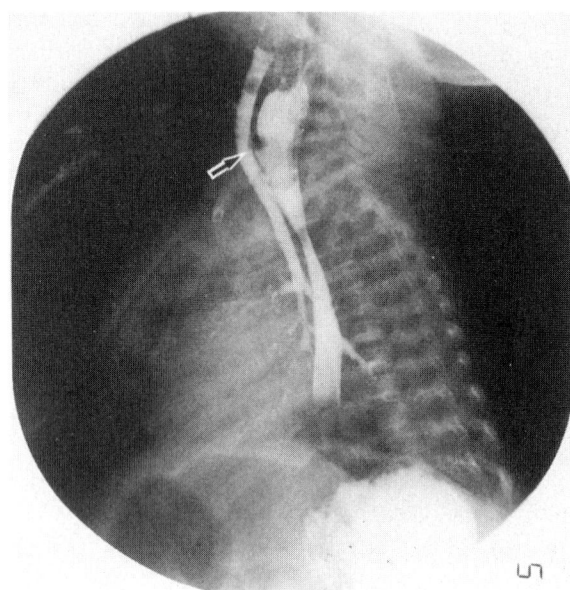

Figure 11.19 *Tracheo-oesophageal fistula. 'H' type fistula (arrow) with contrast entering the trachea and bronchial tree.*

- Air in gastrointestinal tract implies a distal fistula.
- Gasless abdomen with no TOF or proximal TOF.
- Aspiration pneumonia.

Prenatal US

- With the widespread use of US in obstetric care oesophageal atresia and TOF may be suspected prenatally.
- Polyhydramnios.
- Absence of fluid-filled stomach.
- Distended pouch of atretic oesophagus may be identified on high quality scans.

'H-Type' TOF

- Plain films are often normal.

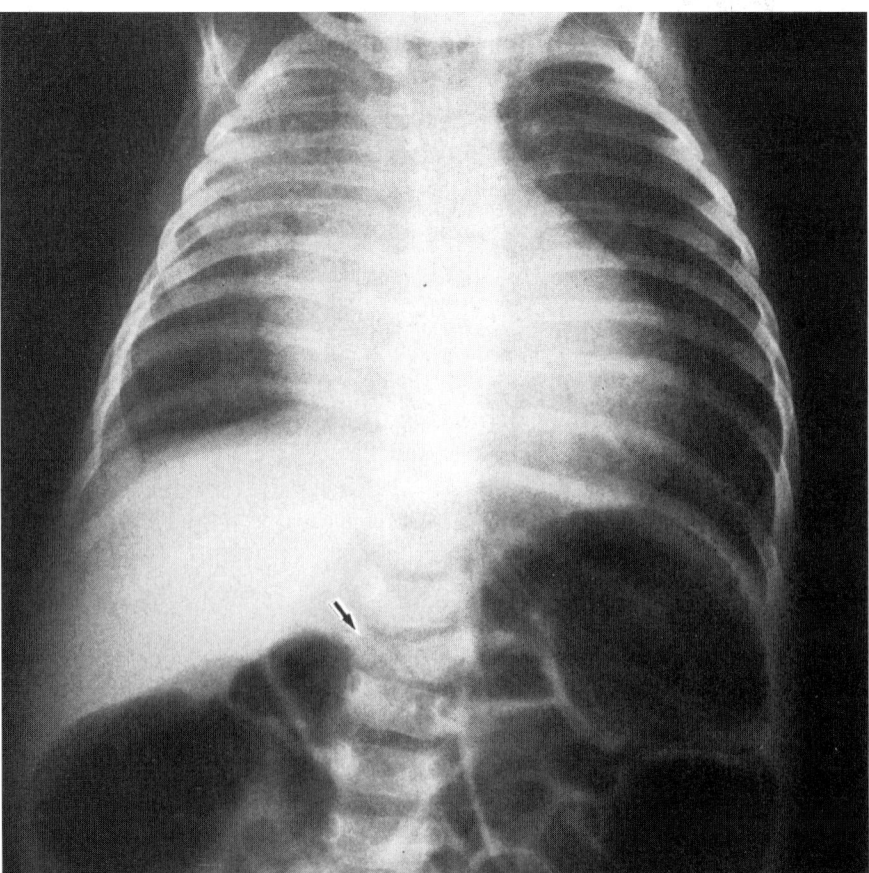

Figure 11.20 *'VACTERL' association.*
This is the same patient as Figure 11.19. Note the following features:
- *vertebral anomalies (arrow)*
- *large heart due to complex anomaly*
- *right upper lobe consolidation due to aspiration through 'H' fistula*
- *on US examination a left multicystic dysplastic kidney was found.*
The 'VACTERL' association consists of Vertebral, Anorectal, and Cardiac anomalies, Tracheo-Esophageal fistula, Renal and Limb anomalies.

- Contrast studies are very important as the fistula may be very small and difficult to image.

- Water soluble contrast is used through a tube in the upper oesophagus with the patient prone or lateral (*Fig. 11.19*).

Associated anomalies

- Approximately 25% of cases (*Fig. 11.20*).

- Vertebral anomalies.

- Anorectal atresia; duodenal atresia.

- Renal anomalies, e.g. MCDK, renal agenesis.

- Cardiac anomalies, e.g. VSD, ASD, PDA.

- Radial dysplasia and other limb anomalies.

- Right sided aortic arch seen in 5% of cases; important to diagnose pre-operatively.

- All patients should have a renal ultrasound and an echocardiogram.

Post-operative complications: plain films and contrast studies

- Oesophageal leak: pneumomediastinum, pneumothorax, pleural effusion.

- Oesophageal stricture.

- Tracheomalacia.

- Recurrent fistula.

Gut obstruction and/or bile-stained vomiting in the neonate

Plain films: AXR

- In some cases AXR is sufficient for diagnosis, e.g. duodenal obstruction.

- In other cases AXR may be normal, e.g. malrotation, or may have non-specific appearances, e.g. Hirschsprung disease.

Contrast studies: upper GI series, contrast enema

- Contrast studies are often required for diagnosis particularly in malrotation and in large bowel disorders.

Duodenal obstruction

- Duodenal atresia is the most common cause of congenital duodenal obstruction.

- Other causes include stenosis, web, annular pancreas.

- Associated anomalies (60%):
  - (i)   Oesophageal atresia.
  - (ii) Imperforate anus.
  - (iii) Renal anomalies.
  - (iv) Congenital heart disease.
  - (v)   Down's syndrome in 30%.

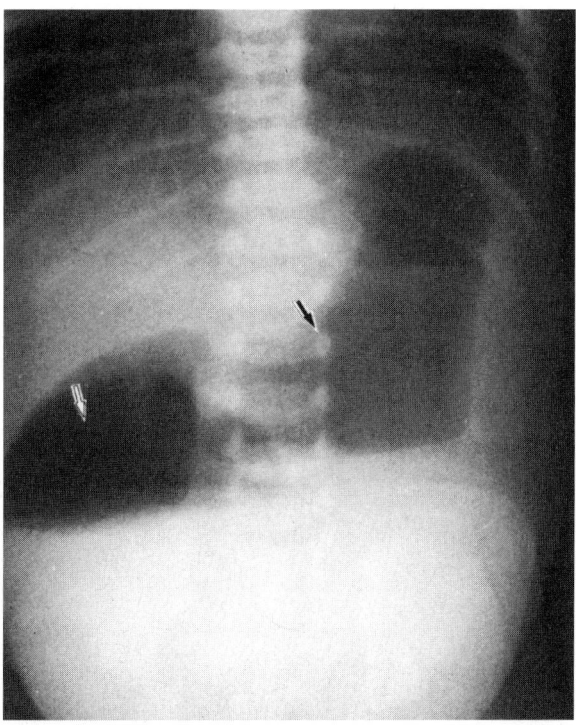

Figure 11.21 *Duodenal atresia.*
Classic 'double-bubble' appearance due to distended stomach (solid arrow) and duodenal cap (hollow arrow). Note lack of gas in distal bowel.

(a) *Prenatal US:*
- Polyhydramnios.

- Double bubble in upper abdomen due to dilated fluid-filled stomach and duodenal cap.

(b) *AXR:*
- Classic double bubble sign due to gas in distended stomach and duodenal cap (*Fig. 11.21*).

- Absence of gas in distal bowel.

- 'Triple bubble' may be seen with gas in the gallbladder.

Jejuno-ileal atresia

(a) *AXR:*
- Dilated small bowel (*Fig. 11.22*).

- Occasional calcification due to meconium peritonitis.

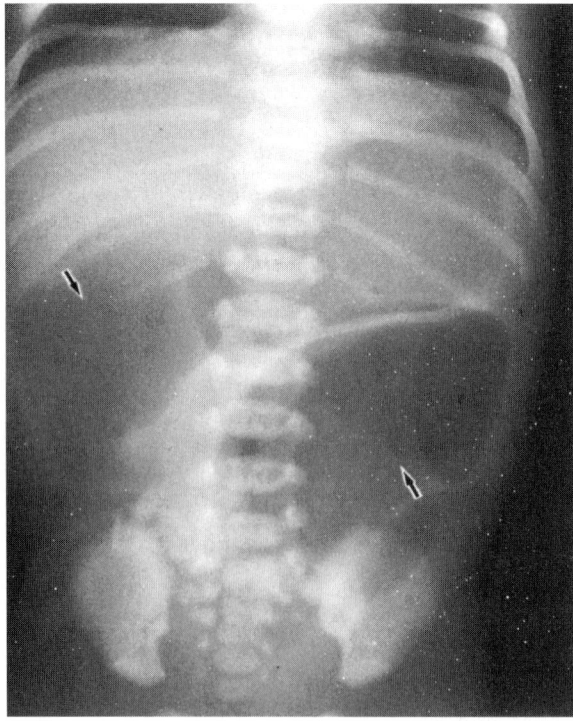

Figure 11.22 *Jejunal atresia.*
Markedly distended duodenum and proximal jejenum (arrows) with no passage of gas into the distal bowel. (Courtesy of Dr E J Stockdale, Aberdeen.)

(b) Contrast enema:
- Small colon.

Anorectal atresia

- Classified into low and high anomaly.

- *Low anomaly:* bowel ends below levator sling.

- *High anomaly:* bowel end above levator sling; fistula into vagina or posterior urethra.

(a) *AXR:*
- Lateral rectal view to classify lesion by relation of most distal part of bowel to pelvic floor (*Fig. 11.23*).

- Gas in bladder/vagina in the presence of a fistula.

- Associated sacral anomalies: failure of sacral segmentation, sacral agenesis.

(b) *US:*
- US of the perineum may determine the distance between the anal dimple on the perineal surface and the distal bowel end.

Hirschsprung disease

- Aganglionic segment of distal large bowel due to arrest of craniocaudal migration of neuroblasts.

- Distal short aganglionic segment most common form.

- Total colonic aganglionosis in 5%; sparing of rectum with more proximal involvement very rare.

(a) *AXR:*
- Dilated bowel loops.

(b) *Contrast enema:*
- Transition zone from small aganglionic bowel distally to dilated innervated bowel (*Fig. 11.24*).

Meconium ileus

- Associated with cystic fibrosis (mucoviscidosis).

(a) *Prenatal US:*
- Polyhydramnios.

- Hyperechoic contents in small bowel.

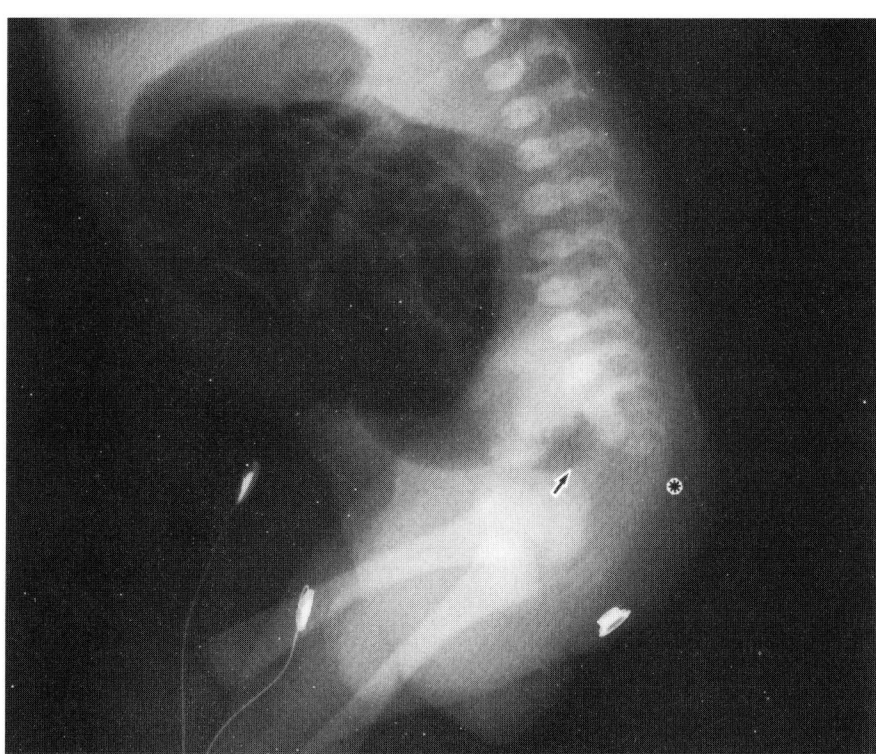

Figure 11.23 *Anorectal malformation.*
A high lesion with the most distal part of the bowel (arrow) well above the pelvic floor. Note:
- *absence of distal sacrum and coccyx (*)*
- *metal marker on perineum.*
(Courtesy of Dr M Hendry, Edinburgh.)

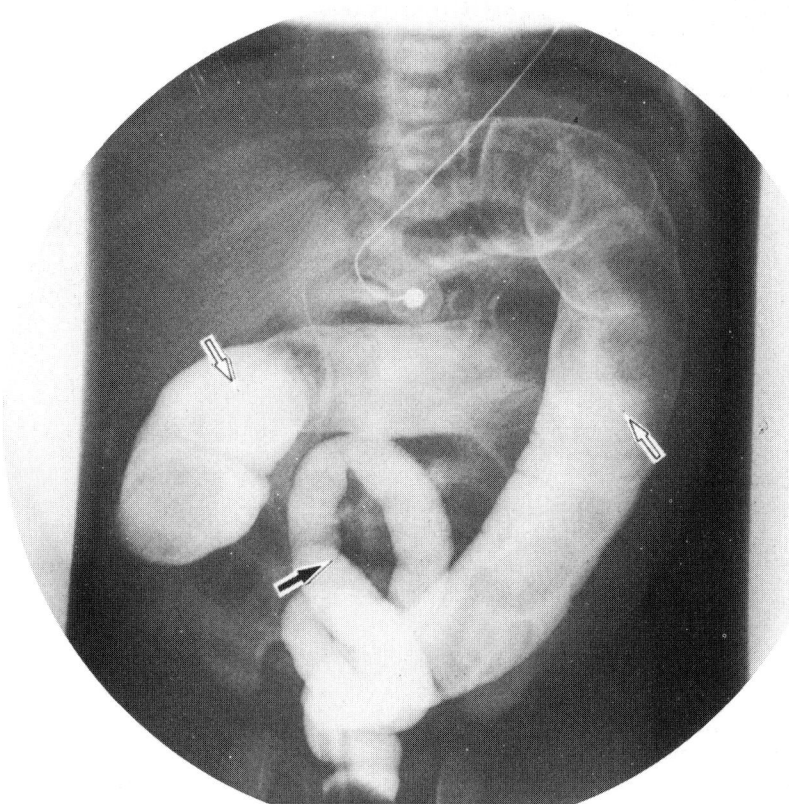

Figure 11.24 *Hirschsprung disease.*
The rectum and sigmoid colon are of normal calibre (solid arrow). The remainder of the bowel was dilated and contains retained faecal material (hollow arrows).
(Courtesy of Dr M Hendry, Edinburgh.)

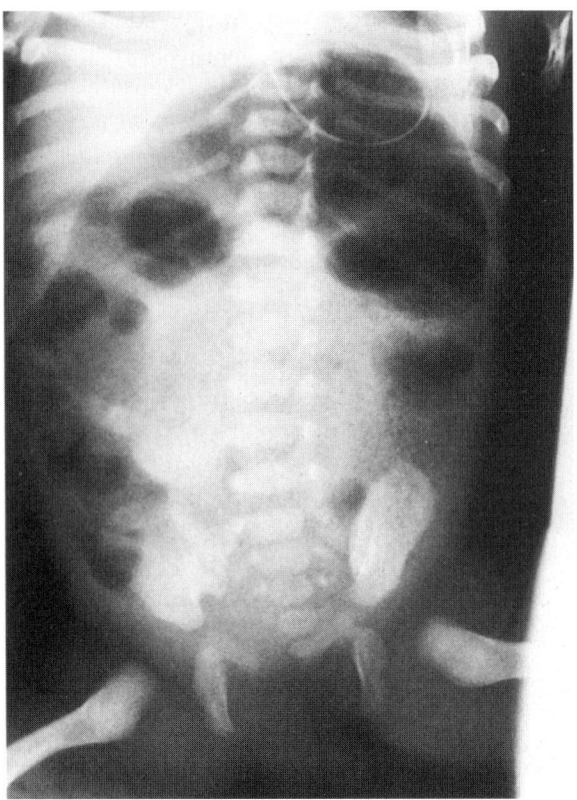

Figure 11.25 *Meconium ileus.*
Grossly dilated small bowel loops contain a mixture of air and viscous meconium giving the characteristic 'soap bubble' appearance. (Courtesy of Dr M Hendry, Edinburgh.)

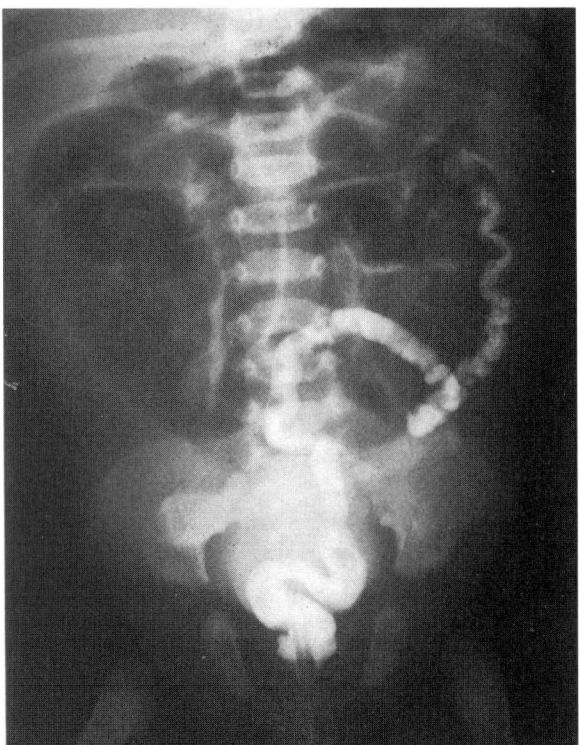

Figure 11.26 *Meconium ileus – contrast enema.*
The colon is of very small calibre and is incompletely opacified i.e. microcolon. Note the distended small bowel loops.

(b) *AXR:*
- 'Soap bubble' appearance in right lower quadrant.

- Dilated small bowel loops of variable calibre with no fluid levels on the erect view (*Fig. 11.25*).

(c) *Contrast enema:*
- Microcolon (*Fig. 11.26*).

- Large distal ileum with filling defects due to meconium.

Meconium plug syndrome

- Inspissated meconium causing distal large bowel obstruction; not related to meconium ileus.

(a) *AXR:*
- Dilated small bowel loops.

(b) *Contrast enema:*
- Often therapeutic.

- Dilated rectum.

- Large filling defects in the colon.

Small left colon syndrome

(a) *AXR:*
- Dilated bowel loops.

(b) *Contrast enema:*
- Normal distensible rectum.

- Small sigmoid and descending colon.

- Transition to dilated colon at splenic flexure.

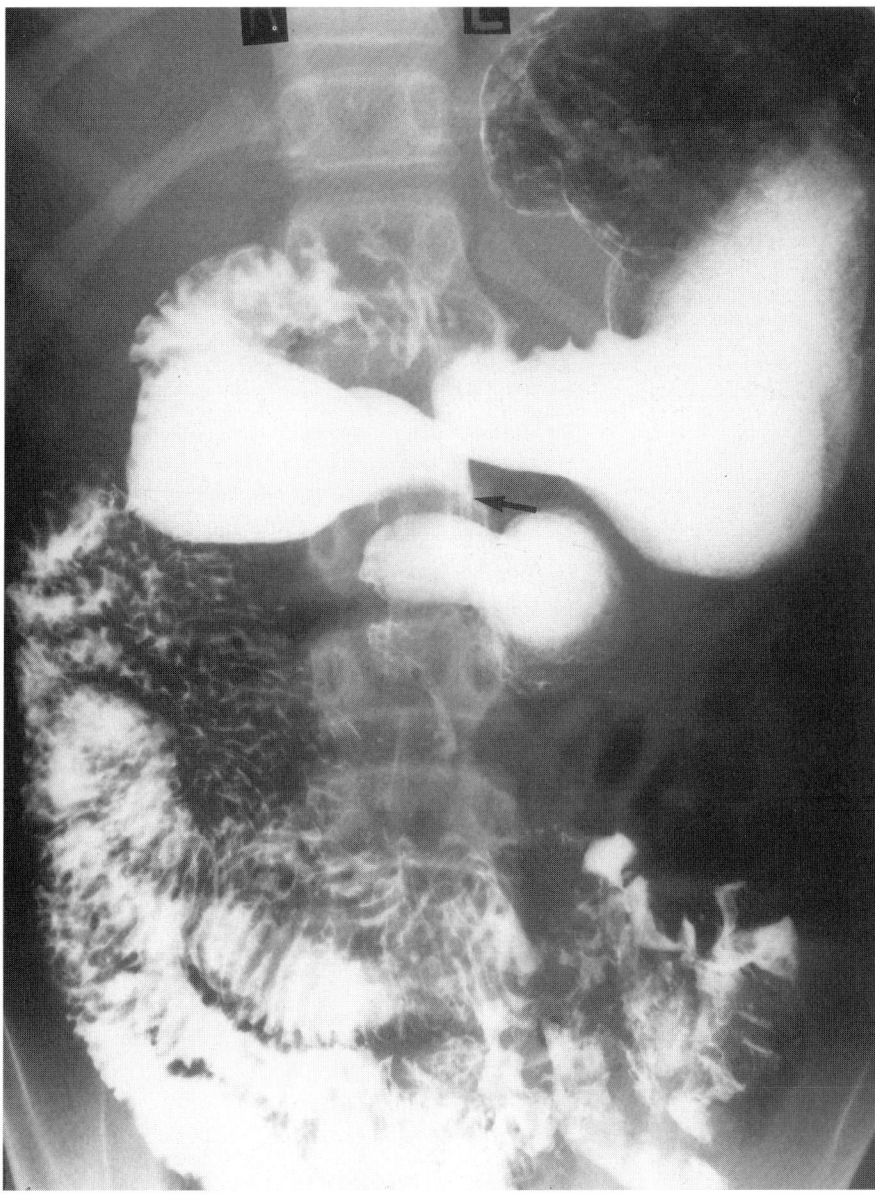

Figure 11.27 *Malrotation – barium meal.*
An 11-year-old child with repeated bile-stained vomiting. Note the features of volvulus of the duodenum:
- *dilated upper duodenum with 'beaked' ending (arrow)*
- *the duodenum has a 'twisted ribbon' or 'corkscrew' appearance.*

Note also that the jejunum lies in an abnormal position to the right of midline.

Malrotation and midgut volvulus

- Malrotation refers to a wide spectrum of anatomical variants, the common feature being abnormal rotation of the gut.

(a) *Anatomical variations include:*
- Duodenum and duodenojejunal flexure to the right of midline.

- Colon to the left of midline.

- Caecum in the left upper abdomen.

- Transverse colon lying posterior to the superior mesenteric artery.

- Peritoneal (Ladd) bands which cross and may compress the duodenum.

- Internal paraduodenal hernia.

- Shortened small bowel mesenteric attachment.

(b) *Complications:*
- Volvulus of the small bowel and duodenum.
- Intestinal obstruction due to Ladd bands or paraduodenal hernia.

(c) *Two types of clinical presentation:*
- Severe bile-stained vomiting in neonates.
- Intermittent symptoms in older children: vomiting, nausea, abdominal pain.

(d) *AXR:*
- Often normal.
- May show dilated duodenum.

(e) *Upper GI series:*
- Preferable to contrast enema as initial investigation.
- Duodenal obstruction.
- Proximal jejunum lies on the right with abnormally positioned duodenojejunal flexure.
- 'Corkscrew' appearance of small bowel loops (*Fig. 11.27*).
- Abnormally high caecum on follow-through films.

(f) *US:*
- Superior mesenteric vein lies abnormally to the left of the superior mesenteric artery.

Further Reading

1. Brindle MJ. Children with urinary tract infection; a critical diagnostic pathway. *Clinical Radiology* 1990; **41**:95–97.

2. Daneman A, Alton DJ. Intussusception: issues and controversies related to diagnosis and reduction. *Radiological Clinics of North America* 1996; **34**:743–756.

3. Gordon I. Urinary tract infection in paediatrics: the role of diagnostic imaging. *British Journal of Radiology* 1990; **63**:507–511.

4. McAlister WH, Kronemer KA. Emergency gastrointestinal radiology of the newborn. *Radiological Clinics of North America* 1996; **34**:819–844.

5. Morrison SC. Controversies in abdominal imaging. *Pediatric Clinics of North America* 1997; **44**:555–574.

6. Tonkin ILD, Wrenn EL, Hollabaugh RS. The continued value of angiography in planning surgical resection of benign and malignant hepatic tumours in children. *Pediatric Radiology* 1988; **18**:35–44.

7. Zerin JM. Hydronephrosis in the neonate and young infant: current concepts. *Seminars in US, CT, and MRI* 1994; **15**:306–316.

12 Staging of malignancy

The roles of imaging in malignancy include:

- Tumour detection.
- Staging.
- Biopsy guidance.
- Planning of surgery and radiotherapy.
- Monitoring of response to therapy.
- Diagnosis of complications of therapy.

Two factors need to be considered in planning a logical approach to imaging in the staging of the various types of malignancy: (a) local growth, and (b) pattern of distant spread.

(a) Local growth

Imaging depends on the pattern of local growth and on factors likely to change management, e.g. invasion of organ capsule, invasion of local structures.

(b) Distant spread

Imaging depends on the typical pattern of spread, e.g. via lymph channels or blood-borne metastases, and will be aimed at detecting or excluding the more usual types of metastases for each tumour.

First, a few general comments.

(a) Cross-sectional imaging and lymph node size

- US, CT, and MRI are generally unable to visualise the internal architecture of lymph nodes.
- As such, size alone remains the only criterion for lymph node involvement with malignancy.
- Lymph nodes of 1.0 cm or greater are considered positive (*Fig. 12.1*).
- Limitations:
  (i) Nodes less than 1.0 cm may have microscopic tumour deposits.

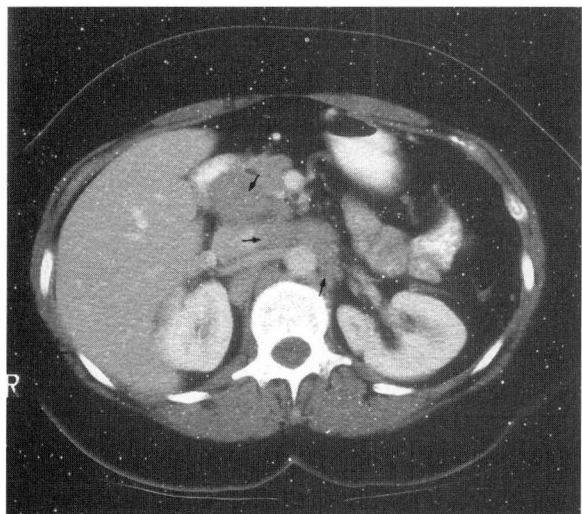

Figure 12.1 *Malignant lymphadenopathy. Multiple enlarged lymph nodes are seen around the aorta and anterior to the IVC (arrows) in a patient with lymphoma.*

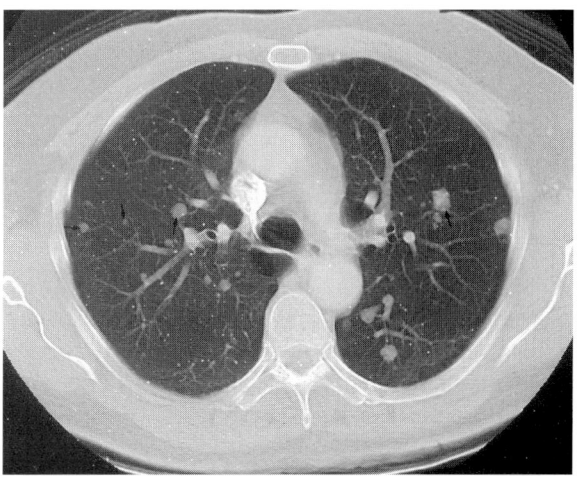

Figure 12.2 *Pulmonary metastases – CT. Multiple soft tissue masses throughout both lungs. Note that these masses are of variable size; this is a typical feature of metastases (arrows).*

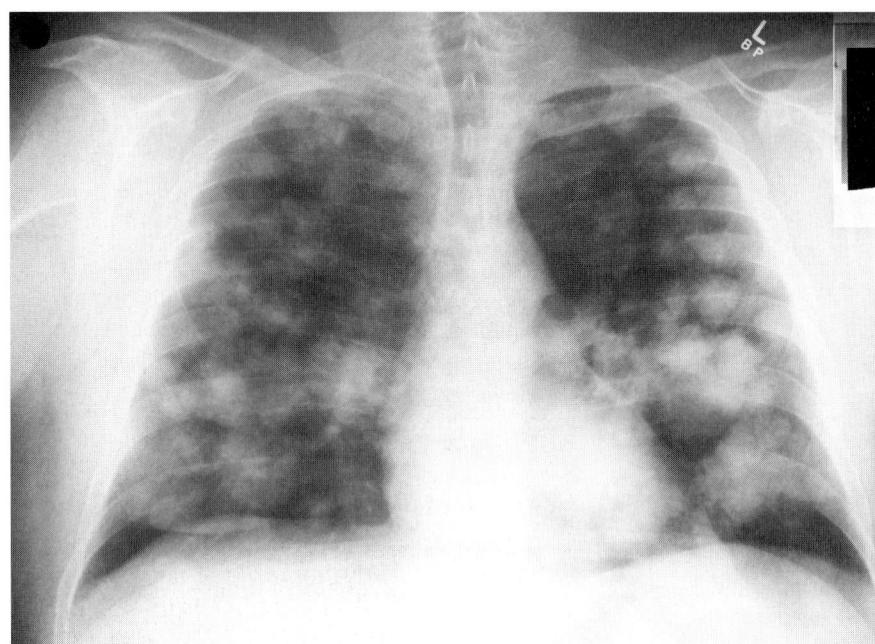

Figure 12.3 *Pulmonary metastases.*
Note multiple, well-defined masses throughout both lungs. Metastases tend to be more numerous peripherally due to haematogenous dissemination.

(ii) Nodes greater than 1.0 cm are not necessarily malignant.

(b) Lung metastases

- CT has a higher pick-up rate than CXR for pulmonary metastases and as such may be used in the initial investigation of tumour with a high incidence of spread to the lungs, e.g. testicular carcinoma (*Fig. 12.2*).

- CXR should also be performed for baseline appearances and subsequent follow-up (*Fig. 12.3*).

(c) Liver metastases

- US, CT, MRI, and scintigraphy may all be used for the detection of liver metastases.

- Helical CT with a dual-phase technique is the most sensitive method for detection of liver metastases:
  (i) Arterial phase for hypervascular metastases.
  (ii) Portal-venous phase for the vast majority of hypovascular metastases.

- Arterial portography may be used in patients being assessed for possible liver resection.

(d) Bone metastases

- Bone scintigraphy (^{99m}Tc-MDP) is the most sensitive technique for detection of bone metastases (*Fig. 12.4*).

- Plain films and occasionally CT may be used to assess abnormal or doubtful findings.

- The exception to the above is multiple myeloma in which plain films are more sensitive than scintigraphy.

Colorectal carcinoma (CRC)

Probably the most widely used classification of CRC is Kirklin's modification of Dukes' original system as below:

- Stage A   Tumour confined to mucosa.

- Stage B1   Tumour extension into, but not through, muscularis propria.

- Stage B2   Tumour extension through muscularis propria but confined to bowel wall.

- Stage C   Stage B1 or B2 with lymph node metastases.

As can be seen, the two most critical factors influencing survival data are depth of invasion of the bowel wall and presence or absence of lymph node metastases. Unfortunately, two major limitations of imaging

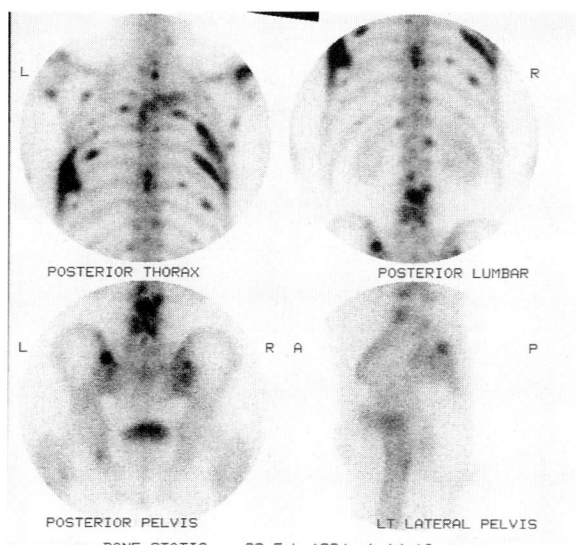

Figure 12.4 *Bone metastases – scintigraphy. Note multiple areas of increased uptake of radiopharmaceutical in the pelvis, spine and ribs. This indicates multiple sites of increased osteoblastic activity in a pattern typical of disseminated skeletal metastases, in this case from a prostate primary.*

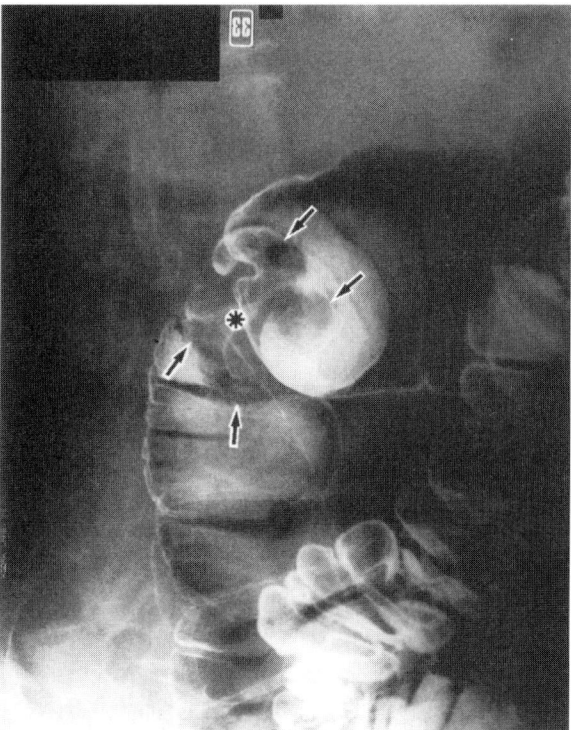

Figure 12.5 *Carcinoma of the colon – barium enema. Classic 'apple-core' stricture (*) of an annular carcinoma. Note rolled, elevated margins (arrows).*

of CRC are assessment of depth of wall invasion and detection of microscopic metastases in non-enlarged lymph nodes.

Whilst accurate pre-treatment staging of CRC is probably useful for planning of surgery, radiotherapy, and chemotherapy, it remains controversial due to the limitations of imaging plus the fact that most patients with CRC will have surgery for cure or palliation.

(a) Local growth

1. Colonoscopy/barium enema:

Both of these investigations are most useful for initial detection of CRC and adenomatous polyps and in localisation, characterisation, and diagnosis of multiple lesions. Colonoscopy is more accurate than barium enema for detection of small and sessile polyps and has the added advantages of biopsy and polyp removal at the time of examination. Barium enema remains a highly accurate and relatively non-invasive technique. It is particularly useful for assessment of an elongated, tortuous colon where redundant loops may not be amenable to negotiation with a colonoscope (*Fig. 12.5*).

2. CT:

- CRC seen as a mass or thickening of the bowel wall.

- Invasion beyond bowel wall (*Fig. 12.6*).

- Invasion of adjacent structures.

- CT unable to assess depth of wall invasion and to detect small metastases in non-enlarged lymph nodes.

- Therefore, CT is accurate for advanced disease though less so for earlier non-invasive disease.

3. Transrectal ultrasound (TRUS):

- Layers of rectal wall are well seen therefore able to evaluate depth of wall invasion.

- Guided biopsy of perirectal lymph nodes.

- Limitations include overstaging due to peritumoral inflammation mimicking invasion beyond the muscularis propria, as well as understaging due to

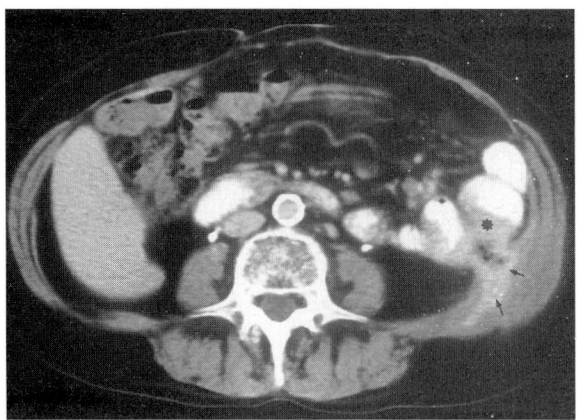

Figure 12.6 *Carcinoma of the colon – CT.*
There is a carcinoma of the descending colon seen on
CT as a soft tissue mass (*). Note spread beyond the
bowel wall with direct invasion of the lateral
abdominal wall (arrows).

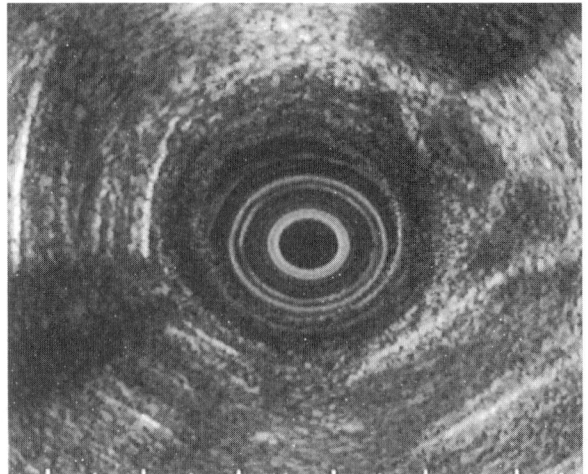

Figure 12.7 *Carcinoma of the oesophagus –*
transoesophageal ultrasound.
The tumour is seen as symmetrical thickening of the
oesophageal wall, surrounding the central circular
ultrasound probe. Note the irregularity of the
oesophageal wall at the top of the picture indicating
local invasion into the adventitia. (Courtesy of Dr W
Lees, London.)

microscopic tumour invasion too small to be seen
with TRUS.

(b) Distant spread

- Liver: CT.

- Lung: CXR/CT.

- Bone: Scintigraphy/plain films.

Carcinoma of the oesophagus

(a) Local growth

1. Endoscopy and biopsy

2. Barium swallow:

- Useful for initial tumour detection rather than
  actual staging.

- Appearances depend on pattern of tumour growth
  and include: intraluminal mass, irregular stricture,
  mucosal irregularity and ulceration, sinus and
  fistula formation.

3. Endoscopic ultrasound:

- Able to directly visualise the layers of the
  oesophageal wall and therefore accurately assess
  depth of tumour invasion (*Fig. 12.7*).

- Invasion of mediastinal structures.

- Mediastinal lymphadenopathy.

- Biopsy guidance is particularly useful for equivocal
  lymph nodes.

- Main limitations are inability to traverse a tight
  stenotic lesion, and inability to visualise distant
  metastases due to a limited field of view.

4. CT:

- Mediastinal lymphadenopathy.

- Invasion of mediastinal structures as evidenced by
  loss of surrounding fat planes.

- Much less accurate for tumours at the gastro-
  oesophageal junction.

- Cannot assess depth of tumour invasion in the
  oesophageal wall.

5. Suggested protocol based on the above:

- *Primary diagnosis:* Barium swallow; endoscopy; biopsy.

- *Staging:* CT. If no distant metastases then perform
  endoscopic ultrasound.

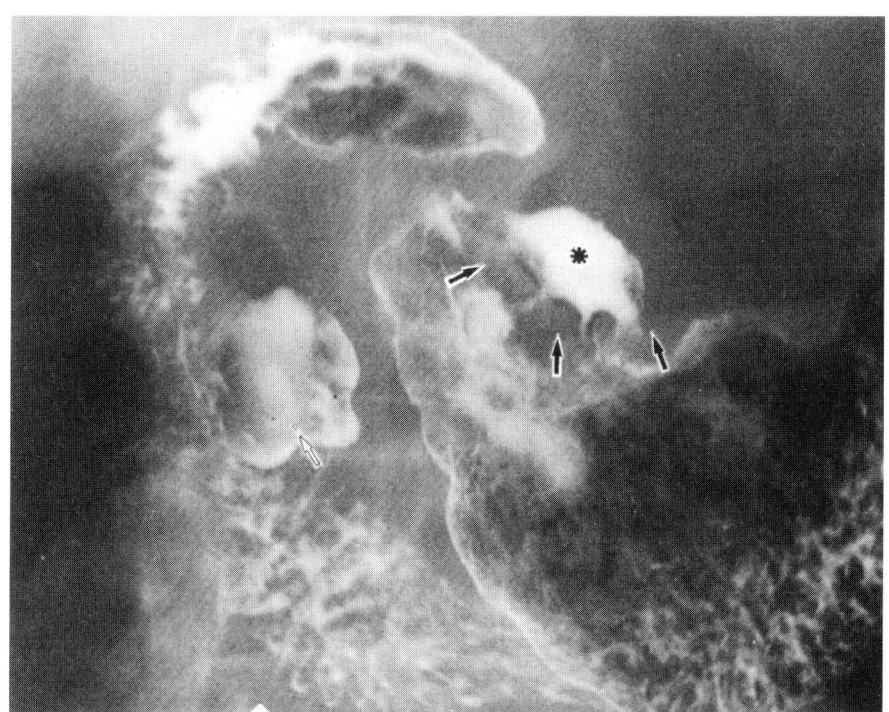

Figure 12.8 *Gastric carcinoma – barium meal. Tumour of the gastric antrum shown as heaped-up folds of soft tissue (black arrows) surrounding a large central ulcer crater (*). A diverticulum of the 2nd part of the duodenum is also shown (white arrow).*

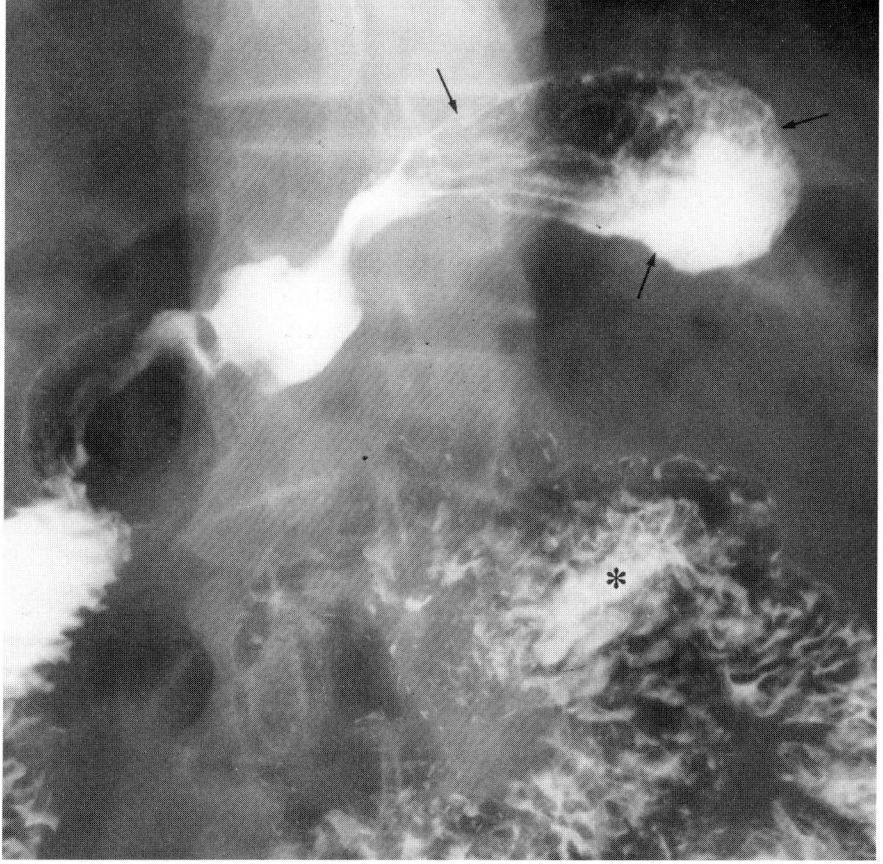

Figure 12.9 *Linitis plastica – barium meal. Small, contracted stomach which fails to distend despite double-contrast technique (arrows). There is rapid passage of contrast and gas into the small bowel (*).*

(b) Distant spread

- Lung: CXR/CT.

- Liver: CT.

- Bone: Scintigraphy/plain films.

Carcinoma of the stomach

(a) Local growth

- Endoscopy and biopsy.

- Barium meal:
  (i)   Appearance of tumour depends on pattern of growth.
  (ii) Gastric mass producing an irregular filling defect.
  (iii) Ulcer, usually with elevated margins (*Fig. 12.8*).
  (iv) Mucosal infiltration with gastric fold thickening, mucosal irregularity, and distorted gastric outline.
  (v)   'Linitis plastica': small non-distensible stomach (*Fig. 12.9*).

(b) Distant spread

- Liver: CT.

- Lung: CXR/CT.

- Bone: Scintigraphy/plain films.

Adenocarcinoma of the pancreas

(a) Local growth

CT:
- Local extension beyond pancreas.

- Invasion of adjacent structures, i.e. duodenum, stomach, left adrenal gland, spleen, mesentery.

- Encasement of mesenteric vessels.

(b) Distant spread

Lymphadenopathy; liver metastases: CT.

- Lung: CXR/CT.

- Bone: Scintigraphy/plain films.

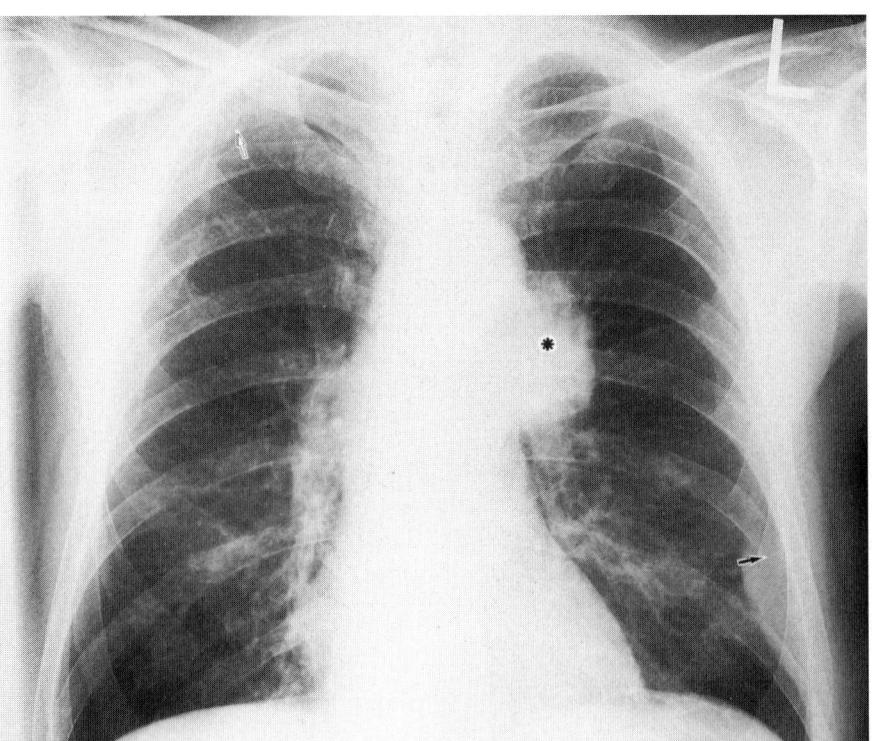

Figure 12.10 *Bronchogenic carcinoma.*
Mass at the left hilum (*). Note also multiple rib metastases with destruction of the lateral aspect of the 9th rib and associated soft tissue mass (solid arrow), and less obvious destruction of the posterior aspect of the right 4th rib (hollow arrow).

Breast carcinoma

(a) Local growth

- Mammography.

- Ultrasound.

(b) Distant spread

- Lung: CXR/CT.

- Bone: Scintigraphy/plain films.

- Liver: CT.

Lung: bronchogenic carcinoma

(a) Local growth

1. CXR:

- Pulmonary mass: smooth or irregular margin; usually containing no calcification; cavitation; progressive increase in size on serial CXR.

- Hilar mass: increased hilar size and density; altered hilar contour (*Fig. 12.10*).

- Mediastinal mass.

- Lobar collapse and/or consolidation.

- Pleural/pericardial effusion.

- Note that the combination of lobar collapse plus pleural effusion in an elderly person is strongly suggestive of underlying malignancy.

- Invasion of chest wall: soft tissue mass with rib destruction (*Fig. 12.11*).

- Pulmonary metastases.

- Rib metastases.

2. CT:

- CT is more accurate than CXR in staging bronchogenic carcinoma especially for the following: mediastinal lymphadenopathy, hilar lymphadenopathy, mediastinal invasion and chest wall invasion (*Figs 12.12 and 12.13*).

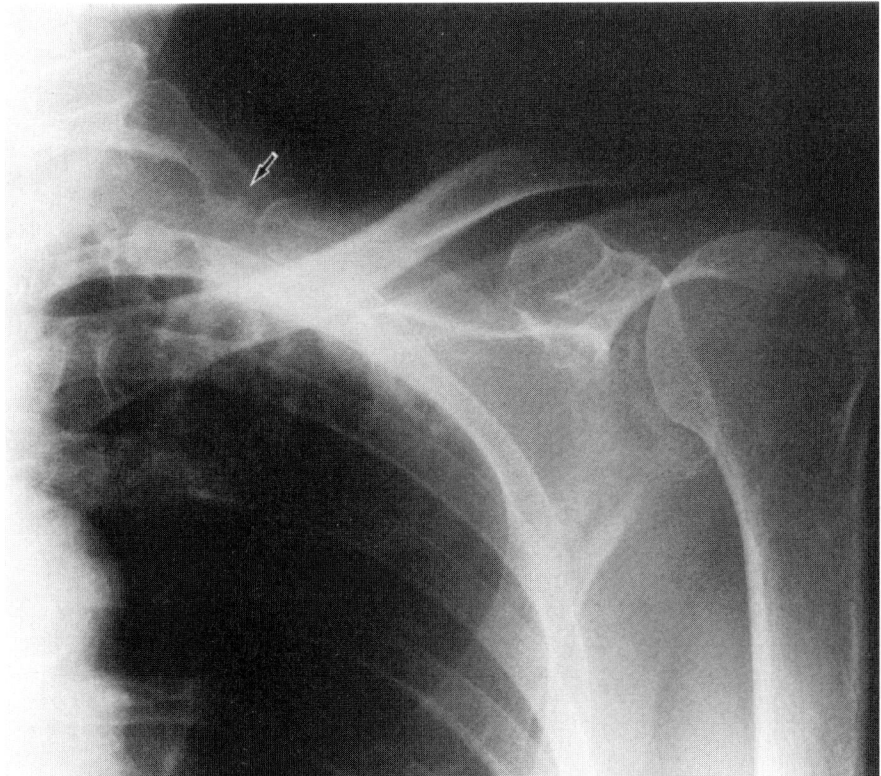

Figure 12.11 *Pancoast tumour.*
Localised view showing a soft tissue mass at the apex of the left lung with destruction of the underlying 1st and 2nd ribs (arrow).

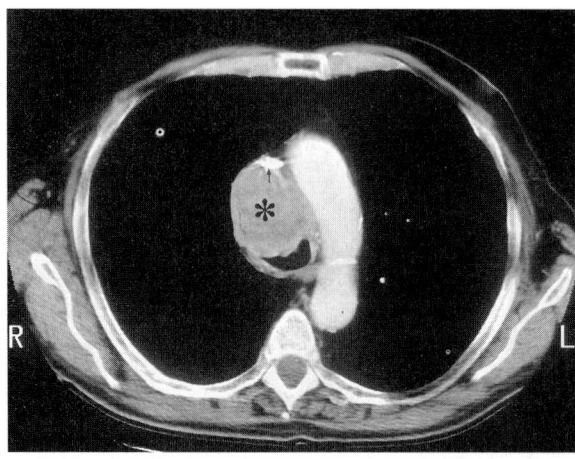

Figure 12.12 *Mediastinal lymphadenopathy – CT. Metastatic spread from bronchogenic carcinoma. A markedly enlarged mediastinal lymph node (*) is seen to the right of the aorta. Note compression of the SVC anteriorly (arrow).*

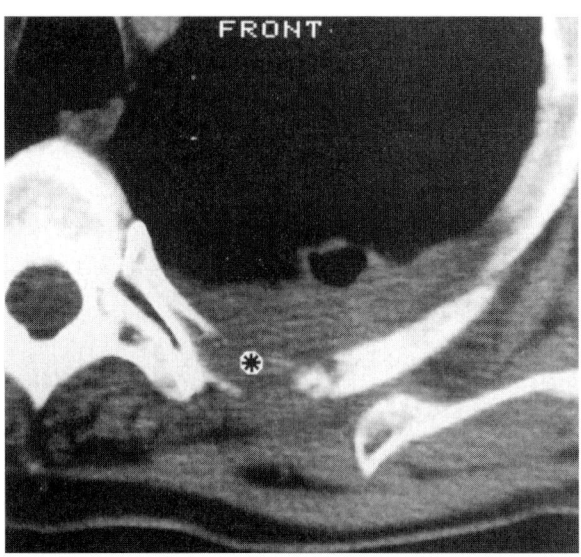

Figure 12.13 *Bronchogenic carcinoma – CT. Peripherally situated squamous cell carcinoma seen as a chest wall mass with destruction of the underlying rib (*).*

- CT may also be used for primary diagnosis, i.e. where the CXR is negative and the presence of a tumour is suspected on clinical grounds, e.g. haemoptysis, sputum cytology, paraneoplastic syndrome.

(b) Distant spread

- Bone: Scintigraphy/plain films.
- Liver and adrenals: CT.
- Brain: CT/MRI.

Kidney: renal cell carcinoma

(a) Local growth

CT/US:

- Invasion of adjacent structures.
- Lymphadenopathy.
- Contralateral kidney (*Fig. 12.14*).
- Venous invasion.

(b) Distant spread

- Liver: CT

- Lung: CXR/CT
    Unusual patterns may be seen: solitary large metastasis; multiple large (cannon ball) metastases; metastases appearing years after resection of the primary tumour.

- Bone:
    (i) *Scintigraphy:* Renal cell metastases may occasionally be 'cold' on bone scan.
    (ii) *Plain films:* Renal cell metastases may produce lytic and expansile bone lesions.

Bladder: transitional cell carcinoma

(a) Local growth

- Cystoscopy.
- CT: Local invasion; pelvic lymphadenopathy.

(b) Distant spread

- Other sites in urinary tract: IVP.
- Retroperitoneal lymph nodes/liver: CT.
- Bone: scintigraphy, plain films.
- Lung: CXR.

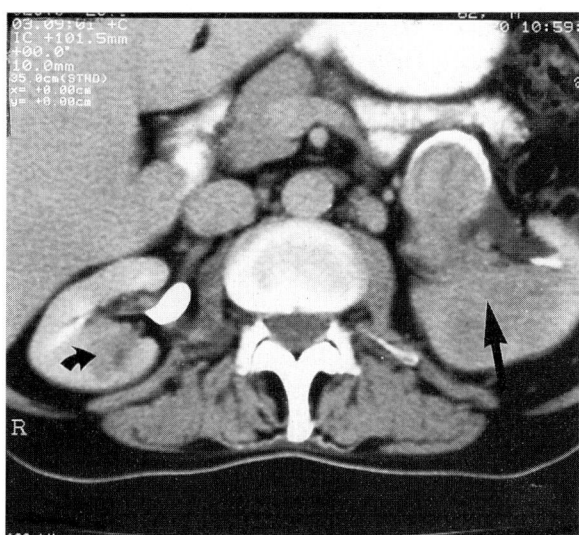

Figure 12.14 *Renal cell carcinoma – CT.*
Note:
- *irregular mass arising from the left kidney (straight arrow)*
- *small contralateral tumour in the right kidney (curved arrow).*

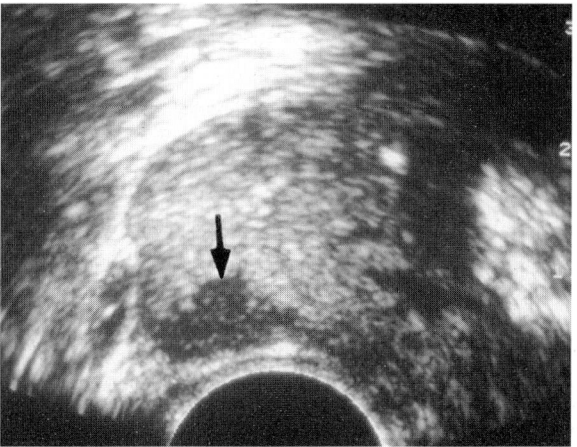

Figure 12.15 *Carcinoma of the prostate – transrectal ultrasound (TRUS).*
A small carcinoma of the prostate is seen on TRUS as a focal hypoechoic mass in the peripheral zone (arrow). Note that the adjacent capsule is smooth and that the tumour is confined to the prostate gland, i.e. stage A. Diagnosis was confirmed by TRUS-guided biopsy.

Prostate: adenocarcinoma

(a) Local growth

1. Transrectal ultrasound (TRUS) and biopsy:
- Particularly useful for Stage A and B tumours not seen on CT (*Fig. 12.15*).

- Malignancies may appear as focal hypoechoic areas in the peripheral zone of the gland.

- As TRUS is poorly sensitive for imaging of tumour confined to the gland it is usually accompanied by biopsy.

- TRUS-guided biopsy of hypoechoic lesions plus sextant biopsy are used for assessing extent and distribution of tumour within the prostate gland.

- TRUS is highly sensitive for subtle signs of local invasion not detectable on CT, i.e. invasion of the gland capsule; early invasion of seminal vesicles.

2. CT:
- Pelvic lymphadenopathy.

- Invasion of pelvic side wall (*Fig. 12.16*).

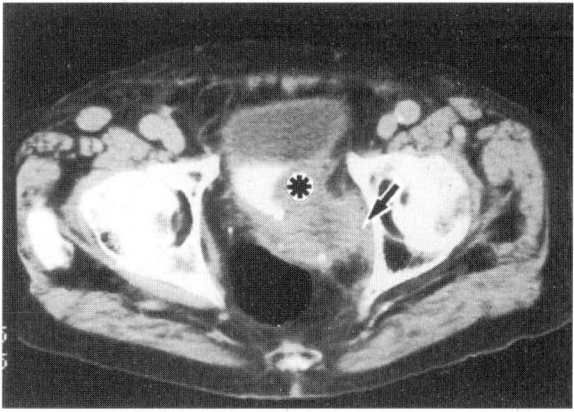

Figure 12.16 *Prostatic carcinoma – CT.*
Irregular mass invading the left base of the bladder (*) and extending to the side wall of the pelvis (arrow).

- Invasion of seminal vesicles.

3. MRI:

MRI using an endorectal coil provides excellent visualisation of the intraglandular architecture of the prostate gland and may be useful for Stage A and B tumours.

(b) Distant spread

- Bone: scintigraphy; plain films.
- Retroperitoneal lymph nodes/liver: CT.
- Lungs: CXR.

Testicular tumours

(a) Local growth

US:

- Intratesticular mass: over 90% of intratesticular masses are malignant exceptions being abscess, TB, infarct, sarcoidosis and benign tumour.
- Usually hypoechoic.
- Occasionally hyperechoic especially when complicated by haemorrhage or calcification.
- Extensive testicular tumour may be seen as hypoechoic expansion of the testicle with no recognisable normal testicular tissue.

(b) Distant spread

- Retroperitoneal lymph nodes: CT.
- Lung and mediastinal lymph nodes: CT/CXR.

Ovarian tumours

(a) Local growth

US:

- Ovarian tumours are usually cystic with solid components such as septa, soft tissue masses, or irregular wall thickening.
- Fluid contents may be clear (anechoic) or may have internal echoes due to mucin, haemorrhage or fat.
- Occasionally ovarian tumours are solid masses, e.g. fibroma, Brenner tumour.
- Pelvic ultrasound may be transabdominal or transvaginal; the two techniques are complementary.
- Transabdominal scanning has a large field of view so that other organs, e.g. kidneys and liver may be assessed.

- Transvaginal scanning has excellent resolution and is therefore highly accurate for tumour characterisation; it does however have a relatively small field of view and probe size may be inappropriate in very young or elderly patients.

(b) Distant spread

- Ascites, lymphadenopathy, liver metastases: CT.
- Lung: CXR/CT.

Carcinoma of the cervix

(a) Local growth

- Colposcopy.
- CT: Invasion of surrounding structures and pelvic side wall; pelvic lymphadenopathy.

(b) Distant spread

- Retroperitoneal lymph nodes, liver: CT.
- Lung: CXR/CT.
- Bone: scintigraphy/plain films.

Endometrial carcinoma

(a) Local growth

- Transvaginal ultrasound.

(b) Distant spread

- Lungs: CXR/CT.

Thyroid carcinoma

(a) Local growth

CT:

- Size of tumour.
- Invasion of surrounding structures: laryngeal cartilages, blood vessels, sternomastoid muscle.
- Compression/displacement of trachea/oesophagus (*Fig. 12.17*).

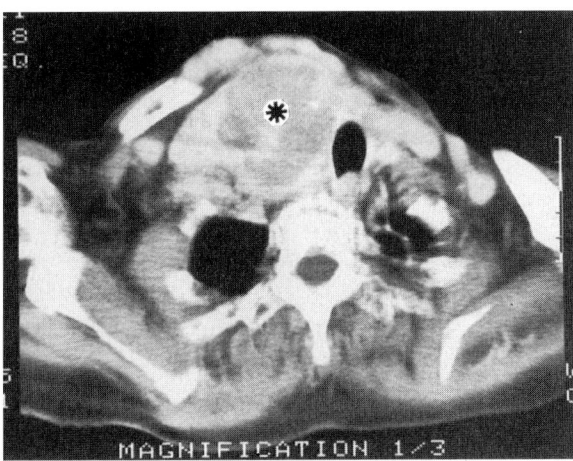

Figure 12.17 *Thyroid carcinoma – CT.*
Large masses of heterogeneous attenuation (*) occupying the right lobe of the thyroid gland with displacement of the trachea to the left.

- Cervical lymphadenopathy.

(b) Distant spread

- Lung, mediastinum: CT/CXR.

- Bone: scintigraphy/plain films; note that thyroid metastases are usually lytic and often expansile.

Carcinoma of the larynx

(a) Local growth

1. Laryngoscopy:
- Assessment of mucosal surface.

- CT is required to assess submucosal and deeper tissues.

2. CT:
- Complementary to laryngoscopy.

- Site and anatomy of tumour: high attenuation mass causing asymmetry of the airway and anatomical distortion with obliteration of surrounding fat planes (*Fig. 12.18*).

- Invasion of surrounding fat planes.

- Invasion of surrounding structures, e.g. cartilages.

- Cervical lymphadenopathy.

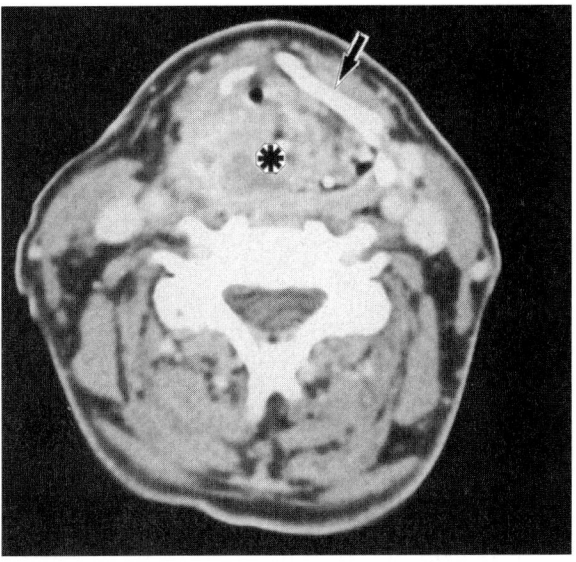

Figure 12.18 *Laryngeal carcinoma – CT.*
Large mass with almost complete occlusion of the airway (*). The tumour has destroyed the right lamina of the thyroid cartilage; the left lamina is intact (arrow). (Courtesy of Dr W Lun, Brisbane.)

(b) Distant spread

- Lung, mediastinum: CXR/CT.

Lymphoma

The type of investigation used will depend on clinical presentation and suspected areas of involvement. Accurate staging is prognostically more significant for Hodgkin's disease, whereas in non-Hodgkin's lymphoma, it is the cell type that largely dictates the clinical course. Nevertheless, accurate staging is still important in all types of lymphoma, especially when assessing response to therapy and incidence of recurrence.

A staging protocol should be planned using the following general principles:

- Commonly involved sites are screened routinely, i.e. chest and abdomen.

- Less commonly involved sites are investigated depending on symptomatic presentation, e.g. testes, brain, bone.

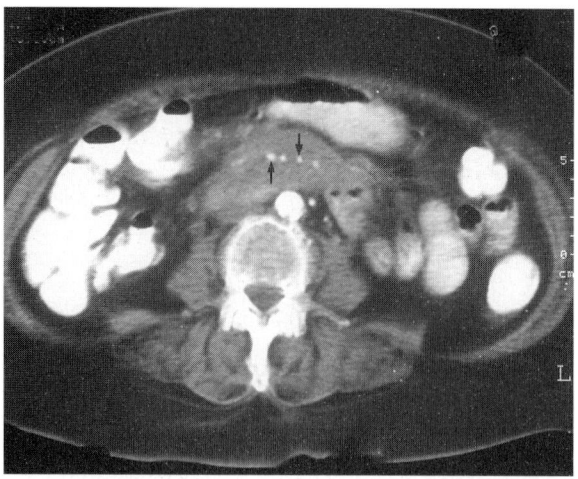

Figure 12.19 *Lymphoma – CT.*
There is a large lymph node mass anterior to the aorta.
Note that the mesenteric vessels (arrows) are encased by
tumour. Such encasement may also be seen with
advanced pancreatic tumours.

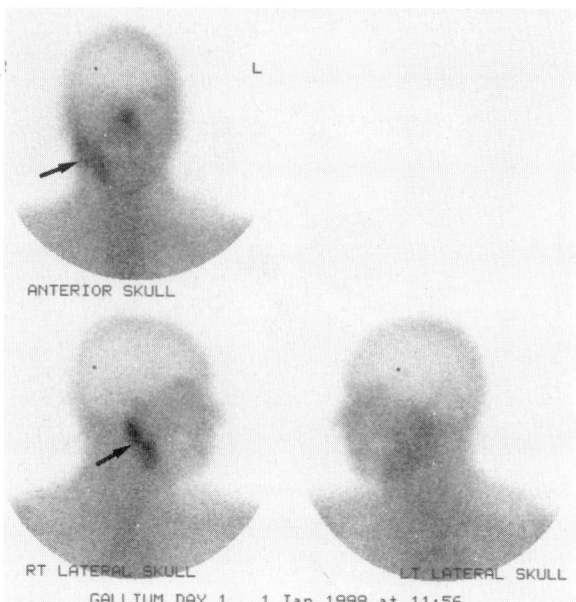

Figure 12.20 *Lymphoma – gallium scan.*
Recurrent non-Hodgkin's lymphoma of the right cervical
lymph nodes is well shown as an oval-shaped area of
gallium uptake in the right side of the neck.

(a) Chest

1. CT:

* More sensitive than CXR.

* Mediastinal lymphadenopathy.

* Hilar lymphadenopathy.

* Direct lung involvement: pulmonary mass; interstitial or alveolar shadowing.

* Pleural/pericardial effusion.

* Anterior mediastinal mass is a common presentation of Hodgkin's disease.

2. CXR:

* Less sensitive than CT, particularly for mediastinal and hilar lymphadenopathy.

* Useful as an inexpensive method of follow-up and for assessing complications of therapy, i.e. pneumonitis/fibrosis following radiotherapy, cardiac failure, atypical infections.

(b) Abdomen

1. CT:

* Most sensitive method for assessing liver and spleen, retroperitoneum and kidneys.

* Generally the only criterion of lymph node involvement is enlargement although necrotic lymph nodes may also show central low attenuation.

* < 1.0 cm: normal; 1.0–1.5 cm: equivocal; > 1.5 cm: abnormal (*Figs 12.19 and 12.1*).

* The exception to these size criteria is the retrocrural group where > 6 mm is considered abnormal.

* Signs of liver involvement: multiple low-attenuation masses of varying size, hepatomegaly.

* Signs of splenic involvement: splenomegaly, multiple low-attenuation masses or small nodules.

* In general, imaging for liver and spleen involvement is neither sensitive nor specific: one-third of enlarged spleens in Hodgkin's disease patients are not neoplastic whilst one-third of normal sized spleens do have neoplastic involvement.

2. US:

* Not as accurate as CT in detection of lymphadenopathy.

* May be useful for follow-up, particularly in children.

(c) Extranodal disease

1. Investigations dictated by clinical suspicion of involvement:

- Gastrointestinal tract.

- Barium studies/CT.

- Distal ileum and caecum are common sites of involvement though lymphoma may involve any part of the gastrointestinal tract.

- Localised or diffuse areas of wall thickening.

- Soft tissue masses.

- May be complicated by intussusception, especially in children where intussusception may occasionally be the initial presenting complaint.

2. Bone:

- Scintigraphy/plain films.

3. CNS:

- CT/MRI.

(d) Scintigraphy: gallium citrate

Gallium-67 (^{67}Ga) binds to transferrin and is taken up by leucocytes and some bacteria. Uptake in the lymphomas is variable though sensitivity is greater for Hodgkin's disease (90%) than for non-Hodgkin's lymphoma (50%). The exception to this variability is Burkitt's lymphoma which shows virtually 100% uptake.

Over 50% of patients with a complete response to treatment have a residual mass on CT due to necrotic tissue and fibrosis. ^{67}Ga Scintigraphy is highly sensitive and specific for differentiating such masses from resid-ual malignancy. It is also highly sensitive for the diagnosis of early recurrence, often months prior to CT (*Fig. 12.20*).

Therefore, gallium scanning has been found to be more useful for monitoring response to treatment than for primary diagnosis and remains a worthwhile investigation in lymphoma treatment.

Further Reading

1. Botet JF, Lightdale CJ, Zauber AG *et al.* Preoperative staging of esophageal cancer: comparison of endoscopic US and dynamic CT. *Radiology* 1991; **181**:419–425.

2. Front D, Bar–Shalom R, Israel O. The continuing clinical role of gallium 67 scintigraphy in the age of receptor imaging. *Seminars in Nuclear Medicine* 1997; **23**:68–74.

3. Garnick MB. Prostate cancer: screening, diagnosis, and management. *Annals of Internal Medicine* 1993; **118**:804–818.

4. Ott DJ, Wolfman NT. Integrated imaging in colorectal cancer. *Seminars in Roentgenology* 1996; **31**:166–169.

5. Reznek H, Husband JE. The radiology of lymphoma. *Current Imaging* 1990; **2**:9–17.

6. Slonim SM, Cuttino JT, Johnson CJ *et al.* Diagnosis of prostatic carcinoma: value of random transrectal sonographically guided biopsies. *AJR* 1993; **161**:1003–1006.

7. Thompson WM (ed.). Staging neoplasms. *Radiological Clinics of North America* 1994; **32**(1).

8. Wolfman NT, Ott DJ. Endoscopic ultrasonography. *Seminars in Roentgenology* 1996; **31**:154–161.

Index

Page numbers in **bold type** refer to figures; *italic* page numbers indicate tables.